Environmental, Health and Economic Conditions during the COVID-19 Pandemic

Environmental, Health and Economic Conditions during the COVID-19 Pandemic

Editor

Dirga Kumar Lamichhane

MDPI • Basel • Beijing • Wuhan • Barcelona • Belgrade • Manchester • Tokyo • Cluj • Tianjin

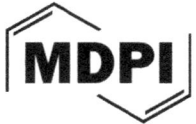

Editor
Dirga Kumar Lamichhane
Occupational and
Environmental Medicine
Inha University
School of Medicine
Incheon
Korea, South

Editorial Office
MDPI
St. Alban-Anlage 66
4052 Basel, Switzerland

This is a reprint of articles from the Special Issue published online in the open access journal *International Journal of Environmental Research and Public Health* (ISSN 1660-4601) (available at: www.mdpi.com/journal/ijerph/special_issues/pandemic_economic).

For citation purposes, cite each article independently as indicated on the article page online and as indicated below:

LastName, A.A.; LastName, B.B.; LastName, C.C. Article Title. *Journal Name* **Year**, *Volume Number*, Page Range.

ISBN 978-3-0365-3492-3 (Hbk)
ISBN 978-3-0365-3491-6 (PDF)

© 2022 by the authors. Articles in this book are Open Access and distributed under the Creative Commons Attribution (CC BY) license, which allows users to download, copy and build upon published articles, as long as the author and publisher are properly credited, which ensures maximum dissemination and a wider impact of our publications.

The book as a whole is distributed by MDPI under the terms and conditions of the Creative Commons license CC BY-NC-ND.

Contents

About the Editor vii

Preface to "Environmental, Health and Economic Conditions during the COVID-19 Pandemic" ix

Dirga Kumar Lamichhane, Sabina Shrestha and Hwan-Cheol Kim
District-Level Risk Factors for COVID-19 Incidence and Mortality in Nepal
Reprinted from: *Int. J. Environ. Res. Public Health* **2022**, *19*, 2659, doi:10.3390/ijerph19052659 . . . 1

Katarzyna Sekścińska, Agata Trzcińska, Daniel Pankowski, Ewa Pisula and Kinga Wytrychiewicz-Pankowska
Financial Factors and Psychological Distress during the COVID-19 Pandemic in Poland
Reprinted from: *Int. J. Environ. Res. Public Health* **2022**, *19*, 1798, doi:10.3390/ijerph19031798 . . . 15

Dongyi Zhou and Rui Zhou
ESG Performance and Stock Price Volatility in Public Health Crisis: Evidence from COVID-19 Pandemic
Reprinted from: *Int. J. Environ. Res. Public Health* **2021**, *19*, 202, doi:10.3390/ijerph19010202 . . . 35

Feng Wang and Min Wu
The Impacts of COVID-19 on Chinarsquo;s Economy and Energy in the Context of Trade Protectionism
Reprinted from: *Int. J. Environ. Res. Public Health* **2021**, *18*, 12768, doi:10.3390/ijerph182312768 . 51

Jan Schmidt, Vojtech Perina, Jana Treglerova, Nela Pilbauerova, Jakub Suchanek and Roman Smucler
COVID-19 Prevalence among Czech Dentists
Reprinted from: *Int. J. Environ. Res. Public Health* **2021**, *18*, 12488, doi:10.3390/ijerph182312488 . 75

Ammar Javed, Farheen Aamir, Umar Farooq Gohar, Hamid Mukhtar, Muhammad Zia-Ul-Haq and Modhi O. Alotaibi et al.
The Potential Impact of Smog Spell on Humans' Health Amid COVID-19 Rages
Reprinted from: *Int. J. Environ. Res. Public Health* **2021**, *18*, 11408, doi:10.3390/ijerph182111408 . 91

Yaping Zhang, Jianjun Zhang, Ke Wang and Xia Wu
An Empirical Perception of Economic Resilience Responded to the COVID-19 Epidemic Outbreak in Beijing–Tianjin–Hebei Urban Agglomeration, China: Characterization and Interaction
Reprinted from: *Int. J. Environ. Res. Public Health* **2021**, *18*, 10532, doi:10.3390/ijerph181910532 . 111

Jan Schmidt, Eliska Waldova, Stepanka Balkova, Jakub Suchanek and Roman Smucler
Impact of COVID-19 on Czech Dentistry: A Nationwide Cross-Sectional Preliminary Study among Dentists in the Czech Republic
Reprinted from: *Int. J. Environ. Res. Public Health* **2021**, *18*, 9121, doi:10.3390/ijerph18179121 . . . 129

Ourania S. Kotsiou, Georgios K. D. Saharidis, Georgios Kalantzis, Evangelos C. Fradelos and Konstantinos I. Gourgoulianis
The Impact of the Lockdown Caused by the COVID-19 Pandemic on the Fine Particulate Matter ($PM_{2.5}$) Air Pollution: The Greek Paradigm
Reprinted from: *Int. J. Environ. Res. Public Health* **2021**, *18*, 6748, doi:10.3390/ijerph18136748 . . . 143

Xiaozhen Lai, Hongguo Rong, Xiaochen Ma, Zhiyuan Hou, Shunping Li and Rize Jing et al.
The Economic Burden of Influenza-Like Illness among Children, Chronic Disease Patients, and the Elderly in China: A National Cross-Sectional Survey
Reprinted from: *Int. J. Environ. Res. Public Health* **2021**, *18*, 6277, doi:10.3390/ijerph18126277 . . . **155**

Nadia Yusuf and Lamia Saud Shesha
Economic Role of Population Density during Pandemics—A Comparative Analysis of Saudi Arabia and China
Reprinted from: *Int. J. Environ. Res. Public Health* **2021**, *18*, 4318, doi:10.3390/ijerph18084318 . . . **171**

Diego Galvan, Luciane Effting, Hágata Cremasco and Carlos Adam Conte-Junior
Can Socioeconomic, Health, and Safety Data Explain the Spread of COVID-19 Outbreak on Brazilian Federative Units?
Reprinted from: *Int. J. Environ. Res. Public Health* **2020**, *17*, 8921, doi:10.3390/ijerph17238921 . . . **189**

About the Editor

Dirga Kumar Lamichhane

Ph.D., Medicine, is research professor at the Department of Occupational and Environmental Medicine, Inha University School of Medicine, South Korea. He has been a visiting faculty at the graduate school of economics, Nagoya University, Nagoya, Japan, where he teaches courses in environmental health and health economics. His research focuses on the health effects of environmental toxins such as air pollution, household chemicals, and heavy metals on adverse birth outcomes, mental disorders, and idiopathic interstitial pneumonia and chronic diseases including, lung cancer, chronic obstructive pulmonary diseases, and asthma and socioeconomic inequalities in health outcomes. His research involves applying geographic information system modeling, biomonitoring techniques, environmental measurements, and statistical models to provide comprehensive and quantitative assessments of exposure to combinations of traditional and emerging environmental contaminants. He has published over 45 journal and conference papers, books, and technical guidelines related to health and environment. He has presented over 20 multi-day training courses for I/NGOs on infectious diseases and guidelines for preparedness and response to disaster.

Preface to "Environmental, Health and Economic Conditions during the COVID-19 Pandemic"

The spread of coronavirus disease 2019 (COVID-19), which started at the end of 2019, has evolved as a global pandemic. Since the start of the pandemic, COVID-19 has overwhelmed health systems worldwide, from crippling health resources to causing paradigms shifts in healthcare delivery. The various strategies taken to control viral transmission including testing process, quarantine, and isolation have had dire psychological and financial implications on individuals and institutions. Furthermore, many countries have implemented lockdowns and other restrictions to curb the virus's spread resulted in disrupted formal education, unplanned fiscal costs on emergency reliefs, and decreased productivity. Although these strategies to control viral transmission are widely debated, the relative success of these strategies may depend on the concerted multi-sectoral efforts of public health agencies across all level in a coordinated manner. Although the costs of enforcing these control measures are enormous, the ongoing pandemic may have some indirect positive impacts. Among them, locking down cities has brought a sudden drop in air pollution and carbon emissions. These declines are mainly due to the close-down of transport, constructional works, and industrial activities. The purpose of this Special Issue is to explore the environmental, health, and economic dimensions of the effect of COVID-19, considering the multiple interactions between atmospheric emissions, outdoor and indoor air quality, and health and economic conditions. In this context, the most important issues in need of discussion are risk factors for transmission, disease severity, and COVID-19 related deaths, effects of urban environments on the transmission and fatality of COVID-19, impact of COVID-19 on health and economic outcomes, and impact of COVID-19 control measure on air quality.

Dirga Kumar Lamichhane
Editor

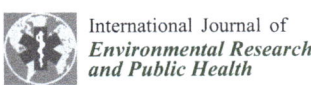 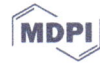

Article

District-Level Risk Factors for COVID-19 Incidence and Mortality in Nepal

Dirga Kumar Lamichhane [1,*], Sabina Shrestha [2] and Hwan-Cheol Kim [1]

[1] Department of Occupational and Environmental Medicine, School of Medicine, Inha University, Incheon 22212, Korea; carpediem@inha.ac.kr
[2] Department of Community and Global Health, Graduate School of Medicine, The University of Tokyo, Tokyo 113-0033, Japan; sabinashrestha2001@yahoo.com
* Correspondence: dirgalamichhane@gmail.com

Abstract: The recent global pandemic of the novel coronavirus disease 2019 (COVID-19) is affecting the entire population of Nepal, and the outcome of the epidemic varies from place to place. A district-level analysis was conducted to identify socio-demographic risk factors that drive the large variations in COVID-19 mortality and related health outcomes, as of 22 January 2021. Data on COVID-19 extracted from relevant reports and websites of the Ministry of Health and Population of Nepal, and the National Population and Housing Census and the Nepal Demographic and Health Survey were the main data sources for the district-level socio-demographic characteristics. We calculated the COVID-19 incidence, recovered cases, and deaths per 100,000 population, then estimated the associations with the risk factors using regression models. COVID-19 outcomes were positively associated with population density. A higher incidence of COVID-19 was associated with districts with a higher percentage of overcrowded households and without access to handwashing facilities. Adult literacy rate was negatively associated with the COVID-19 incidence. Increased mortality was significantly associated with a higher obesity prevalence in women and a higher smoking prevalence in men. Access to health care facilities reduced mortality. Population density was the most important driver behind the large variations in COVID-19 outcomes. This study identifies critical risk factors of COVID-19 outcomes, including population density, crowding, education, and hand hygiene, and these factors should be considered to address inequities in the burden of COVID-19 across districts.

Keywords: COVID-19; district-level analysis; risk factors; Nepal

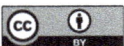

1. Introduction

The spread of coronavirus disease 2019 (COVID-19), which is caused by severe acute respiratory syndrome coronavirus 2 (SARS-CoV-2), has evolved as a global pandemic [1]. As of 17 December 2021, more than 271 million confirmed cases were reported worldwide, and more than 5.3 million people have died due to COVID-19 [2]. This pandemic has posed further threats to people due to the emergence of the number of novel SARS-CoV-2 strains with unknown original hosts [3,4]. Several studies have been conducted to better understand the risk factors associated the spread and severity of COVID-19 infections. Research indicates that the risk of disease spread and deaths are influenced by several characteristics, such as socio-demographic factors [5], behavioral traits [6], and pre-existing health conditions [7]. However, the risk factors impacting the spread and severity of COVID-19 infections are inconsistent across studies, and they vary from place to place [8,9]. Therefore, studies focused on the local-level transmission of this disease are necessary for identifying the main drivers of disease spread that are suitable to contain the current pandemic in this specific region.

In Nepal, the first case of COVID-19 was confirmed on 23 January 2020 in a 32-year-old Nepalese man who had recently returned from Wuhan, China [10]. On 24 March 2020, the Government of Nepal implemented a strict lockdown, including business closures, restrictions on movement within the country, and flights in and out of the country [11]. The rate of spread of the disease was relatively low until mid-July 2020 [12], possibly because of the early nationwide lockdown. The government aggressively initiated a border screening policy to quarantine people traveling to Nepal from abroad, and provincial governments put in place targeted action on quarantine facilities and travel protocols. Nepal has faced multiple epidemic waves, with three distinct surge periods of COVID-19 cases: low (20 May to 25 June 2020), medium (22 July to 20 September 2020), and high (post-16 September 2020); these waves were due to an increase in susceptible population flow following the border opening (~20 May 2020), lockdown ending (~21 July 2020), and countrywide travel opening (~20 September 2020), respectively [13]. There was a rapid increase in the number of confirmed COVID-19 cases following the lifting of travel restrictions in many districts. As of 16 September 2020, a total of 58,327 cases were reported, and cases reached 268,948 on 22 January 2021 (end of the study) [14]. Despite a rapid spread of COVID-19, Nepal had high recovery rate, about 98%, as of 22 January 2021 [15], and a relatively low case fatality rate (CFR); the CFR was 0.6% up to 8 October 2020 [16].

The Nepalese government ended a country-wide lockdown on 21 July 2020 [13] and called for various preventive interventions on hand hygiene, health, and social distancing to be designed and implemented [17], possibly prioritizing areas at elevated risk. Washing hands with soap and running water is one of the best preventive measures to protect individuals and prevent the community from COVID-19 transmission [18]. In addition, population density and household crowding have emerged as important risk factors for COVID-19 transmission [8,9,19]. A previous study reported geographic variation in the pandemic trends in Nepal and suggested regional strategies along with the national-level strategy to control the local spread of COVID-19 [13]. Therefore, it is critical to understand the risk factors at the district level that are associated with widespread infection, severity of illness, and mortality. Representative data on the risk factors for COVID-19 mortality are lacking in Nepal. However, a recent nationally representative household survey and census data can be leveraged to find the risk factors for both the spread and severity of COVID-19 infections.

This study aims to examine the district-level socio-economic and demographic risk factors associated with the spread and severity of COVID-19 in Nepal. Identification of such risk factors can assist health policy makers in resource allocation decisions, provide evidence regarding the effectiveness of population health measures, and assist in developing a targeted, evidence-based response strategy to reduce the risk of subsequent waves of infection at a local level.

2. Materials and Methods

2.1. Data Extraction

Publicly available information on COVID-19-related health outcomes, consisting of the total number of cases, recovered cases, and deaths in all districts of Nepal, were assessed from the official websites of the different ministries of Nepal and previous studies [14,15,20,21]. For this study, we considered one year after the first case of COVID-19 was detected in Nepal (23 January 2020) as the final data capture point (22 January 2021).

Data for socio-demographic and health-related characteristics for each district were captured through various sources. These included per capita income based on purchasing power parity (2011) [22], the total population projection for 2021 [23], the age and gender distribution of the population [24], the population density (people per km^2) [24], the adult literacy rate (2011) [22], and sanitation coverage (2011) [22].

For health indicators, we utilized data from the Nepal Demographic and Health Survey 2016 (NDHS 2016), a cross-sectional survey of 12,862 women and 4063 men in 11,040 households with a response rate of 98% of women and 96% of men. Details of the 2016 NDHS have been previously published [25]. Briefly, the survey was conducted from 19 June 2016 to 31 January 2017, and the sampling frame was based on the National

Population and Housing Census 2011 (NPHC 2011), which was conducted by Nepal Central Bureau of Statistics [24]. The NPHC 2011 and NDHS 2016 were based on the 75 districts of Nepal. The eligible study population for the NDHS 2016 included all men or women aged 15–49 years who were permanent residents of the selected household or visitors who stayed the night in the households the night before the survey. The NDHS sampling and sample size were guided by the need to produce indicators that were representative at the district level. The survey included various socio-demographic, health, and family planning indicators. The survey used a two-stage stratified sampling design in rural areas and a three-stage design in urban areas. In both rural and urban areas, wards formed the primary sampling units (PSUs). Households were selected from the sample PSUs in rural areas, whereas one enumeration area (EA) was selected from each PSU in urban areas, and then households were selected from the sample EAs. PSUs were selected with a probability proportional to size, and households were selected using systematic sampling. We included only 73 districts for this study, as the health indicator data for the remaining two districts were not available.

2.2. COVID-19 Incidence and Mortality

The outcome variables of interest were the COVID-19 confirmed cases, recovered cases, and deaths as of 22 January 2021. For all districts of Nepal, we computed the total counts of confirmed cases per 100,000 persons (i.e., incidence), recovered cases per 100,000 persons, and deaths per 100,000 persons using the district-level population for the year 2021, which was projected from the census of 2001 and 2011 [23]. The district-level CFR was calculated by dividing the number of coronavirus deaths in the district by the total number of district cases.

2.3. Social Risk Factors

District-level social factors included population density, household crowding, sex ratio, proportion of elderly people, adult literacy rate, and per capita income. Population density was defined as persons per square kilometer in each district. Population density is considered as a proxy for the increased likelihood of crowded living environments and may increase the risk of COVID-19 transmission at a regional level [19]. According to the World Health Organization (WHO), household crowding is defined as the presence of more than three people per habitable room [26]. Household crowding has emerged as an important risk factor since spending a long period of time in close vicinity of an infected person significantly increases the risk of COVID-19 transmission [27]. In line with the WHO definition, we defined household crowding as the percentage of the households of a district who lived in homes with more than three people per room for sleeping. In our study, the percentage of household crowding was created using two variables from the household questionnaire of the NDHS 2016: the number of usual household members and visitors and the number of rooms used for sleeping. Furthermore, the sex composition of a population is indicated by the sex ratio, which was calculated as a ratio of total number of males to that of females multiplied by 100, indicating males per 100 females. In addition, we calculated the percentage of the total population of a district that was 60 years and above using the NPHC 2011. Older people are at higher risk of complications from COVID-19 [28]. In Nepal, 58.7% of deaths due to COVID-19 (data cutoff of 22 January 2021) were observed in elderly people ($\geq$60 years) [15].

The level of literacy is a key social and economic indicator and has an important role in health communication. We obtained district-level adult literacy rates for 2011 from the Nepal Human Development Report by the United Nations Development Program (UNDP) [22]. The adult literacy rate was calculated as the ratio of literates, who can read and write, aged 15 years and above, by the corresponding age group of the population. In addition, the district-level per capita income in terms of purchasing parity per person (PPP) for 2011 was used to indicate the economic status of people and was obtained from the Nepal Human Development Report by the UNDP [22].

2.4. Factors Related to Hand Hygiene

Hand hygiene has become important in preventing the spread of COVID-19. In general, handwashing prevents germs from entering the body when people touch their eyes, nose, and mouth, as well as food and drinks [29]. The lack of access to handwashing facilities was defined as the percentage of the population of a district with no access to basic handwashing facilities at home, including soap and water [30]. We used the NDHS 2016 to estimate the percentage of the whole sample without basic handwashing facilities. The variable was constructed using three household questions related to handwashing facilities: (1) whether a handwashing facility was observed in the dwelling, (2) whether water was present at the handwashing facility, and (3) whether soap or detergent was present at the handwashing facility. We created a binary variable from these questions, and coded "1" if the handwashing facility was not observed or if there was either no water or no soap present and "0" otherwise. We estimated the absolute counts of people without access to handwashing facilities in each district. The percentage of people without access to handwashing facilities was calculated by dividing the absolute counts in each district by the number of the whole NDHS sample in each district multiplied by 100.

2.5. Health-Related Factors

The biomarker questionnaire of the NDHS 2016 collected measures of blood pressure (using an Omron Blood Pressure Monitor), height, and weight. We defined obesity as the percentage of eligible men or women (% of 15–49 years old) in a district with a body mass index, which was calculated as the ratio of weight in kilograms by the square of height in meters, equal or greater than 30. Hypertension was defined as the percentage of eligible men or women (% of 15 years and above) in a district that had systolic blood pressure > 140 mm Hg or diastolic blood pressure > 90 mm Hg. We excluded implausible values for blood pressures, such as systolic blood pressure above 250 or below 60 or diastolic blood pressure above 140 or below 40. We also obtained information on the access to health facilities at a district level using the NDHS 2016, which was defined as the percentage of households within 30 min walking distance of a government health facility. The access to a health facility reflects the availability of healthcare services in an emergency. In addition, we defined smoking as the percentage of men or women (% of 15–49 years old) who smoked cigarettes daily (manufactured or hand-rolled). The NDHS 2016 recorded daily cigarette smoking for all participants aged 15–49 years who were interviewed. In order to estimate the percentage of these risk factors (i.e., obesity, hypertension, access to a health facility, and smoking) at district level, we created a binary variable for each risk factor, indicating whether an individual experiences the risk factor. We calculated the percentage of a risk factor by dividing the number of people experiencing the risk factor in each district by the sample size for the risk factor in each district multiplied by 100.

2.6. Statistical Analysis

The unit of analysis was district in our analysis, and the baseline information on each district was reported as means, standard deviations, and proportions. A locally weighted scatterplot smoothing (LOWESS) curve was plotted to show the relationships between potential risk factors and COVID-19 outcomes per 100,000 people.

We applied a multiple linear regression to estimate the best fit regression equations and to assess the amount of variation that can be explained by the risk factors, assuming independent noise terms, all with an identical normal distribution. We built several main effects multivariable regression models to identify the factors significantly associated with the COVID-19 cases, recovered cases, and deaths per 100,000 people. In order to reduce overfitting caused by the limited sample size (n = 73 districts), the potential predictors for model development were first identified by a univariable screening process with a pre-set p-value of 0.25. This approach is recommended for removing weak predictors [31]. Then, we used a backward stepwise elimination approach, based on a likelihood ratio test, to select the final set of covariates for retention in the COVID-19 outcome models. All models were robust to heteroskedasticity (Breusch–Pagan test), and multicollinearity was not observed, as measured by the variance inflation factor (VIF < 3).

A Poisson regression model is typically used to evaluate count data. In our study, an initial assessment of the outcome variables indicated considerable overdispersion, meaning that the variance exceeded the mean. Therefore, a negative binomial regression model was used to estimate the rate ratio (RR) of the risk factors for COVID-19 outcomes. The outcome variables were the total number of COVID-19 cases, recovered cases, and deaths. The population size for each district was included as an offset to estimate the standardized RR: a value < 1 indicates a decreased likelihood and a value > 1 indicates an increased likelihood of the event under investigation. We assessed overdispersion in each model using a likelihood ratio test, which compares the negative binomial model to a Poisson model. A statistically significant p-value for chi-square with one degree of freedom indicates the presence of overdispersion.

Furthermore, we employed restricted cubic spline models to examine potential non-linear associations between the covariate that explain large variations in the linear regression model, COVID-19 case rates, and other outcomes. To provide enough flexibility to the model and to make the model less sensitive to the smallest fluctuations, we prespecified the use of three knots [32].

Additionally, to validate the model, we randomly split the data into training and validation sets using a 60/40 split and evaluated the model in both the training and validation sets. Adjusted R^2 and McFadden's pseudo R^2 were used to assess the model performance in the linear regression and negative binomial regression, respectively. All the statistical analyses were conducted using Stata v.17.0 (Stata Corp., College Station, TX, USA).

3. Results

The descriptive statistics of the outcome and exposure variables for the 73 districts are summarized in Table 1. As of 22 January 2021, the average rates for case fatality and recovery were 1.2% and 97.2%, respectively. The proportion of the population aged 60 and above was 6.1%, and it ranged between 1.8% and 13.7% among the districts of Nepal. The population density (number of persons per square kilometer) varied from 4.7 in Dolpa district to 4415.8 in Kathmandu district. Household crowding, across districts, ranged between 3.3% and 37.9%, while the adult literacy rate ranged from 16.0% to 66.1%. A wide variation across districts was observed for the prevalence of individuals who did not have access to a handwashing facility (mean 60.9%; range 9.8% to 100%). Furthermore, the prevalences of obesity in women and smoking in men were 3.6% and 18.9%, respectively.

Table S1 presents confirmed, recovered, and deceased cases by district for the entire study period (23 January 2020 to 22 January 2021). As of 22 January 2021, 268,948 COVID-19-positive cases were reported, with 263,546 recovered, and 1986 deaths. The confirmed cases of COVID-19 were distributed throughout the country in all the administrative districts. Among the 73 districts included in the analysis, the total number of confirmed cases was highest in Kathmandu district (n = 103,523), followed by Lalitpur (n = 16,106) and Morang (n = 13,236) districts, and was lowest in Mugu (n = 37), Humla (n = 44), and Dolpa (n = 60) districts. The highest number of cases was reported in the age group 21–40 years (53.18%, n = 143,039) (Figure 1A); however, the number of deaths was higher in the age group 61–80 (Figure 1B).

In Nepal, the overall rate of cases, recovered cases, and deaths were 881.04, 863.35, and 6.51 per 100,000 people (Table S1), indicating that 11.18 cases per 100,000 people had continuing illness when the data collection was stopped. The distribution of COVID-19 outcomes varied across districts in Nepal (Figure 2). The top 10% of districts by incidence accounted for 36% of the cases, whereas the lowest 10% of districts by incidence accounted for only 1.8% (Figure 2A). The highest COVID-19 incidence was 4499 per 100,000 (Table S1). The top 10% of districts by mortality accounted for 35% of all COVID-19 deaths (Figure 2C). The highest rate of COVID-19 mortality was 32 per 100,000 (Table S1). In addition, we conducted an analysis using province-level data to show interprovincial variation in the

COVID-19 outcomes. Among the provinces, Bagmati province had the highest average rate of confirmed cases (1191 per 100,000), recovered cases (1164 per 100,000), and deaths (9 per 100,000) in Nepal, followed by Gandaki and Lumbini (Figure 2D–F).

Table 1. District-level characteristics of the study population.

Characteristics	Mean	SD	Min	Max
COVID-19 infection characteristics				
Number of cases	3756.37	12,240.46	37	1035.23
Number of recovered cases	3677.27	11,902.28	35	1005.84
Number of deaths	27.18	86.66	0	738
Cases per 100,000 population	552.29	649.21	56.83	4499.26
Recovered cases per 100,000 population	540.26	635.53	53.76	4371.53
Deaths per 100,000 population	4.55	4.94	0.00	32.07
Case fatality rate (%) [a]	1.20	1.46	0.00	9.09
Recovery rate (%) [a]	97.21	2.53	84.09	99.72
Socio-demographic and health-related characteristics				
Population density (people per km^2)	320.59	595.48	4.65	4415.80
Household crowding (%)	17.05	7.48	3.33	37.93
Sex ratio (number of males/females × 100)	91.99	7.77	76.02	109.84
Percentage aged ≥ 60 years	6.13	2.38	1.82	13.74
Obesity prevalence (%)				
Women	3.59	3.98	0.00	19.30
Men	1.86	2.12	0.00	8.43
Smoking prevalence (%)				
Women	5.36	5.37	0.00	20.93
Men	18.85	10.53	0.00	61.54
No access to handwashing facilities (%)	60.90	20.19	9.76	100
Adult literacy rate (%)	42.76	11.42	15.96	66.11
Access to a health facility (%)	39.85	24.70	0.00	84.62
Per capita income (USD)	1039.71	360.30	487.00	2764.00

[a] Calculated by dividing the number of events by the total number of reported cases. USD, United States Dollar.

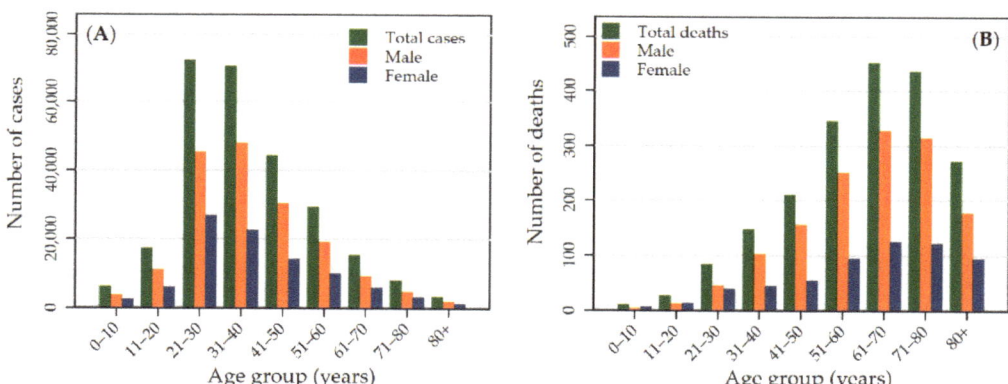

Figure 1. Age and gender distributions of confirmed COVID-19 cases (**A**) and deaths (**B**) in Nepal up to 22 January 2021.

The COVID-19 incidence and mortality per 100,000 are plotted as a function of district-level predictors using the bivariate smoother ("LOWESS") for each predictor (Figure 3). The five predictors, including population density, obesity in women, sex ratio, no access to handwashing facilities, and per capita income, showed positive associations with the COVID-19 incidence and mortality per 100,000 people.

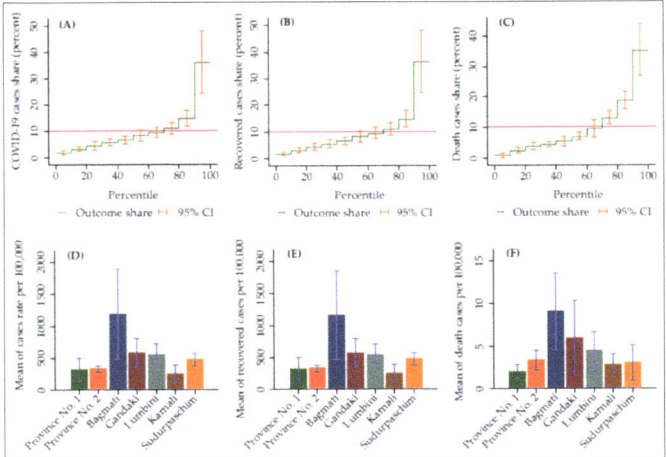

Figure 2. District incidence (**A**), recovery (**B**), and mortality (**C**) per 100,000 population, ranked by district percentile. Figures (**D**), (**E**), and (**F**) present the provincial distributions of COVID-19 outcomes.

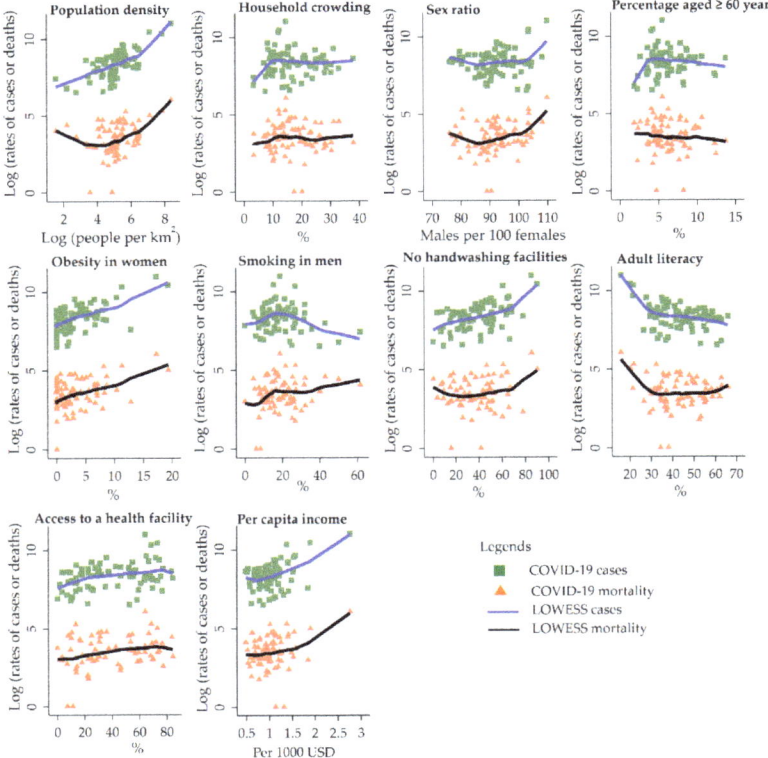

Figure 3. Bivariate analysis for the risk factors of COVID-19 cases and deaths per 100,000 population using LOWESS (locally weighted scatterplot smoothing) in the 73 districts.

The findings of the multivariable regression analysis to identify factors associated with COVID-19 incidence and recovered cases are presented in Table 2. The predictors significantly associated with the COVID-19 incidence in both the linear and negative binomial regressions were population density, household crowding, obesity prevalence in women, and adult literacy; access to basic handwashing facilities at home was significantly associated with the COVID-19 incidence per 100,000 people only in the linear regression model. There was a positive association of COVID-19 incidence rate with the population density (RR = 1.38; 95% CI: 1.09, 1.76), household crowding (RR = 1.04; 95% CI: 1.01, 1.06), and the prevalence of obesity in women (RR = 1.07; 95% CI: 1.02, 1.13), where higher values of these variables were associated with a higher number of detected cases. In contrast, those with higher levels of literacy had a significantly lower incidence rate (RR = 0.97; 95% CI: 0.96, 0.99). When the analysis was continued with the outcome variable of recovered cases, population density (RR = 1.63; 95% CI: 1.18, 2.24) and adult literacy (RR = 1.03; 95% CI: 1.00, 1.06) were positively associated with an increased number of recovered cases (Table 2). When COVID-19 mortality was assessed, variables significantly associated with an increased COVID-19 mortality rate were population density, obesity in women, and smoking in men (Table 3). The linear regression model showed that geographic accessibility to healthcare facilities was negatively associated with deaths per 100,000 people.

Table 2. Multivariable linear regression and negative binomial regression analyses on COVID-19 case diagnosis and successful resolution of disease.

Variables	Linear Regression β (95% CI)	Negative Binomial Regression RR (95% CI)
Incidence [a]		
Population density	0.689 (0.571, 0.806) ***	1.38 (1.09, 1.76) [c] **
Household crowding (%)	15.18 (5.86, 24.51) **	1.04 (1.01, 1.06) **
Obesity prevalence in women (%)	45.74 (13.87, 77.60) **	1.07 (1.02, 1.13) **
Smoking in men (%)	3.00 (−1.65, 7.66)	1.00 (0.98, 1.01)
No access to handwashing facilities (%)	5.52 (0.698, 10.35) *	1.00 (0.99, 1.01)
Adult literacy (%)	−15.32 (−22.43, −8.22) ***	0.97 (0.96, 0.99) **
Percentage aged ≥ 60 years	−11.86 (−34.61, 10.90)	0.98 (0.93, 1.03)
R^2/McFadden's Pseudo R^2	0.874	0.047
Recovered cases [b]		
Population density	0.752 (0.618, 0.887) ***	1.63 (1.18, 2.24) **
Sex ratio	3.92 (−13.59, 21.44)	1.01 (0.98, 1.01)
Adult literacy (%)	16.42 (0.744, 32.09) *	1.03 (1.00, 1.06) *
Access to a health facility (%)	−0.073 (−2.83, 2.68)	1.00 (0.99, 1.01)
Per capita income (USD)	0.198 (−0.104, 0.500)	1.08 (0.53, 2.22) [d]
Percentage aged ≥ 60 years	−7.42 (−39.80, 24.97)	0.99 (0.92, 1.07)
R^2/McFadden's Pseudo R^2	0.826	0.037

* $p < 0.05$, ** $p < 0.01$, *** $p < 0.001$. [a] Dependent variable: cases per 100,000 population in the linear regression model and the number of confirmed cases in the negative binomial regression model. [b] Dependent variable: recovered cases per 100,000 population in the linear regression model and the number of recovered cases in the negative binomial regression model. [c] For every 1000 population. [d] For every thousand dollars increase in per capita income.

Older age (aged ≥ 60 years) was not a significant factor in the multivariable models that included population density, sex ratio, obesity in women, smoking in men, access to a health facility, and per capita income as explanatory variables (Table 3). However, after omitting the lifestyle factors (smoking and obesity), the association between older age and COVID-19 mortality became significant in the negative binomial regression model (RR = 1.16; 95% CI: 1.01, 1.32). Further analysis revealed significant interactions between older age and sex ratio in COVID-19 mortality (p for interaction = 0.047).

Furthermore, we assessed the demographic and health-related indicators that had significant predictive power in our model. The correlation analysis (Table S2) suggested that population density was the most important explanatory variable in the model. Indeed, it independently explained 76% of the variation in COVID-19 incidence (per 100,000 population) in the linear regression model (Table S3). However, a significantly superior fit was obtained by adding the remaining explanatory variables (Table 2). This model accounted for 87% of the variation in the incidence. Population density continued to be the main determinant of the recovered cases and deaths per 100,000 people (Table S3). The multiplicative interaction between population density and household crowding was not significant for deaths per 100,000 population ($p = 0.960$), and the interaction terms showed a marginal level of significance for cases and recovered cases per 100,000 population ($p = 0.080$ and 0.078, respectively).

Table 3. Multivariable linear regression and negative binomial regression analyses on COVID-19 mortality.

Variables	Linear Regression [a]	Negative Binomial Regression [b]
	β (95% CI)	RR (95% CI)
Population density	0.006 (0.004, 0.007) ***	1.42 (1.07, 1.88) [c] *
Sex ratio	−0.047 (−0.191, 0.096)	0.99 (0.97, 1.03)
Obesity prevalence in women (%)	0.293 (−0.033, 0.618) +	1.06 (1.00, 1.14) *
Smoking in men (%)	0.073 (−0.002, 0.148) +	1.01 (1.00, 1.03) *
Percentage aged ≥ 60 years	−0.107 (−0.506, 0.293)	0.97 (0.88, 1.06)
Access to a health facility (%)	−0.040 (−0.080, −0.001) *	1.00 (0.99, 1.004)
Per capita income (USD)	0.001 (−0.003, 0.004)	1.20 (0.54, 2.65) [d]
R^2/McFadden's Pseudo R^2	0.566	0.030

+ $p < 0.1$, * $p < 0.05$, *** $p < 0.001$. [a] Dependent variable: deaths per 100,000 population. [b] Dependent variable: number of deaths due to COVID-19. [c] For every 1000 population. [d] For every thousand dollars increase in per capita income.

We found a linear association between population density and COVID-19 cases, recovered cases, and deaths per 100,000 population (Figure 4). Figure 4A displays the relative increase in the incidence associated with the population density. In the study period, the incidence was higher in the areas with high density, and a rapid increase in the incidence was observed in the areas with a population density over 153.3 (log population density = 5.03). Figure 4C presents the number of deaths per 100,000 people and its association with population density. COVID-19 mortality risk was positively associated with population density; a significant increase in mortality was observed in the areas with a population density over 153.3.

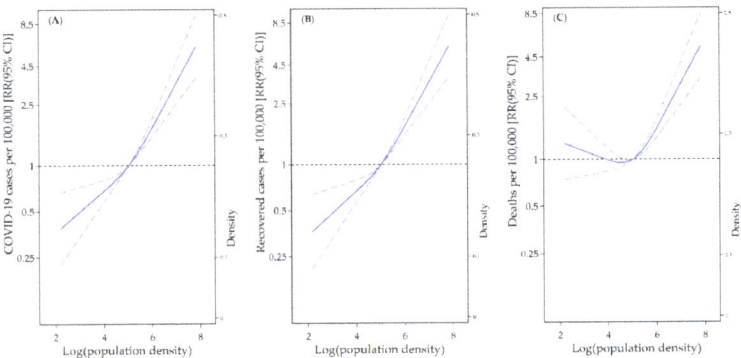

Figure 4. Associations of log-transformed population density with COVID-19 cases (**A**), recovered cases (**B**), and deaths (**C**) per 100,000 people using a restricted cubic spline with three knots. The solid line represents the relative risk (RR), and the long-dashed lines represent the confidence intervals. The reference population density for these plots (with RR fixed as 1.0) is 5.03. The histograms show the distribution of the log-transformed population density.

Evaluation of the prediction model on the training and validation data using the linear regression model is shown in Figure 5. The scatter plots show that the model performed well in both datasets. However, the performance was better for training data, with adjusted R^2 of 0.914, 0.894, and 0.584 for COVID-19 cases, recovered cases, and deaths (per 100,000 people), respectively. The scatter plots of the observed counts against the model-predicted counts using a negative binomial regression are shown in the Supplementary Materials (Figure S1). The values of the adjusted Pseudo R^2 indicated that the model performance was better for training data, which is consistent with the linear regression model.

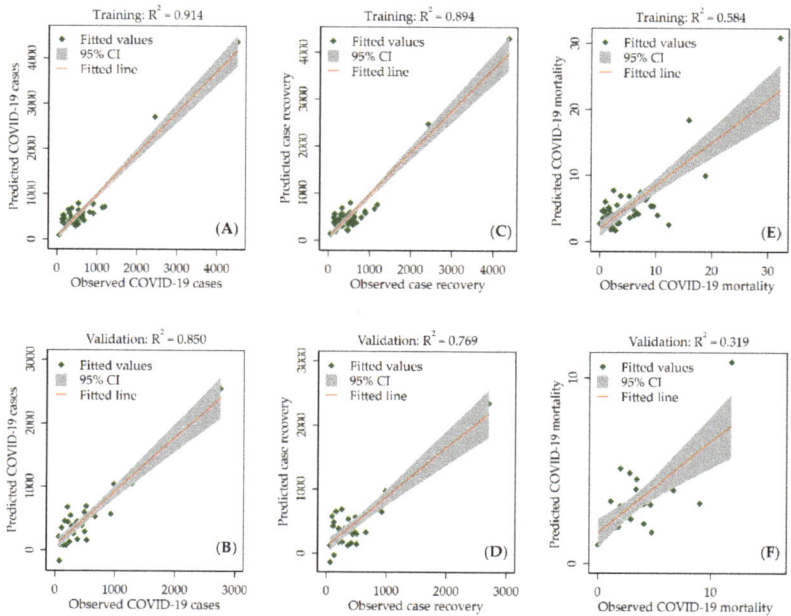

Figure 5. Scatter plot of the observed and predicted COVID-19 cases (**A**,**B**), recovered cases (**C**,**D**), and mortality (**E**,**F**) per 100,000 people for the training and validation datasets using the linear regression model. R^2 is the adjusted R^2 values.

4. Discussion

This is the first study to examine the risk factors associated with COVID-19-related health outcomes in Nepal. We found the districts that were vulnerable to the spread of COVID-19 in the study period due to high population density, the percentage of people living in crowded households, the percentage of people without access to basic handwashing facilities in their homes, and the percentage of adult literacy. Furthermore, higher COVID-19 transmission was associated with obesity in women. The mortality risk of COVID-19 was also generally higher in high-density areas. In addition, higher prevalences of obesity in women and smoking in men were associated with higher mortality rates, whereas access to a health facility was associated with a lower mortality rate. Population density was identified as the most important demographic variable associated with the large variation in COVID-19 transmission in our study.

Our finding of a positive association between population density and COVID-19 transmission is consistent with the existing literature [8,33]. The underlying mechanism for the association with population density is related to increased transmission of saliva, respiratory droplets, and or aerosol between individuals when people are in close physical proximity [34,35]. Furthermore, we found that household crowding was associated with higher COVID-19 transmission. Relatively few studies have examined the impact of household crowding, as opposed to household size. In the United States, an analysis of data from 91 counties in New York, New Jersey, and Connecticut found that people with more crowded households were more likely to contract COVID-19 infections [8]. Household crowding can increase the risk of exposure to coughs, sneezes, and food sharing, which have been considered as dominant risk factors for COVID-19 transmission [36]. Overcrowding is a common residential situation in Nepal due to small housing units, particularly for urban residents and large families. Therefore, improvement of overcrowded living conditions would reduce the high transmission of COVID-19.

We found a positive association between the lack of access to handwashing facilities and COVID-19 transmission. Limited access to handwashing facilities increases the risk of transmission from hands to eyes or mouth and may promote the spread and magnitude of the COVID-19 pandemic. Previous research showed that handwashing could reduce the transmission of respiratory viruses by 45−55% [37]. According to the WHO and UNICEF [38], the frequent washing of hands using water and soap could help contain the spread of COVID-19. Therefore, it is crucial to distribute hand sanitizers to those districts without access to handwashing facilities. Furthermore, our finding showed that areas with higher adult literacy rates were less vulnerable to COVID-19 spread. Potential reasons for the association might include higher rates of compliance with COVID-19 preventive measures among literate people, which may slow COVID-19 transmission [39].

Health-related lifestyle factors, such as obesity in women and smoking in men were significantly associated with the mortality rate in our study. Obesity has been identified as one of the key risk factors associated with COVID-19 deaths [40]. Our finding is consistent with a previous study that suggested a stronger risk of COVID-19 mortality in obese women than men [41]. Furthermore, we found a higher frequency of deaths in districts with a higher smoking prevalence in men. This finding is consistent with research showing higher risks of COVID-19-related death among current smokers [42]. In our study, the prevalences of obesity in men and smoking in women were not significantly associated with COVID-19 mortality; however, we cannot fully explore gender-specific differences in obesity and smoking for COVID-19 outcomes with this data, and further research should investigate how gender differences in COVID-19 outcomes vary regionally.

In addition, our study showed that the physical accessibility of medical services, which indicates the capability of a population to obtain health care services [43,44], was significantly associated COVID-19 mortality: areas with a lower percentage of health facilities within 30 min walking distance were likely to have a higher mortality rate. Previous research reported that limited or poor access to healthcare was associated with increased COVID-19 deaths [45]. People in areas with poor access to health facilities may delay receiving COVID-19 testing and diagnosis or even forgo being tested, and may, consequently, turn to medical care only in the advanced stages, which may result in poor outcomes.

Previous studies suggested that mortality due to COVID-19 was significantly higher in older people [46,47]. In our study, older age was significantly associated with a higher risk of COVID-19 mortality in the model adjusted for population density, sex ratio, access to a health facility, and per capita income. When the model was additionally adjusted for lifestyle factors, the association remained insignificant. In addition, the interactions between older age and sex ratio were significant in COVID-19 mortality. Our findings suggested a complex interplay of age, sex, and lifestyle factors in explaining the high mortality rate of COVID-19. Previous research highlighted a differential risk of COVID-19 mortality according to age, sex, and lifestyle factors [48,49]. However, further study using individual-level data are needed to confirm how age, sex, and lifestyle factors and their interactions contribute to the variations in the COVID-19 outcomes.

There are several limitations to this study. First, our study used district-level determinants. Therefore, the results of this study can only suggest associations between risk factors and COVID-19 outcomes at the district level but cannot be interpreted as the associations at the individual level. Second, the patient-level information was unavailable. Thus, the spread pattern of COVID-19 among specific sub-populations, such as among age, sex, and ethnicity subgroups, which might be associated differently with the other risk factors, could not be determined. Third, because of data limitations, we could not estimate district-specific data on the prevalence of clinical risk factors of COVID-19, including asthma, congestive heart failure, and cerebrovascular diseases. However, using the NDHS 2016 data, we provided available clinical risk correlates related to hypertension and obesity across districts. It should be noted that the estimates presented for these risk factors only apply to adults aged 15–49 years in the district, and not the entire district population. Finally, there is a possibility of bias due to the time elapsed between the current crisis and the collection of our data. However, the NPHC 2011 and NDHS 2016 are the main data sources in this study and are the most reliable data on the district-level demographic characteristics of Nepal, and major changes in the relative distributions of these measures are unlikely.

5. Conclusions

This study using district-level data from Nepal suggests that populations living in high-density areas may be more vulnerable to COVID-19 spread, as well as mortality. In addition, health- and sanitation-related population features, such as smoking prevalence, obesity rate, and access to a health facility and handwashing facility, may be contributing factors to the disparities in COVID-19 outcomes across districts. This study can provide a baseline for evaluating local level epidemic factors and designing policies for the control of local COVID-19 outbreaks.

Supplementary Materials: The following supporting information can be downloaded at: https://www.mdpi.com/article/10.3390/ijerph19052659/s1. Table S1: COVID-19 cases in Nepal by district, Table S2: Correlation coefficients among the variables, Table S3: Linear regression results with population density as the single explanatory variable. Figure S1. Scatter plot of observed and predicted COVID-19 cases (A and B), recovered cases (C and D), and mortality (E and F) for training and validation datasets using the negative binomial regression.

Author Contributions: Conceptualization, D.K.L.; methodology, D.K.L. and S.S.; software, S.S.; validation, D.K.L., S.S. and H.-C.K.; formal analysis, D.K.L.; investigation, D.K.L.; resources, S.S. and H.-C.K.; data curation, S.S.; writing—original draft preparation, D.K.L.; writing—review and editing, D.K.L., S.S. and H.-C.K.; visualization, S.S.; supervision, D.K.L. and H.-C.K. All authors have read and agreed to the published version of the manuscript. Figure S1. Scatter plot of observed and predicted COVID-19 cases (A and B), recovered cases (C and D), and mortality (E and F) for training and validation datasets using the negative binomial regression.

Funding: This research received no external funding.

Institutional Review Board Statement: Procedures and questionnaires for standard Demographic and Health Surveys (DHS) have been reviewed and approved by the ICF International Institutional Review Board (IRB). The NDHS obtained ethical approvals from Nepal Health Research Council, Kathmandu, Nepal. The first author communicated with MEASURE DHS/ICF International, and permission was granted to download the data for the study.

Informed Consent Statement: Informed consent was obtained from all NDHS participants. COVID-19 data were obtained from routinely collected clinical data and, therefore, consent was not individually collected.

Data Availability Statement: The data presented in this study are available upon request from the corresponding author.

Conflicts of Interest: The authors declare no conflict of interest.

References

1. World Health Organization. Coronavirus Disease 2019 (COVID-19) Situation Report 51. 2020. Available online: https://www.who.int/docs/default-source/coronaviruse/situation-reports/20200311-sitrep-51-covid-19.pdf?sfvrsn=1ba62e57_10 (accessed on 1 November 2021).
2. World Health Organization. WHO Coronavirus Disease (COVID-19) Dashboard. Available online: https://covid19.who.int (accessed on 17 December 2021).

3. Centers of Disease Control and Prevention. New Variants of the Virus that Causes COVID-19. Available online: https://www.cdc.gov/coronavirus/2019-ncov/transmission/variant.html (accessed on 10 December 2021).
4. Mackenzie, J.S.; Smith, D.W. COVID-19: A novel zoonotic disease caused by a coronavirus from China: What we know and what we don't. *Microbiol. Aust.* **2020**, *41*, 45–50. [CrossRef]
5. Davies, N.G.; Klepac, P.; Liu, Y.; Prem, K.; Jit, M.; CMMID COVID-19 working group; Eggo, R.M. Age-dependent effects in the transmission and control of COVID-19 epidemics. *Nat. Med.* **2020**, *26*, 1205–1211. [CrossRef]
6. Ochi, S.; So, M.; Hashimoto, S.; Denda, K.; Sekizawa, Y. Behavioral factors associated with COVID-19 risk: A cross-sectional survey in Japan. *Int. J. Environ. Res. Public Health* **2021**, *18*, 12184. [CrossRef] [PubMed]
7. Treskova-Schwarzbach, M.; Haas, L.; Reda, S.; Pilic, A.; Borodova, A.; Karimi, K.; Koch, J.; Nygren, T.; Scholz, S.; Schönfeld, V.; et al. Pre-existing health conditions and severe COVID-19 outcomes: An umbrella review approach and meta-analysis of global evidence. *BMC Med.* **2021**, *19*, 212. [CrossRef] [PubMed]
8. Lee, W.; Kim, H.; Choi, H.M.; Heo, S.; Fong, K.C.; Yang, J.; Park, C.; Kim, H.; Bell, M.L. Urban environments and COVID-19 in three Eastern states of the United States. *Sci. Total Environ.* **2021**, *779*, 146334. [CrossRef] [PubMed]
9. Federgruen, A.; Naha, S. Crowding effects dominate demographic attributes in COVID-19 cases. *Int. J. Infect. Dis.* **2021**, *102*, 509–516. [CrossRef]
10. Government of Nepal, COVID-19 Nepal. Available online: https://covidnepal.org (accessed on 5 December 2021).
11. United Nations. COVID-19 Nepal: Preparedness and Response Plan (NPRP) April-2020. Available online: https://www.who.int/docs/default-source/nepal-documents/novel-coronavirus/covid-19-nepal-preparedness-andresponse-plan-(nprp)-draft-april-9.pdf?sfvrsn=808a970a_2 (accessed on 5 December 2021).
12. Epidemiology and Diseases Control and Division, Nepal. Epidemiological Update on COVID 19 (17 July 2020). Available online: http://edcd.gov.np/news/download/epidemiological-update-on-covid-19-17-july-2020 (accessed on 5 December 2021).
13. Pantha, B.; Acharya, S.; Joshi, H.R.; Vaidya, N.K. Inter-provincial disparity of COVID-19 transmission and control in Nepal. *Sci. Rep.* **2021**, *11*, 13363. [CrossRef]
14. Ministry of Health and Population, Government of Nepal. COVID-19 Update (2020). Available online: https://covid19.mohp.gov.np/ (accessed on 13 December 2021).
15. Basnet, B.B.; Bishwakarma, K.; Pant, R.R.; Dhakal, S.; Pandey, N.; Gautam, D.; Ghimire, A.; Basnet, T.B. Combating the COVID-19 pandemic: Experiences of the first wave from Nepal. *Front. Public Health* **2021**, *9*, 613402. [CrossRef]
16. Shah, M.R.T.; Ahammed, T.; Anjum, A.; Chowdhury, A.A.; Suchana, A.J. Finding the real COVID-19 case-fatality rates for SAARC countries. *Biosaf. Health* **2021**, *3*, 164–171. [CrossRef]
17. Sapkota, K.; Dangal, G.; Koirala, M.; Sapkota, K.; Poudel, A.; Dhital, S.R. Strategies for prevention and control of COVID-19 in Nepal. *J. Patan Acad. Health Sci.* **2020**, *7*, 85–88. [CrossRef]
18. Bedford, J.; Enria, D.; Giesecke, J.; Heymann, D.L.; Ihekweazu, C.; Kobinger, G.; Lane, H.C.; Memish, Z.; Oh, M.D.; Sal, A.A.; et al. COVID-19: Towards controlling of a pandemic. *Lancet* **2020**, *395*, 1015–1018. [CrossRef]
19. Rubin, D.; Huang, J.; Fisher, B.T.; Gasparrini, A.; Tam, V.; Song, L.; Wang, X.; Kaufman, J.; Fitzpatrick, K.; Jain, A.; et al. Association of social distancing, population density, and temperature with the instantaneous reproduction number of SARS-CoV-2 in counties across the United States. *JAMA Netw. Open* **2020**, *3*, e2016099. [CrossRef]
20. Ministry of Health and Population, Government of Nepal. Coronavirus Disease Outbreak Updates and Resources Materials. Available online: https://heoc.mohp.gov.np/update-on-novel-corona-virus-covid-19/ (accessed on 13 December 2021).
21. National Disaster Risk Reduction and Management Authority, Government of Nepal. Nepal COVID-19 Dashboard. Available online: https://covid19.ndrrma.gov.np/ (accessed on 13 December 2021).
22. Government of Nepal National Planning Commission; United Nations Development Programme. *Nepal Human Development Report 2014 Beyond Geography, Unlocking Human Potential*; Government of Nepal National Planning Commission: Kathmandu, Nepal, 2014.
23. Government of Nepal National Planning Commission, Central Bureau of Statistics. *National Population and Housing Census 2011 (Population Projection 2011–2031)*; Central Bureau of Statistics: Kathmandu, Nepal, 2014.
24. Government of Nepal National Planning Commission, Central Bureau of Statistics. *National Population and Housing Census 2011 (National Report)*; Central Bureau of Statistics: Kathmandu, Nepal, 2012.
25. Ministry of Health, Nepal; New ERA; ICF. *Nepal Demographic and Health Survey 2016*; Ministry of Health: Kathmandu, Nepal, 2017.
26. World Health Organization. *WHO Housing and Health Guidelines*; World Health Organization: Geneva, Switzerland, 2018.
27. Ge, Y.; Martinez, L.; Sun, S.; Chen, Z.; Zhang, F.; Li, F.; Sun, W.; Chen, E.; Pan, J.; Li, C.; et al. COVID-19 transmission dynamics among close contacts of index patients with COVID-19: A population-based cohort study in Zhejiang province, China. *JAMA Intern. Med.* **2021**, *181*, 1343–1350. [CrossRef]
28. Romero Starke, K.; Petereit-Haack, G.; Schubert, M.; Kämpf, D.; Schliebner, A.; Hegewald, J.; Seidler, A. The age-related risk of severe outcomes due to COVID-19 infection: A rapid review, meta-analysis, and meta-regression. *Int. J. Environ. Res. Public Health* **2020**, *17*, 5974. [CrossRef]
29. Centers for Disease Control and Prevention. Show Me the Science—Why Wash Your Hands? Available online: https://www.cdc.gov/handwashing/whyhandwashing.html (accessed on 15 October 2021).

30. United Nations Children's Fund; World Health Organization. *Progress on Drinking Water, Sanitation and Hygiene in Schools: Special Focus on COVID-19*; United Nations Children's Fund and World Health Organization: New York, NY, USA, 2020.
31. George, S.L. Identification and assessment of prognostic factors. *Semin. Oncol.* **1988**, *15*, 462–471.
32. Durrleman, S.; Simon, R. Flexible regression models with cubic splines. *Stat. Med.* **1989**, *8*, 551–561. [CrossRef]
33. Tamrakar, V.; Srivastava, A.; Saikia, N.; Parmar, M.C.; Shukla, S.K.; Shabnam, S.; Boro, B.; Saha, A.; Debbarma, B. District level correlates of COVID-19 pandemic in India during March–October 2020. *PLoS ONE* **2021**, *16*, e0257533. [CrossRef]
34. Bahl, P.; Doolan, C.; de Silva, C.; Chughtai, A.A.; Bourouiba, L.; MacIntyre, C.R. Airborne or droplet precautions for health workers treating COVID-19? *J. Infect. Dis.* **2020**, jiaa189. [CrossRef]
35. van Doremalen, N.; Bushmaker, T.; Morris, D.H.; Holbrook, M.G.; Gamble, A.; Williamson, B.N.; Tamin, A.; Harcourt, J.L.; Thornburg, N.J.; Gerber, S.I.; et al. Aerosol and Surface Stability of SARS-CoV-2 as compared with SARS-CoV-1. *N. Engl. J. Med.* **2020**, *382*, 1564–1567. [CrossRef]
36. Cook, T.M. Personal protective equipment during the coronavirus disease (COVID) 2019 pandemic—A narrative review. *Anaesthesia* **2020**, *75*, 920–927. [CrossRef]
37. Jefferson, T.; Del Mar, C.B.; Dooley, L.; Ferroni, E.; Al-Ansary, L.A.; Bawazeer, G.A.; van Driel, M.L.; Jones, M.A.; Thorning, S.; Beller, E.M.; et al. Physical interventions to interrupt or reduce the spread of respiratory viruses. *Cochrane Database Syst. Rev.* **2020**, *11*, CD006207.
38. World Health Organization; United Nations Children's Fund. Water, Sanitation, Hygiene, and Waste Management for the COVID-19 Virus: Interim Guidance, 19 March 2020. Available online: https://apps.who.int/iris/handle/10665/331499 (accessed on 20 December 2021).
39. Sharif, N.; Alzahrani, K.J.; Ahmed, S.N.; Opu, R.R.; Ahmed, N.; Talukder, A.; Nunia, R.; Chowdhury, M.S.; Nodi, I.J.; Saha, T.; et al. Protective measures are associated with the reduction of transmission of COVID-19 in Bangladesh: A nationwide cross-sectional study. *PLoS ONE* **2021**, *16*, e0260287. [CrossRef]
40. Williamson, E.J.; Walker, A.J.; Bhaskaran, K.; Bacon, S.; Bates, C.; Morton, C.E.; Curtis, H.J.; Mehrkar, A.; Evans, D.; Inglesby, P.; et al. Factors associated with COVID-19-related death using OpenSAFELY. *Nature* **2020**, *584*, 430–436. [CrossRef]
41. Peters, S.A.E.; MacMahon, S.; Woodward, M. Obesity as a risk factor for COVID-19 mortality in women and men in the UK biobank: Comparisons with influenza/pneumonia and coronary heart disease. *Diabetes Obes. Metab.* **2021**, *23*, 258–262. [CrossRef] [PubMed]
42. Clift, A.K.; von Ende, A.; Tan, P.S.; Sallis, H.M.; Lindson, N.; Coupland, C.A.C.; Munafò, M.R.; Aveyard, P.; Hippisley-Cox, J.; Hopewell, J.C. Smoking and COVID-19 outcomes: An observational and Mendelian randomisation study using the UK Biobank cohort. *Thorax* **2022**, *77*, 65–73. [CrossRef] [PubMed]
43. Kelly, C.; Hulme, C.; Farragher, T.; Clarke, G. Are differences in travel time or distance to healthcare for adults in global north countries associated with an impact on health outcomes? A systematic review. *BMJ Open* **2016**, *6*, e013059. [CrossRef]
44. Bhattarai, S.; Parajuli, S.B.; Rayamajhi, R.B.; Paudel, I.S.; Jha, N. Clinical health seeking behavior and utilization of health care services in eastern hilly region of Nepal. *JCMS Nepal* **2015**, *11*, 8–16.
45. Gesesew, H.A.; Koye, D.N.; Fetene, D.M.; Woldegiorgis, M.; Kinfu, Y.; Geleto, A.B.; Melaku, Y.A.; Mohammed, H.; Alene, K.A.; Awoke, M.A.; et al. Risk factors for COVID-19 infection, disease severity and related deaths in Africa: A systematic review. *BMJ Open* **2021**, *11*, e044618. [CrossRef] [PubMed]
46. Mehraeen, E.; Karimi, A.; Barzegary, A.; Vahedi, F.; Afsahi, A.M.; Dadras, O.; Moradmand-Badie, B.; Seyed Alinaghi, S.A.; Jahanfar, S. Predictors of mortality in patients with COVID-19—A systematic review. *Eur. J. Integr. Med.* **2020**, *40*, 101226. [CrossRef] [PubMed]
47. Ho, F.K.; Petermann-Rocha, F.; Gray, S.R.; Jani, B.D.; Katikireddi, S.V.; Niedzwiedz, C.L.; Foster, H.; Hastie, C.E.; Mackay, D.F.; Gill, J.M.R.; et al. Is older age associated with COVID-19 mortality in the absence of other risk factors? General population cohort study of 470,034 participants. *PLoS ONE* **2020**, *15*, e0241824. [CrossRef]
48. Cifuentes, M.P.; Rodriguez-Villamizar, L.A.; Rojas-Botero, M.L.; Alvarez-Moreno, C.A.; Fernández-Niño, J.A. Socioeconomic inequalities associated with mortality for COVID-19 in Colombia: A cohort nationwide study. *J. Epidemiol. Community Health* **2021**, *75*, 610–615. [CrossRef]
49. Ahmadi, M.N.; Huang, B.H.; Inan-Eroglu, E.; Hamer, M.; Stamatakis, E. Lifestyle risk factors and infectious disease mortality, including COVID-19, among middle aged and older adults: Evidence from a community-based cohort study in the United Kingdom. *Brain Behav. Immun.* **2021**, *96*, 18–27. [CrossRef]

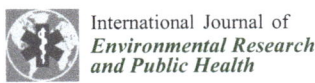 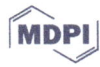

Article

Financial Factors and Psychological Distress during the COVID-19 Pandemic in Poland

Katarzyna Sekścińska [1,*], Agata Trzcińska [1], Daniel Pankowski [1,2], Ewa Pisula [1] and Kinga Wytrychiewicz-Pankowska [1,2]

[1] Faculty of Psychology, University of Warsaw, 00-183 Warsaw, Poland; atrzcinska@psych.uw.edu.pl (A.T.); daniel.pankowski@psych.uw.edu.pl (D.P.); ewa.pisula@psych.uw.edu.pl (E.P.); kwytrychiewicz@gmail.com (K.W.-P.)
[2] Institute of Psychology, University of Economics and Human Sciences in Warsaw, 01-043 Warsaw, Poland
* Correspondence: ks@psych.uw.edu.pl

Abstract: During the COVID-19 pandemic, many factors have simultaneously affected people's psychological distress (PD). The most commonly studied types of factors have been those relating to health risks involving SARS-CoV-2 infection and sociodemographic factors. However, financial changes at both the national and global levels and these changes' influences on people's personal finances constitute another group of factors with the potential to cause symptoms of anxiety and depression. A correlation study of 1135 working adults in Poland was conducted to analyze the roles of a wide range of financial variables in explaining the extent of people's PD during the pandemic. Three groups of financial factors predicted PD over and above sociodemographic variables and COVID-19 health-related factors: a person's objective financial situation, their subjective financial situation, and their individual financial disposition, the last of these being the most important. The present study adds to the current state of knowledge by showing that financial variables explain a significant portion of variance in PD over and above sociodemographic and COVID-19 health-related factors. Moreover, the study also identified individual financial variables that were capable of predicting people's psychological distress during the pandemic.

Keywords: psychological distress; depression symptoms; anxiety symptoms; financial variables; COVID-19 pandemic

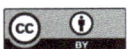

1. Introduction

The COVID-19 pandemic has had a significant impact on almost all areas of people's lives. In addition to the threat it has posed to people's physical health and lives, it has been associated with a number of other burdens. In response to the developing health threat, governments have introduced numerous measures, such as social distancing, closing borders, banning gatherings, closing selected industries, and mandating remote learning and working. Moreover, the circumstances surrounding the pandemic have directly and indirectly affected people's mental health. It has already been shown that the pandemic has increased psychological distress (PD) [1,2], which is commonly defined as a state of emotional suffering characterized by symptoms of depression and anxiety [3]. The stress–distress model postulates that PD occurs when a stressful event threatens a person's physical or mental health and they are unable to cope with the stressor effectively, emotional discomfort being the result of this ineffective coping [4]. The COVID-19 pandemic has been one such stressful event. A meta-analysis conducted by Cénat et al. [1] showed depression to be over three times more prevalent during the pandemic (occurring in 15.97% of people) than it was prior to the pandemic (4.4% of people) and the prevalence of anxiety to be four times higher (15.15% compared to 3.6%). Given these observations, to understand the pandemic's effects on PD, it is important to determine the factors that may provide protection or constitute a threat with respect to people's susceptibility to experiencing symptoms of depression and anxiety.

During the pandemic, many different factors may have had a simultaneous influence on psychological distress. Previous research has shown that a higher infection risk (e.g., the number of suspected/confirmed COVID-19 cases in a geographical location) and increased risk of developing a severe infection (having a pre-existing physical condition or worse general health) are predictive of a greater severity of PD [5]. Experience with COVID-19 is also an important risk factor for PD, and a study of Cai [6] showed that the severity of PD is particularly high in people who have developed COVID-19.

Moreover, other research has identified the important roles of sociodemographic variables such as gender, age, place of residence, and educational level in explaining people's tendency to experience symptoms of depression and anxiety [5,7–9]. Studies have indicated that women have been at increased risk of developing psychopathological symptoms during the pandemic [7,10] and that this may be related to the fact that they are more likely than men to work in positions with a high risk of SARS-CoV-2 infection (the virus that causes COVID-19), e.g., nurses, shop assistants, kindergarten teachers, beauticians, and hairdressers. Previous work also showed that being of an older age was protective against psychological distress during the pandemic [11], and it is likely that losing a job and/or uncertainty resulting from the restrictions introduced may have been particularly stressful for people under 40 years of age due to the increased likelihood of them being caretakers of children or older family members. Moreover, emerging adults (18–29 year olds) may have been particularly at risk of PD, because mandatory social distancing, isolation from people outside their household, and restrictions on movement and travel are likely to have interfered with their need to build their autonomy and maintain friendships and romantic relationships [8]. Place of residence is a further sociodemographic factor that has been connected with PD during the pandemic, the research indicating that people living in rural areas have been at greater risk of PD compared to those living in urban areas [5]; this may be because of inferior medical, economic, and educational infrastructure in rural areas [12]. Another factor that may be indirectly related to the greater incidence of PD in people living in rural areas is socioeconomic status, including lower levels of education; the meta-analysis of Wang et al. [5] showed that less well-educated people are likely to have been at risk of developing symptoms of depression and anxiety during the pandemic.

As shown above, both COVID-19 health-related variables (number of suspected/confirmed COVID-19 cases and increased risk of developing severe COVID-19) and sociodemographic variables have been extensively investigated as predictors of psychological distress during the pandemic. However, despite the fact that the restrictions introduced by governments during the pandemic have had significant negative financial consequences for many people, and the likelihood that this will have been the cause of increased psychological distress in such people, there has been a lack of research identifying the extent to which various financial variables can augment sociodemographic and health threat-related variables in explaining the psychological distress that has occurred during the pandemic. The present study aimed to fill this gap. As in other countries, high levels of anxiety and depression symptoms were observed in Poland (where our study was conducted) during the pandemic [8]. Given the potential long-term consequences of temporarily elevated psychological distress, it is important to determine factors other than the commonly studied COVID-19 health-related variables and sociodemographic variables that may have contributed to or been protective against anxiety and depression.

1.1. Financial Variables and Psychological Distress

As mentioned above, the coronavirus pandemic has increased anxiety and depression symptoms among people across the globe. This may be partly due to the effects that government-imposed restrictions have had on countries' economies and workforces (for example, people's income and job security—see, e.g., Reference [13]). A number of studies have shown that various financial factors can be associated with psychological distress [14–16] and that people's mental health may be associated both with their objective financial situations (income, level of savings, and level of liabilities including debt—e.g., References [17–19] and their subjective perceptions of their financial situations (perceived income, sense of financial security, and job security—e.g., References [13,14,20]. Additionally, studies have shown that psychological distress may be associated with individual financial dispositions such as materialism, economic optimism, and the propensity to take financial risks [21–23].

1.1.1. Objective Financial Situations and Psychological Distress

The effect that a household's objective financial situation can have on the risk that its members will experience anxiety and depression is well-documented [15,24,25]. For example, Orpana et al. [16] demonstrated that a lower income is associated with a higher risk of becoming psychologically distressed. Additionally, using British Household Panel Survey data, Wildman [19] found that a person's financial situation and changes in their situation to be associated with depression, and conversely, research conducted in Sweden has shown that a high household income may be protective against symptoms of depression [26]. Moreover, Gambin et al. [8] showed that, during the COVID-19 pandemic, continuity in Polish people's incomes and their financial situations has had a significant effect on experiencing symptoms of anxiety and depression.

In addition to household income, the objective level of a person's debt has also been shown to be related to their mental health. Brown, Taylor and Wheatley Price [27] observed that debt is associated with increased levels of psychological distress and that a household's psychological well-being is adversely affected by large amounts of unsecured debt (but not secured debt, such as a mortgage on a house). Additionally, there is a positive relationship between the amount of debt and the experiencing of mental health problems [18], and both Skapinakis et al. [28] and Jenkins et al. [29] showed that excessive debt and problems in paying it off make it more likely that a person will become depressed. Finally, Drentea [30] showed that anxiety increases as the ratio of credit card debt to income increases.

At the same time, researchers have emphasized that savings can act as a type of buffer against psychological distress. For example, Brown, Taylor and Wheatley Price [27] showed that people who save (or whose households save) on a regular basis are more likely to report complete psychological well-being than non-savers. Additionally, Bridges and Disney [17] noted that the number of savings accounts that a person had (which was associated with having greater savings) was indirectly associated with a lowered incidence of self-reported symptoms of depression. Moreover, Gardner and Oswald [31] found that positive 'shocks' (medium-sized lottery wins) to the financial well-being of a household tended to be associated with improvements in psychological well-being.

1.1.2. Subjective Financial Situations and Psychological Distress

Bridges and Disney [17] noted that objective indicators of a household's financial situation are not sufficient in understanding the impact of economic factors on psychological distress. These authors found that positive relationships between depression symptoms and self-reported problems of indebtedness and financial stress arise irrespective of objective indicators of a household's financial situation. Thus, when investigating economic sources of psychological distress, one should pay attention not only to the objective financial factors but also to how individuals perceive their financial situation. In fact, research conducted as long as forty years ago showed that perceptions of economic hardship in acquiring the necessities of life dispose people toward depression [32], and more recent research by Dijkstra-Kersten et al. [14] showed financial strain to be associated with having a depressive and/or anxiety disorder, over and above the effects of income.

O'Neill et al. [33] noted that people are happier when they are financially secure, and Ferrie et al. [20] showed that differences in self-reported financial insecurity are important determinants of differences in the incidence of depression. The COVID-19 pandemic has caused many people to worry more about their financial security and experience greater financial concerns, and the research by Wilson et al. [13] showed that, among people saying that the pandemic is posing a significant threat to their personal finances (e.g., those expecting their financial situation to worsen over the next 12 months), 57% of people reported experiencing moderate and high levels of psychological distress, including symptoms of depression and anxiety. Furthermore, it should be noted that, while a sense of financial security and financial concerns are largely related to job security, perceived job insecurity is a stressful experience in itself and is related to greater symptoms of depression and anxiety, as shown by Wilson et al. [13].

1.1.3. Individual Financial Dispositions and Psychological Distress

The studies described above show that psychological distress may depend on both a person's objective financial situation and how they perceive their financial situation. However, many previous studies have shown that an individual's mental health is related not only to their financial situation (whether objective or subjective) but also to their individual financial dispositions: their psychological characteristics with respect to financial issues [34]. Examples of these include materialism, economic optimism, and the tendency to take financial risks. Probably, the most frequently analyzed financial disposition in the context of well-being and psychological distress is materialism, this being defined as "the importance a person places on possessions and their acquisition as a necessary or desirable form of conduct to reach desired end states, including happiness" [35] (p. 307). Materialism has been linked to mental health problems, particularly depression and anxiety [23,36–38], and a meta-analysis of several hundred studies by Dittmar et al. [39] showed clear negative relationships between a broad array of types of personal well-being (including depression and anxiety) and people's materialistic values.

In addition to materialism, a second financial disposition that is associated with PD is economic optimism. Optimists see positive aspects of current situations and events and believe that things will turn out to be positive in the future as well. One recent study of people's economic optimism (often referred to as consumer confidence or consumer sentiment) by van Giesen and Pieters [40] recently showed that the more optimistic people are about economic issues, the less personal stress they experience, this applying irrespective of whether the economic issues involved are on a global, national, or personal level. Additionally, research by Kahle et al. [21] showed that economic optimism is negatively associated with depression.

Another financial disposition that may be related to psychological distress is a propensity for financial risk-taking. Here, studies have shown that risk avoidance is associated with high anxiety [22,41]. In these studies, and in other studies on emotions and risk-taking [42,43], researchers have assumed that emotions such as anxiety trigger risk-averse behaviors. However, given that a propensity for risk-taking is strongly rooted in personality [44] and is a relatively constant individual trait, the relationship between a propensity for financial risk-taking and emotional variables is probably bidirectional. Such an assumption is consistent with the results of Gutter and Copur [34], who showed that an unwillingness to take any financial risks at all is negatively related to financial well-being (which is likely to be related to general well-being). Moreover, in this study, people characterized by a greater than average willingness to take financial risks reported higher levels of financial well-being. This suggests that a higher propensity to take financial risks may translate into lower levels of psychological distress.

In summary, all the above studies of the role of economic variables in generating psychological distress provide evidence that financial factors may be important in explaining PD during the COVID-19 pandemic and that such factors are worth considering in the search for factors that may have a protective function or present a threat with respect to people's susceptibility to experiencing symptoms of depression and anxiety. Due to the deteriorating economic situation, it can be assumed that the financial effects of the pandemic will affect more and more people over time and be one of the most important sources of PD in the short- to medium-term future.

1.2. The Current Study

During the COVID-19 pandemic, financial changes on both the global and national scale have affected many people's personal finances, and this is likely to have caused people to experience symptoms of anxiety and depression. Therefore, one of the present study's main goals was to explore whether financial variables could explain the variance in people's psychological distress (PD) over and above the sociodemographic and COVID-19 health-related variables.

The study's second aim was to ascertain which financial factors are the most important predictors of PD. While previous studies have established links between various financial factors and PD, these studies have tended to analyze each financial variable in isolation without simultaneously analyzing the financial status (both objective and subjective) and financial disposition variables' relationships with symptoms of anxiety and depression. Therefore, to date, studies have been unable to determine the relative importance of various financial factors in predicting PD, and this is particularly important in the context of the COVID-19 pandemic. Thus, our research considered a wide spectrum of financial factors as predictors of PD during the pandemic. We analyzed the role of financial factors on three levels, which allowed us to answer three research questions: (1) Taken together, can financial variables explain the variance in the levels of people's depression and anxiety symptoms over and above the variance explained by sociodemographic and COVID-19 health-related factors? (2) Which category of financial factors (people's objective financial situation, their subjective financial situation, or their individual financial dispositions) explains the largest proportion of variance in PD symptoms? (3) Which specific financial variables in the aforementioned three categories are the strongest predictors of variance in PD symptoms?

2. Materials and Methods

2.1. Participants

A nationwide sample of working age (18+ year olds) Polish adults, diversified in terms of age, sex, place of residence, and educational level, were recruited online from the ARIADNA research panel. ARIADNA is a Polish online research panel with over 150,000 registered Polish users. For any particular study, ARIADNA randomly recruits voluntary participants from its panel (registered users), collects data, and then provides the anonymized data to the party conducting the research. Respondents were awarded points for their participation, which they could later exchange for rewards from a pool of several hundred products offered by ARIADNA. Panel studies may have some limitations, for example: the incentive structure makes web panels more attractive to low-income respondents, research is limited to internet users, and data integrity concerns may arise. Nevertheless, the sociodemographic profiles of people registered in the ARIADNA panel corresponds with the profiles of Polish Internet users, and recruitment to the panel is carried out continuously. The panel has a current and valid Interviewer Quality Control Programme (PKJPA) certificate confirming the high quality of the research services provided, issued on the basis of an independent audit carried out annually by the Polish Association of Public Opinion and Marketing Research Firms. Only genuine persons of a verified identities participate in research on the ARIADNA panel.

A total of 1135 working people (732 women and 403 men, aged between 18 and 87 years-old; M = 38.68 years, SD = 11.59 years) participated in the study. More detailed socioeconomic data for the participants are presented in Table 1. A sensitivity analysis using G*Power [45] revealed that the sample provided 80% power for detecting effect sizes of $f^2 = 0.01$ to $f^2 = 0.02$ (depending on the model tested).

Table 1. Descriptive statistics for the socioeconomic variables.

Variable	Category	n (%)
Education	Primary education	79 (7.0)
	Secondary education	304 (26.8)
	Post-secondary	140 (12.3)
	Higher education—bachelor's/engineer's degree	149 (13.1)
	Higher education—master's degree	463 (40.8)
Place of residence	Countryside	196 (17.3)
	Small town (<20,000 inhabitants)	130 (11.5)
	Medium town (20,000–99,000 inhabitants)	263 (23.2)
	Large city (100,000–500,000 inhabitants)	297 (26.2)
	Very large city (>500,000 inhabitants)	249 (21.9)
Household net income per capita	Less than PLN 1000	43 (3.8)
	PLN 1001–2000	174 (15.3)
	PLN 2001–3000	285 (25.1)
	PLN 3001–4000	197 (17.4)
	PLN 4001–5000	113 (10.0)
	More than PLN 5000	165 (14.5)
	Refused to answer *	158 (13.9)

* Taking into account the data on wages and inflation in the Polish population [46], it can be assumed that those who refused to answer the question about income were evenly distributed in each of the above groups.

2.2. Materials

2.2.1. Psychological Distress

Anxiety symptoms. Participants' current levels of anxiety symptoms were measured using a Polish version (MAPI Institute; www.phqscreeners.com) of the General Anxiety Disorder—7 scale (GAD-7) [47]. This self-rating questionnaire consists of seven items that have response options ranging from "not at all" to "nearly every day". The total scores range from 0 to 21, with higher scores reflecting greater anxiety. The scale was shown to exhibit high reliability in the present study, the Cronbach's α being 0.95.

Depression symptoms. Symptoms of depression were measured by a Polish version (MAPI Institute; www.phqscreeners.com) of the Patient Health Questionnaire—9 (PHQ-9) [48]. This self-rating questionnaire contains nine items measuring the severity of symptoms of depression. Each item is scored on a four-point Likert scale ranging from 0 (not at all) to 3 (nearly every day). A total score is computed by summing the scores for all the items, with higher scores reflecting a greater severity of depression. A Cronbach's α of 0.93 revealed a high reliability for the present study.

2.2.2. Financial Variables

Sixteen financial variables were included in the study. These variables fell into three categories: objective financial situation, subjective financial situation, and individual financial dispositions.

Objective financial situation variables:

Monthly net income per capita for household—participants indicated their net household income on the following scale: 1—lower than PLN 1000~USD 264; 2—PLN 1001 to 2000~USD 265 to 528; 3—PLN 2001 to 3000~USD 529 to 792; 4—PLN 3001 to 4000~USD 793 to 1056; 5—PLN 4001 to 5000~USD 1057 to 1320; 6—>PLN 5000~>USD 1320.

Possession of savings was measured using one question where participants indicated whether they currently had (answer "yes") or did not have (answer "no") savings.

Saving money before the COVID-19 pandemic was measured using one question where participants indicated whether they had saved money during the last six months before the COVID-19 pandemic (answer "yes") or not (answer "no").

Financial liabilities were measured using two questions: one relating to the holding of loans/credit (scaled yes/no) and one concerning the size of monthly commitments relating to any such loans/credits (measured as the percentage of monthly household income allocated to debt repayments and scaled as follows: 1–15%, 16–30%, 46–65%, 66–80%, 81–95%, and more than 95%).

Subjective financial situation variables:

Subjective assessment of the current household financial situation—participants answered the following question: How do you rate the current financial situation of your household? To answer, they provided a rating on a scale from 1 (very bad) to 7 (very good).

Subjective change in household financial situation—measured by asking participants to give a subjective assessment of the financial change in their household's situation during the COVID-19 pandemic on a scale from 1 (significantly deteriorated) to 7 (significantly improved).

Financial security—participants answered the following question: How financially secure do you feel today? They responded on a scale from 1 (definitely insecure) to 7 (definitely secure).

Perceived job security—participants answered the following question: In the current pandemic situation, can you be sure of keeping your job? Possible responses were "yes" and "no".

Individual financial dispositions:

Materialism: general materialism was measured using the short version of the Material Values Scale (MVS) developed by Richins and Dawson [35]. The short version of the MVS is a three-dimensional self-reporting measure consisting of nine statements to which answers are given on a scale from 1 (definitely no) to 5 (definitely yes). The instrument provides a total score (general materialism) and subscale scores: centrality (e.g., I like a lot of luxury in my life), happiness (e.g., I'd be happier if I could afford to buy more things), and success (e.g., The things I own say a lot about how well I'm doing in life). Presently, only a total general materialism score was computed by summing participants' responses to all nine items. Richins [49] conducted a meta-analysis of 15 studies, thus confirming the reliability and empirical utility of the MVS. The tool's reliability was acceptable in the present study (Cronbach's α = 0.83).

A general propensity to take financial risks was measured using two subscales of the DOSPERT scale [50]. This scale consists of 30 statements relating to four different risk domains: ethical, financial (divided into gambling and investing subdomains), health/safety, and social. In the present study, only the two financial subscales were used. Each of these subscales is comprised of three items (e.g., Betting a day's income at the horse races, and Investing 5% of your annual income in a very speculative stock). Participants were asked to indicate the likelihood that they would engage in the described activity or behavior on a scale from 1 (very unlikely) to 7 (very likely). An indicator of a general propensity to take financial risks was calculated as the sum of the answers given for all six DOSPERT scale items used. For the present data, the measuring was found to exhibit a high degree of reliability (Cronbach's α = 0.91).

Economic optimism was measured on both the national and household levels, and with respect to both short (6 months) and long (18 months) periods, using four questions: Questions 1 and 2 asked participants—How do you think the situation brought about by the pandemic will affect the economic situation in the country at the end of this year (December 2020)/at the end of next year (December 2021) in relation to the economic situation before the outbreak of the pandemic? Questions 3 and 4 asked participants—How do you think the situation brought about by the pandemic will affect your household financial situation at the end of this year (December 2020)/at the end of next year (December 2021) relative to your financial situation before the outbreak of the pandemic? Participants were asked to indicate their answers on a scale from 1 (it will definitely deteriorate) through 4 (it will remain unchanged) to 7 (it will definitely improve).

2.2.3. COVID-19 Health-Related Variables

COVID-19 experience—this variable was coded 1 for participants with experience of COVID-19 and 0 for participants with no experience of COVID-19. Having experience of the disease was measured using four questions: Are you/have you been infected with coronavirus? Has anyone close to you been diagnosed with the coronavirus infection? Does anyone close to you have, or have they had, symptoms of coronavirus infection? Are you, or have you been, subject to home quarantine for suspected coronavirus infection? Participants were considered to have experience of COVID-19 if they answered "yes" to at least one of these questions.

Risk grouping for severe COVID-19—participants were placed into two groups depending on whether they had a medical condition that would be likely to place them at risk of developing severe COVID-19 symptoms if they were to become infected with SARS-CoV-2. Participants giving a positive answer to at least one of the following questions were coded as being at severe risk: Do you suffer from a chronic disease? Are you on immunosuppressive therapy or chemotherapy? Do you need ongoing medical care (e.g., for pregnancy, chemotherapy, dialysis, etc.)? Participants not answering positively to any of these questions were coded as not being at severe risk.

2.2.4. Sociodemographic Data

The sociodemographic questionnaire collected data concerning participants' gender (male/female); age (in years); place of residence (countryside, a small town of less than 20,000 inhabitants, a medium town of 20,000–99,000 inhabitants, a large city of 100,000–500,000 inhabitants, or a very large city of more than 500,000 inhabitants); and the highest level of educational attainment (primary education, secondary education, post-secondary education, bachelor/engineer degree, or Master's degree).

2.3. Procedure

The study was conducted using CAWI methodology to collect data from members of an online panel. Participants completed each of the abovementioned research tools in a rotated order. Data were collected during the first wave of the COVID-19 pandemic in Poland over the period from 5 to 12 May 2020. Previous studies conducted both during the COVID-19 pandemic [51] and during earlier outbreaks of high-risk infectious diseases such as SARS (as caused by SARS-CoV-1), Ebola, and H1N1 influenza [52] showed that psychological distress is at its greatest at the very beginning of a pandemic. Over time, and despite increasing numbers of COVID-19 cases, the degree to which people have exhibited daily preoccupation with topics involving the disease and the pandemic has been shown to have decreased, resulting in decreased subjective perceptions of risk [51]. Thus, the first wave of the pandemic seems to be an appropriate point at which to analyze the pandemic's short-term consequences for people's mental health and to investigate factors that may have a protective function or present a threat with respect to people's susceptibility toward experiencing symptoms of depression and anxiety. Up to the start of the study (5 May 2020), a total of 14,006 SARS-CoV-2 infections and 698 COVID-19 deaths had been confirmed in Poland. At the time the data were collected, the daily number of new Polish cases ranged from 285 to 425 [53], and a study of psychological distress conducted during this time showed that such distress was at a high level among Poles [5].

3. Results

Since they refused to answer questions measuring the monthly net per capita income for their household or the size of their monthly commitments relating to the repayment of any loans/credits, 138 participants were excluded from the analyses. As a result, data for 977 participants were analyzed. Descriptive statistics (means and standard deviations) and zero-order correlations for the analyzed variables are presented in Appendix A (Tables A1 and A2).

3.1. The Specific Role of Financial Variables (in General and When Divided into Three Categories) in Explaining Psychological Distress

Initial hierarchical regression analyses were performed to determine the specific contributions of financial variables in explaining variance in psychological distress (PD) over and above sociodemographic and COVID-19 health-related variables. Further hierarchical regression analyses evaluated the specific contributions of each category of variables in turn (sociodemographic and COVID-19 health-related variables, objective financial variables, subjective financial variables, and individual financial dispositions) in explaining the variance in PD while all the other categories of variables were controlled. Analyses were conducted for depression symptoms and anxiety symptoms as two separate dependent variables (DVs).

First, two hierarchical regression analyses were conducted, one each for anxiety and depression symptoms as DVs. In both analyses, independent variables (IVs) were introduced in the following blocks: Block 1—sociodemographic variables (gender (with females coded as 1), age, place of residence, and educational level); Block 2—COVID-19 health-related variables (COVID-19 risk grouping (with high risk coded as 1) and COVID-19 experience (with experience coded as 1)); Block 3—objective financial situation: monthly net per capita income for household, possession of savings (with possession of savings coded as 1), saving money before the COVID-19 pandemic (with having saved money coded as 1), loan/credit holding (with holding of debt coded as 1), and amount of monthly commitments related to loans/credits; Block 4—subjective financial situation: subjective assessment of current household financial situation, subjective change in financial situation, financial security, and perceived job security; Block 5—individual financial dispositions: materialism, general propensity to take financial risks, economic optimism at a household level (two variables: short-term and long-term optimism) and economic optimism at a national level (two variables: short-term and long-term optimism).

Table 2 presents the results of the hierarchical regression analyses for the two psychological distress DVs and shows cumulative statistics for all the IVs included in the models at a given step. These results indicated that financial variables made statistically significant contributions to explaining the variance in each PD measure. With sociodemographic variables and COVID-19 health-related variables already included in the models, financial variables accounted for around 15 percentage points of the additional variance in both depression and anxiety symptom scores. Moreover, the results showed that individual financial dispositions accounted for around 10 percentage points of additional variance in the two DVs over and above the sociodemographic variables, COVID-19 health-related variables, and participants' objective and subjective financial situations.

Table 2. Results of two hierarchical regression analyses predicting psychological distress from categories of variables.

Dependent Variable	Independent Variable	R	R^2	Adjusted R^2	R^2 Change	F Change	F of the Model
Anxiety symptoms	Sociodemographic variables	0.223	0.050	0.046	0.050	12.658 ***	$F(4, 972) = 12.658$ ***
	COVID-19 health-related variables	0.254	0.065	0.059	0.015	7.851 ***	$F(6, 970) = 11.175$ ***
	Objective financial situation	0.303	0.092	0.082	0.027	5.820 ***	$F(11, 965) = 8.892$ ***
	Subjective financial situation	0.348	0.121	0.107	0.029	7.960 ***	$F(15, 961) = 8.832$ ***
	Individual financial dispositions	0.468	0.219	0.202	0.098	19.953 ***	$F(21, 955) = 12.756$ ***
Depression symptoms	Sociodemographic variables	0.228	0.052	0.048	0.052	13.361 ***	$F(4, 972) = 13.361$ ***
	COVID-19 health-related variables	0.256	0.065	0.060	0.013	6.848 ***	$F(6, 970) = 11.297$ ***
	Objective financial situation	0.308	0.095	0.084	0.029	6.262 ***	$F(11, 965) = 9.176$ ***
	Subjective financial situation	0.344	0.119	0.105	0.024	6.517 ***	$F(15, 961) = 8.620$ ***
	Individual financial dispositions	0.465	0.217	0.199	0.098	19.911 ***	$F(21, 955) = 12.573$ ***

*** $p < 0.001$.

To obtain a wider picture of the relationships between the variables analyzed, eight additional hierarchical regression analyzes were performed in which, in turn, each variable category not entered last in the first two analyses was entered last to determine the specific contributions that each variable category made to explaining variance in the two PD DVs over and above the other categories. The specific contributions made by the different categories of variables were as follows:

- sociodemographic variables: anxiety symptoms (R^2 change = 0.039, $p < 0.001$); depression symptoms (R^2 change = 0.045, $p < 0.001$).
- COVID-19 health-related variables: anxiety symptoms (R^2 change = 0.009, $p = 0.003$); depression symptoms (R^2 change = 0.009, $p = 0.004$).
- objective financial situation variables: anxiety symptoms (R^2 change = 0.006, $p = 0.235$); depression symptoms (R^2 change = 0.005, $p = 0.308$).
- subjective financial situation variables: anxiety symptoms (R^2 change = 0.029, $p < 0.001$); depression symptoms (R^2 change = 0.027, $p < 0.001$).

From the results of these analyses, it can be concluded that, relative to the roles played by the other two groups of financial variables, individual financial dispositions played the most important role in explaining the extent of people's depression and anxiety symptoms (when sociodemographic and COVID-19 health-related variables were controlled).

3.2. The Specific Role of Each Financial Variable in Explaining Psychological Distress

Next, two stepwise regression analyses were conducted to identify significant individual predictors of the two psychological distress DVs. Here, all the IVs entered in the previous analyses were entered in one block. Table 3 presents the final models for each of the DVs (only significantly predictive IVs are included in the table; full descriptions of the stepwise regression analyses are presented in Appendix A: Tables A3 and A4).

Table 3. The results of two stepwise regression analyses predicting psychological distress from individual variables.

Dependent Variable	Statistically Significant Predictors	B	t
Anxiety symptoms $F(10, 966) = 25.878$ *** $R^2 = 0.211$, Adjusted $R^2 = 0.203$	Materialism	0.233	7.751 ***
	Financial security	−0.134	−3.961 ***
	Gender [a]	0.158	5.244 ***
	General propensity to take financial risks	0.124	3.885 ***
	Economic optimism (short-term)—national level	0.129	3.945 ***
	Perceived job security	−0.086	−2.756 **
	Risk grouping for severe COVID-19	0.092	3.162 **
	Age	−0.096	−3.102 **
	Economic optimism (long-term)—household level	−0.076	−2.289 *
	Amount of monthly commitments related to loans/credits	0.062	2.100 *
Depression symptoms $F(8, 968) = 33.992$ *** $R^2 = 0.204$, Adjusted $R^2 = 0.198$	Materialism	0.204	6.792 ***
	Financial security	−0.185	−5.874 ***
	Economic optimism (short-term)—national level	0.175	5.348 ***
	Gender [a]	0.137	4.547 ***
	General propensity to take financial risks	0.137	4.301 ***
	Age	−0.131	−4.255 ***
	Risk grouping for severe COVID-19	0.094	3.211 ***
	Economic optimism (long-term)—household level	−0.103	−3.130 **

[a] Coded: 1—female, 0—male; * $p < 0.05$; ** $p < 0.01$; *** $p < 0.001$.

Eight financial variables were identified as significant predictors of anxiety symptom severity: materialism, financial security, general propensity to take financial risks, short-term economic optimism at a national level, long-term economic optimism at a household level, perceived job security, and amount of monthly commitments related to the loans/credits. Financial security, perceived job security, and long-term economic optimism at the household level were negative predictors, while the other variables were positive predictors. Moreover, nonfinancial variables such as age, gender, and belonging to the group of people at severe risk from COVID-19 were also significant predictors of anxiety symptoms, age being the only negative predictor.

Six economic variables were also identified as significant predictors of severity of depression symptoms. Materialism, general propensity to take financial risks, and short-term economic optimism at a national level were positively predictive, while financial security and long-term economic optimism at a household level were negatively predictive. Two sociodemographic variables (gender and age) and one COVID-19-related variable (belonging to the group of people at severe risk from COVID-19) were also significant predictors of depression symptoms. Among these, only age was negatively predictive.

4. Discussion

The study analyzed the role of financial factors in explaining psychological distress during the COVID-19 pandemic. To obtain a detailed picture, we considered two outcome variables: levels of depression and anxiety symptoms. With respect to financial factors, we took into account a wide range of variables in three categories: people's objective financial situations, their subjective financial situations, and their individual financial dispositions. This approach to financial factors allowed us to answer three questions concerning relationships between economic variables and psychological distress: (1) Taken together, can financial variables explain variance in the levels of people's depression and anxiety symptoms over and above the variance explained by sociodemographic and COVID-19 health-related factors? (2) Which category of financial factors (people's objective financial situation, their subjective financial situation, or their individual financial dispositions) explains the largest proportion of variance in PD symptoms?; (3) Which specific financial variables are the strongest predictors of the variance in PD symptoms?

The results obtained showed that financial variables made a statistically significant contribution to explaining the variance in both PD variables over and above sociodemographic and COVID-19 health-related variables. While all three financial variable categories (objective financial situation, subjective financial situation, and individual financial dispositions) played an important role in explaining people's depression and anxiety symptoms, the role of individual financial dispositions was identified as the most crucial. Individual financial dispositions accounted for around 10% of the variability in depression and anxiety symptoms over and above the variance accounted for by the sociodemographic and COVID-19 health-related variables and people's objective and subjective financial situations, while (when they were placed in the last block in hierarchical regression analyses) the specific contributions to explaining variance in both PD indicators made by the other financial variable categories were nonsignificant in the case of an objective financial situation and relatively small in the case of a subjective financial situation (2.9% for anxiety symptoms and 2.7% for depression symptoms).

It is worth underlining that the lists of significant predictors of depression and anxiety symptoms are almost the same. While the present methodological design does not permit causal inferences to be made, higher levels of materialism, a general propensity to take financial risks, and short-term economic optimism at a national level may promote depression and anxiety symptoms, while high levels of financial security and long-term economic optimism at a household level may decrease depression and anxiety symptoms and, thus, may be protective factors. Perceived job security (being sure of keeping one's job) and monthly loan/credit repayment amount were the only two predictors that were significantly predictive for anxiety but not for depression, with perceived job security being a potential protective factor and monthly repayment commitments being a factor that may promote anxiety. Additionally, the roles of sociodemographic and COVID-19 health-related variables in explaining the extent of people's depression and anxiety symptoms were similar, with age being a negative predictor (and a possible protective factor) and female gender and belonging to the group of people being at severe risk from COVID-19 being positive predictors.

Most of the preset results for particular financial variables as predictors of PD are in line with those of previous studies [5,13,17,18,23]. However, two results contradict previous studies. The first is related to a propensity for financial risk-taking. While previous studies have shown a negative relationship between financial risk-taking and anxiety symptoms [22,41], we found a financial risk-taking propensity to be a positive predictor of PD during the pandemic. This inconsistency may result from certain mediating factors arising during the pandemic. For example, people prone to taking financial risks might have made risky financial decisions before the pandemic (e.g., they might have made investments), which, because of the pandemic, turned out to be unprofitable or even financially damaging. Any such deteriorations in people's financial situations would be likely to be positively corelated with intensity of depression and anxiety symptoms. Of course, this explanation is speculative, and further research taking into account people's wider financial circumstances is required to obtain a better understanding of the present result.

The second result that is inconsistent with previous research concerns economic optimism. Previous studies have shown that more economically optimistic people experience less stress and exhibit lower levels of depression symptoms [21,40]. Our study showed that, although long-term economic optimism at a household level was negatively predictive of PD, short-term economic optimism at the national level was positively predictive of PD. The results of research by Xie et al. [54] on general optimism and PD during the SARS-CoV-1 pandemic may explain this pattern of results. This research showed that, while optimism can be associated with lower PD, it is also associated with greater pandemic-related vigilance, which, in turn, translates into higher levels of anxiety. Therefore, optimistic people may focus more on a pandemic and, thus, experience greater psychological distress. However, further research is required to obtain a better understanding of why economic optimism at household and national levels, and for different periods of time, is related to psychological distress in different ways.

Although the obtained results seem promising, the current findings and methods have limitations. The main limitation of the research is its cross-sectional character. The obtained data only allowed fundamentally correlational analysis—the research should be followed up by studies using repeated measurements. In terms of COVID-19-related variables, we focused on the physical health variables, but it would also be worth controlling for variables that may influence psychological health, e.g., the extent of reductions in people's social contact and their social isolation. Moreover, in terms of objective financial measures, we focused on income, savings, and financial liabilities, but it would also be worth tracing out the effects of wealth and control for respondents' possessions. It should also be noted that the research sample was randomly selected and diversified in terms of gender, age, level of education, and place of residence; however, the sample was not fully representative of the Polish population. This should be taken into account when trying to generalize the results for the Polish population. For example, in our sample, 53.9% of respondents had higher education, while, in the Polish population, among people working professionally, this percentage is about 37.2% (data from 2020) [55]. Additionally, the percentage of women in our sample was significantly higher (64.5%) than the percentage of women in the Polish population of people working professionally (44.7%) [55].

Moreover, it should be considered that, across the world, there are huge cultural variations between Western; more individualistic nations (such as Poland); and other, more collectivistic cultures (e.g., Korea, Ghana, and Nigeria) [56,57], which may, for example, lead to various reactions to COVID-19-related changes in personal finances. In addition, Western countries differ significantly from non-Western nations on socioeconomic issues, such as income inequalities, social protection systems, and welfare benefits [58]. This means that our results may not be generalizable to other socioeconomic contexts, such as non-Western societies.

5. Conclusions

The present study adds to the current state of knowledge by showing that financial variables explain a significant portion of variance in PD over and above sociodemographic and COVID-19 health-related factors. The study confirmed the predictive role of three categories of financial factors: people's objective financial situation, their subjective financial situation, and individual financial dispositions and showed the latter category to be the most important. Moreover, the study also identified individual financial variables which were capable of predicting people's psychological distress during the pandemic, and showed the roles of financial variables to be similar in predicting the extent of people's depression and anxiety symptoms. The current study found that depression and anxiety symptoms were higher among people with higher levels of materialism and a higher general propensity to take financial risks and short-term economic optimism, while psychological distress was lower among people with higher levels of financial security and long-term economic optimism.

Our study provides valuable insights for individuals, therapists, and policy-makers by revealing the association between various financial factors (especially individual financial dispositions such as materialism, general propensity to take financial risks, and economic optimism) and psychological distress during the outbreak of the COVID-19 pandemic. For example, our results suggest that using various strategies to decrease materialistic values (such as encouraging people to focus more on intrinsic and self-transcendent values/goals [59]) may be helpful in reducing mental health problems during the COVID-19 pandemic.

Author Contributions: Conceptualization, K.S.; methodology, K.S., D.P., E.P. and A.T.; validation, K.S. and A.T.; formal analysis, K.S., D.P. and A.T.; investigation, K.S., A.T. and D.P.; data curation, K.S. and D.P.; writing—original draft preparation, K.S., A.T., D.P. and K.W.-P.; writing—review and editing, K.S., A.T.; supervision, K.S. and E.P.; project administration, K.S.; and funding acquisition, K.S., A.T. and E.P. All authors have read and agreed to the published version of the manuscript.

Funding: This research was funded by the University of Warsaw's Faculty of Psychology to K.S., A.T., and E.P. from 2020 funding awarded by the Polish Ministry of Science and Higher Education aimed at subsidizing the maintenance and development of research potential (501-D125-01-1250000 zlec*5011000221 and 5011000230). The APC was funded by the University of Warsaw (Excellence Initiative- Research University) and the University of Economics and Human Sciences in Warsaw.

Institutional Review Board Statement: The study was conducted in accordance with the Declaration of Helsinki and approved by the Ethics Board of the University of Warsaw's Faculty of Psychology (08.04.2020).

Informed Consent Statement: Informed consent was obtained from all subjects involved in the study.

Data Availability Statement: The complete data for all studies and the original materials used to conduct this research can be found on the Open Science Framework (OSF) website.

Conflicts of Interest: The authors declare no conflict of interest. The funders had no role in the design of the study; in the collection, analyses, or interpretation of the data; in the writing of the manuscript; or in the decision to publish the results.

Appendix A

Table A1. Descriptive statistics for the analyzed variables.

Variable	Percentage/Mean (SD) Total Sample $N = 1135$	Percentage/Mean (SD) Analyzed Sample $N = 977$
Gender (%)		
Male	35.5	36.2
Female	64.5	63.8
Age, mean (SD)	38.68 (11.59)	38.60 (11.64)
Place of residence (%)		
Countryside	17.3	16.8
Small town (<20,000 inhabitants)	11.5	12.3
Medium town (20,000–99,000 inhabitants)	23.2	23.2
Large city (100,000-500,000 inhabitants)	26.2	26.2
Very large city (>500,000 inhabitants)	21.9	21.5
Education (%)		
Primary education	7.0	7.4
Secondary education	26.8	27.1
Post—secondary	12.3	12.4
Higher education—bachelor's/engineer's degree	13.1	13.2
Higher education—master's degree	40.8	39.9
COVID-19 experience (%)		
Yes	7.6	8.1
No	92.4	91.9
Risk group of severe COVID-19 (%)		
Yes	29.2	29.9
No	70.8	70.1
Monthly net income per capita (%)		
Less than PLN 1000	3.8	4.4
PLN 1001–2000	15.3	17.8
PLN 2001–3000	25.1	29.2
PLN 3001–4000	17.4	20.2
PLN 4001–5000	10.0	11.6
More than PLN 5000	14.5	16.9
Refuse to answer	13.9	-
Possession of savings		
Yes	74.8	72.6
No	25.2	27.4
Saving money before the COVID-19 pandemic		
Yes	73.2	71.8
No	26.8	28.2
Amount of monthly commitments related to loans/credits (%)		
No commitments	45.0	43.8
1–15% of household monthly income	14.0	14.5
16–30% of household monthly income	22.6	22.6
31–45% of household monthly income	9.2	9.1
46–50% of household monthly income	5.3	5.6
51–65% of household monthly income	1.4	1.6
66–80% of household monthly income	1.6	1.8
81–95% of household monthly income	0.4	0.3
More than 95% of household monthly income	0.5	0.5
Subjective assessment of current financial situation of household, mean (SD)	4.27 (1.31)	4.27 (1.32)
Subjective change of household financial situation, mean (SD)	3.41 (1.26)	3.41 (1.28)
Financial security, mean (SD)	3.53 (1.55)	3.54 (1.56)
Perceived job security (%)		
Yes	53.0	54.4
No	47.0	45.6

Table A1. Cont.

Variable	Percentage/Mean (SD) Total Sample N = 1135	Percentage/Mean (SD) Analyzed Sample N = 977
Materialism, mean (SD)	27.18 (6.40)	27.42 (6.36)
General propensity to take financial risks, mean (SD)	15.25 (8.47)	15.42 (8.58)
Economic optimism (short-term)—national level, mean (SD)	2.17 (1.47)	2.19 (1.49)
Economic optimism (long-term)—national level, mean (SD)	3.36 (1.67)	3.42 (1.69)
Economic optimism (short-term)—household level, mean (SD)	2.99 (1.38)	3.03 (1.40)
Economic optimism (long-term)—household level, mean (SD)	3.53 (1.42)	3.58 (1.46)
Anxiety symptoms, mean (SD)	14.63 (5.55)	14.71 (5.61)
Depression symptoms, mean (SD)	17.68 (6.45)	17.79 (6.51)

Table A2. Zero-order correlations for the analyzed variables.

	2	3	4	5	6	7	8	9	10	11	12	13	14	15	16	17	18	19	20	21	22
1	−0.26 ***	−0.02	0.10 **	0.01	−0.02	−0.09 **	−0.07 *	0.07 *	0.01	0.02	−0.07 *	−0.04	0.00	0.10 **	−0.10 **	−0.07 *	0.00	−0.06	−0.03	0.19 ***	0.17 ***
2		−0.07 *	0.02	−0.07 *	0.18 ***	0.07 *	0.00	−0.14 ***	0.08 *	−0.04	0.01	−0.03	−0.02	−0.16 ***	−0.13 ***	−0.03	−0.12 ***	−0.03	−0.13 ***	−0.16 ***	−0.19 ***
3			0.09 **	−0.02	−0.02	0.15 ***	0.00	0.01	−0.05	0.02	0.01	0.02	0.02	−0.04	−0.01	−0.04	−0.03	−0.02	0.01	−0.01	0.00
4				−0.06	0.03	0.16 ***	−0.01	0.15 ***	−0.02	0.06	0.02	0.02	0.00	0.03	−0.04	−0.01	−0.11 ***	−0.12 ***	−0.12 ***	−0.11 ***	−0.01	−0.02
5					0.07 *	0.06	−0.03	0.04	−0.01	0.06 *	0.05	0.04	−0.01	0.09 **	0.07 *	0.10 ***	0.07 *	0.08 *	0.08 *	0.09 **	0.07 *
6						−0.01	−0.05	−0.01	0.03	−0.10 **	−0.10 **	−0.07 *	−0.05	−0.04	−0.02	−0.04	−0.04	−0.12 ***	−0.10 **	0.08 *	0.07 *
7							0.00	0.13 ***	0.01	0.34 ***	0.20 ***	0.22 ***	0.13 ***	0.00	0.00	−0.05	−0.02	0.11 **	0.07 *	−0.06	−0.08 *
8								0.10 **	−0.12 ***	0.10 **	0.10 **	0.13 ***	0.00	−0.10 **	−0.03	0.03	−0.03	0.06	0.01	−0.08 *	−0.07 *
9									−0.18 ***	0.27 ***	0.10 **	0.21 ***	0.08 *	−0.01	−0.06	−0.03	0.02	0.09 **	0.07	−0.03	−0.05
10										−0.22 ***	−0.17 ***	−0.20 ***	−0.07 *	0.12 ***	0.04	−0.01	−0.01	−0.13 ***	−0.12 ***	0.130 ***	0.12 ***
11											0.60 ***	0.68 ***	0.28 ***	−0.03	0.06	0.21 ***	0.16 ***	0.42 ***	0.31 ***	−0.16 ***	−0.16 ***
12												0.66 ***	0.36 ***	−0.04	0.17 ***	0.34 ***	0.20 ***	0.60 ***	0.38 ***	−0.14 ***	−0.11 **
13													0.40 ***	−0.05	0.15 ***	0.26 ***	0.18 ***	0.53 ***	0.38 ***	−0.18 ***	−0.18 ***
14														0.00	0.02	0.07 *	0.10 **	0.35 ***	0.23 ***	−0.15 ***	−0.13 ***
15															0.22 ***	0.08 *	0.07 *	0.04	0.08 *	0.31 ***	0.28 ***
16																0.36 ***	0.21 ***	0.19 ***	0.20 ***	0.18 ***	0.20 ***
17																	0.51 ***	0.52 ***	0.37 ***	0.11 **	0.15 ***
18																		0.38 ***	0.62 ***	0.03	0.03
19																			0.63 ***	−0.06	−0.03
20																				−0.07 *	−0.06
21																					0.86 ***

* $p < 0.05$; ** $p < 0.01$; *** $p < 0.001$; 1—Gender (female (1) vs. male (0)); 2—Age; 3—Place of residence (city (1) vs. other (0)); 4—education (higher (1) vs other (0)); 5—COVID-19 experience; 6—Risk group of severe COVID-19; 7—Monthly net income; 8—Possession of savings; 9—Saving money before the COVID-19 pandemic; 10—Amount of monthly commitments related to loans/credits; 11—Subjective assessment of current financial situation of household; 12—Subjective change of household financial situation; 13—Financial security; 14—Perceived job security; 15—Materialism; 16—General propensity to take financial risks; 17—Economic optimism (short-term)—national level; 18—Economic optimism (long-term)—national level; 19—Economic optimism (short-term)—household level; 20—Economic optimism (long-term)—household level; 21—Anxiety symptoms; 22—Depression symptoms.

Table A3. Predictors of anxiety symptoms.

Predictors	R	R^2	Adjusted R^2	Beta	R^2 Change	F Change
Materialism	0.307	0.094	0.093	0.307 ***	0.094	101.495 ***
Materialism Financial security	0.348	0.121	0.120	0.299 *** −0.165 ***	0.027	30.095 ***
Materialism Financial security Gender	0.382	0.146	0.143	0.283 *** −0.160 *** 0.157 ***	0.024	27.585 ***

Table A3. Cont.

Predictors	R	R^2	Adjusted R^2	Beta	R^2 Change	F Change
Materialism Financial security Gender General propensity to take financial risks	0.416	0.173	0.170	0.240 *** −0.187 *** 0.177 *** 0.174 ***	0.027	32.277 ***
Materialism Financial security Gender General propensity to take financial risks Economic optimism (short-term)—national level	0.427	0.183	0.179	0.238 *** −0.209 *** 0.181 *** 0.139 *** 0.108 ***	0.010	11.418 ***
Materialism Financial security Gender General propensity to take financial risks Economic optimism (short-term)—national level Perceived job security	0.436	0.190	0.185	0.241 *** −0.171 *** 0.181 *** 0.136 *** 0.106 *** −0.095 **	0.008	9.037 **
Materialism Financial security Gender General propensity to take financial risks Economic optimism (short-term)—national level Perceived job security Risk group of severe COVID-19	0.444	0.197	0.191	0.244 *** −0.166 *** 0.182 *** 0.136 *** 0.107 *** −0.093 ** 0.083 **	0.007	8.217 **
Materialism Financial security Gender General propensity to take financial risks Economic optimism (short-term)—national level Perceived job security Risk group of severe COVID-19 Age	0.450	0.203	0.196	0.237 *** −0.167 *** 0.162 *** 0.125 *** 0.109 *** −0.093 ** 0.096 *** −0.081 **	0.006	7.049 **
Materialism Financial security General propensity to take financial risks Gender Economic optimism (short-term)—national level Perceived job security Risk group of severe COVID-19 Age Economic optimism (long-term)—household level	0.456	0.208	0.200	0.240 *** −0.146 *** 0.159 *** 0.128 *** 0.131 *** −0.085 ** 0.092 ** −0.090 ** −0.080 *	0.005	5.871 *
Materialism Financial security Gender General propensity to take financial risks Economic optimism (short-term)—national level Perceived job security Risk group of severe COVID-19 Age Economic optimism (long-term)—household level Amount of monthly commitments related to loans/credits	0.460	0.211	0.203	0.233 *** −0.134 *** 0.158 *** 0.124 *** 0.129 *** −0.086 ** 0.092 ** −0.096 ** −0.076 * 0.062 **	0.004	4.410 *

* $p < 0.05$; ** $p < 0.01$; *** $p < 0.001$.

Table A4. Predictors of depression symptoms.

Predictors	R	R^2	Adjusted R^2	Beta	R^2 Change	F Change
Materialism	0.280	0.079	0.078	0.280 ***	0.079	83.187 ***
Materialism Financial security	0.325	0.105	0.104	0.272 *** −0.164 ***	0.027	29.196 ***
Materialism Financial security Economic optimism (short-term)—national level	0.367	0.135	0.132	0.256 *** −0.210 *** −0.179 ***	0.030	33.221 ***
Materialism Financial security Economic optimism (short-term)—national level Gender	0.398	0.159	0.155	0.239 *** −0.208 *** 0.190 *** 0.155 ***	0.024	27.241 ***
Materialism Financial security Economic optimism (short-term)—national level Gender General propensity to take financial risks	0.421	0.177	0.173	0.207 *** −0.219 *** 0.143 *** 0.169 ** 0.151 ***	0.019	21.921 ***
Materialism Financial security Economic optimism (short-term)—national level Gender General propensity to take financial risks Age	0.432	0.187	0.182	0.196 *** −0.222 *** 0.145 *** 0.143 *** 0.137 *** −0.103 ***	0.010	11.378 ***
Materialism Financial security Economic optimism (short-term)—national level Gender General propensity to take financial risks Age Risk group of severe COVID-19	0.443	0.196	0.190	0.199 *** −0.216 *** 0.147 *** 0.140 *** 0.134 *** −0.121 *** 0.099 ***	0.010	11.490 ***
Materialism Financial security Economic optimism (short-term)—national level Gender General propensity to take financial risks Age Risk group of severe COVID-19 Economic optimism (long-term)—household level	0.452	0.204	0.198	0.204 *** −0.185 *** 0.175 *** 0.137 *** 0.137 *** −0.131 *** 0.094 *** −0.103 ***	0.008	9.800 **

** $p < 0.01$; *** $p < 0.001$.

References

1. Cénat, J.M.; Blais-Rochette, C.; Kokou-Kpolou, C.K.; Noorishad, P.G.; Mukunzi, J.N.; McIntee, S.E.; Dalexis, R.D.; Goulet, M.A.; Labelle, P.R. Prevalence of symptoms of depression, anxiety, insomnia, posttraumatic stress disorder, and psychological distress among populations affected by the COVID-19 pandemic: A systematic review and meta-analysis. *Psychiatry Res.* **2021**, *295*, 113599. [CrossRef] [PubMed]
2. Lieberoth, A.; Lin, S.Y.; Stöckli, S.; Han, H.; Kowal, M.; Gelpi, R.; Chrona, S.; Tran, T.P.; Jeftić, A.; Rasmussen, J.; et al. Stress and worry in the 2020 coronavirus pandemic: Relationships to trust and compliance with preventive measures across 48 countries in the COVIDiSTRESS global survey. *R. Soc. Open Sci.* **2021**, *8*, 200589. [CrossRef] [PubMed]
3. Mirowsky, J.; Ross, C.E. *Social Causes of Psychological Distress*; Aldine de Gruyter: Berlin, Germany, 2003.
4. Horwitz, A.V. Distinguishing distress from disorder as psychological outcomes of stressful social arrangements. *Health London.* **2007**, *11*, 273–289. [CrossRef] [PubMed]
5. Wang, Y.; Kala, M.P.; Jafar, T.H. Factors associated with psychological distress during the coronavirus disease 2019 (COVID-19) pandemic on the predominantly general population: A systematic review and meta-analysis. *PLoS ONE* **2020**, *15*, e0244630. [CrossRef]
6. Cai, X.; Hu, X.; Ekumi, I.O.; Wang, J.; An, Y.; Li, Z.; Yuan, B. Psychological Distress and Its Correlates Among COVID-19 Survivors During Early Convalescence Across Age Groups. *Am. J. Geriatr. Psychiatry* **2020**, *28*, 1030–1039. [CrossRef]

7. Ahmed, M.Z.; Ahmed, O.; Aibao, Z.; Hanbin, S.; Siyu, L.; Ahmad, A. Epidemic of COVID-19 in China and associated Psychological Problems. *Asian J. Psychiatry* **2020**, *51*, 102092. [CrossRef]
8. Gambin, M.; Sękowski, M.; Woźniak-Prus, M.; Wnuk, A.; Oleksy, T.; Cudo, A.; Hansen, K.; Huflejt-Łukasik, M.; Kubicka, K.; Łyś, A.E.; et al. Generalized anxiety and depressive symptoms in various age groups during the COVID-19 lockdown in Poland. Specific predictors and differences in symptoms severity. *Compr. Psychiatry* **2021**, *105*, 152222. [CrossRef]
9. Solomou, I.; Constantinidou, F. Prevalence and Predictors of Anxiety and Depression Symptoms during the COVID-19 Pandemic and Compliance with Precautionary Measures: Age and Sex Matter. *Int. J. Environ. Public Health* **2020**, *17*, 4924. [CrossRef]
10. Lei, L.; Huang, X.; Zhang, S.; Yang, J.; Yang, L.; Xu, M. Comparison of Prevalence and Associated Factors of Anxiety and Depression Among People Affected by versus People Unaffected by Quarantine During the COVID-19 Epidemic in Southwestern China. *Med. Sci. Monit.* **2020**, *26*, e924609. [CrossRef]
11. Olagoke, A.A.; Olagoke, O.O.; Hughes, A.M. Exposure to coronavirus news on mainstream media: The role of risk perceptions and depression. *Br. J. Health Psychol.* **2020**, *25*, 865–874. [CrossRef]
12. Cao, W.; Fang, Z.; Hou, G.; Han, M.; Xu, X.; Dong, J.; Zheng, J. The psychological impact of the COVID-19 epidemic on college students in China. *Psychiatry Res.* **2020**, *287*, 112934. [CrossRef] [PubMed]
13. Wilson, J.M.; Lee, J.; Fitzgerald, H.N.; Oosterhoff, B.; Sevi, B.; Shook, N.J. Job Insecurity and Financial Concern During the COVID-19 Pandemic Are Associated With Worse Mental Health. *J. Occup. Environ. Med.* **2020**, *62*, 686–691. [CrossRef] [PubMed]
14. Dijkstra-Kersten, S.M.; Biesheuvel-Leliefeld, K.E.; van der Wouden, J.C.; Penninx, B.W.; van Marwijk, H.W. Associations of financial strain and income with depressive and anxiety disorders. *J. Epidemiol. Community Health* **2015**, *69*, 660–665. [CrossRef] [PubMed]
15. Lorant, V.; Croux, C.; Weich, S.; Deliège, D.; Mackenbach, J.; Ansseau, M. Depression and socio-economic risk factors: 7-year longitudinal population study. *Br. J. Psychiatry* **2007**, *190*, 293–298. [CrossRef]
16. Orpana, H.M.; Lemyre, L.; Gravel, R. Income and psychological distress: The role of the social environment. *Health Rep.* **2009**, *20*, 21–28. [PubMed]
17. Bridges, S.; Disney, R. Debt and depression. *J. Health Econ.* **2010**, *29*, 388–403. [CrossRef]
18. Fitch, C.; Hamilton, S.; Bassett, P.; Davey, R. The Relationship between Personal Debt and Mental Health: A Systematic Review. *Ment. Health Rev. Brighton* **2011**, *16*, 153–166. [CrossRef]
19. Wildman, J. Income related inequalities in mental health in Great Britain: Analysing the causes of health inequality over time. *J. Health Econ.* **2003**, *22*, 295–312. [CrossRef]
20. Ferrie, J.E.; Shipley, M.J.; Stansfeld, S.A.; Smith, G.D.; Marmot, M.; Study, W.I. Future uncertainty and socioeconomic inequalities in health: The Whitehall II study. *Soc. Sci Med.* **2003**, *57*, 637–646. [CrossRef]
21. Kahle, L.R.; Shoham, A.; Rose, G.; Smith, M.; Batra, R. Economic versus Personal Future-Oriented Attitudes as Consumer Shopping Indicators. *J. Euro Mark.* **2003**, *12*, 35–54. [CrossRef]
22. Maner, J.K.; Schmidt, N.B. The role of risk avoidance in anxiety. *Behavioral* **2006**, *37*, 181–189. [CrossRef] [PubMed]
23. Muñiz-Velázquez, J.A.; Gomez-Baya, D.; Lopez-Casquete, M. Implicit and Explicit Assessment of Materialism: Associations with Happiness and Depression. *Pers. Individ. Dif.* **2017**, *116*, 123–132. [CrossRef]
24. Kessler, R.C. A disaggregation of the relationship between socioeconomic status and psychological distress. *Am. Sociol. Rev.* **1982**, *47*, 752–764. [CrossRef]
25. Link, B.G.; Lennon, M.C.; Dohrenwend, B.P. Socioeconomic Status and Depression: The Role of Occupations Involving Direction, Control, and Planning. *Am. J. Sociol.* **1993**, *98*, 1351–1387. [CrossRef]
26. Kosidou, K.; Dalman, C.; Lundberg, M.; Hallqvist, J.; Isacsson, G.; Magnusson, C. Socioeconomic status and risk of psychological distress and depression in the Stockholm Public Health Cohort: A population-based study. *J. Affect. Disord.* **2011**, *134*, 160–167. [CrossRef]
27. Brown, S.; Taylor, K.; Wheatley Price, S. Debt and distress: Evaluating the psychological cost of credit. *J. Econ. Psychol.* **2005**, *26*, 642–663. [CrossRef]
28. Skapinakis, P.; Weich, S.; Lewis, G.; Singleton, N.; Araya, R. Socio-economic position and common mental disorders. Longitudinal study in the general population in the UK. *Br. J. Psychiatry* **2006**, *189*, 109–117. [CrossRef]
29. Jenkins, R.; Bhugra, D.; Bebbington, P.; Brugha, T.; Farrell, M.; Coid, J.; Fryers, T.; Weich, S.; Singleton, N.; Meltzer, H. Debt, income and mental disorder in the general population. *Psychol. Med.* **2008**, *38*, 1485–1493. [CrossRef]
30. Drentea, P. Age, debt and anxiety. *J. Health Soc. Behav.* **2000**, *41*, 437–450. [CrossRef]
31. Gardner, J.; Oswald, A.J. Money and mental wellbeing: A longitudinal study of medium-sized lottery wins. *J. Health Econ.* **2007**, *26*, 49–60. [CrossRef]
32. Pearlin, L.I.; Johnson, J.S. Marital status, life-strains and depression. *Am. Sociol. Rev.* **1977**, *42*, 704–715. [CrossRef] [PubMed]
33. O'Neill, B.; Sorhaindo, B.; Xiao, J.J.; Garman, E.T. Financially Distressed Consumers: Their Financial Practices, Financial Well-being, and Health. *J. Fin. Couns. Plan.* **2005**, *16*, 73–87.
34. Gutter, M.; Copur, Z. Financial Behaviors and Financial Well-Being of College Students: Evidence from a National Survey. *J. Fam. Econ. Issues* **2011**, *32*, 699–714. [CrossRef]
35. Richins, M.L.; Dawson, S. A Consumer Values Orientation for Materialism and Its Measurement: Scale Development and Validation. *J. Consum. Res.* **1992**, *19*, 303–316. [CrossRef]

36. Kasser, T.; Ryan, R.M. A dark side of the American dream: Correlates of financial success as a central life aspiration. *J. Pers. Soc. Psychol.* **1993**, *65*, 410–422. [CrossRef]
37. Ryan, R.M.; Chirkov, V.I.; Little, T.D.; Sheldon, K.M.; Timoshina, E.; Deci, E.L. The American Dream in Russia: Extrinsic Aspirations and Well-Being in Two Cultures. *Pers. Soc. Psychol. Bull.* **1999**, *25*, 1509–1524. [CrossRef]
38. Wang, R.; Liu, H.; Jiang, J.; Song, Y. Will Materialism Lead to Happiness? A Longitudinal Analysis of the Mediating Role of Psychological Needs Satisfaction. *Pers. Individ. Dif.* **2017**, *105*, 312–317. [CrossRef]
39. Dittmar, H.; Bond, R.; Hurst, M.; Kasser, T. The relationship between materialism and personal well-being: A meta-analysis. *J. Pers. Soc. Psychol.* **2014**, *107*, 879–924. [CrossRef]
40. van Giesen, R.I.; Pieters, R. Climbing out of an Economic Crisis: A Cycle of Consumer Sentiment and Personal Stress. *J. Econ. Psychol.* **2019**, *70*, 109–124. [CrossRef]
41. Eisenberg, A.; Baron, J.; Seligman, M.E.P. Individual Differences in Risk Aversion and Anxiety. Available online: https://www.sas.upenn.edu/~{}baron/papers.htm/amyold.html (accessed on 10 March 2021).
42. Kuhnen, C.M.; Knutson, B. The Influence of Affect on Beliefs, Preferences, and Financial Decisions. *J. Fin. Quant. Anal.* **2011**, *46*, 605–626. [CrossRef]
43. Raghunathan, R.; Pham, M.T. All Negative Moods Are Not Equal: Motivational Influences of Anxiety and Sadness on Decision Making. *Organ. Behav. Hum. Decis. Process.* **1999**, *79*, 56–77. [CrossRef] [PubMed]
44. Nicholson, N.; Soane, E.; Fenton-O'Creevy, M.; Willman, P. Personality and Domain-specific Risk Taking. *J. Risk Res.* **2005**, *8*, 157–176. [CrossRef]
45. Faul, F.; Erdfelder, E.; Lang, A.G.; Buchner, A. G*Power 3: A flexible statistical power analysis program for the social, behavioral, and biomedical sciences. *Behav. Res. Methods* **2007**, *39*, 175–191. [CrossRef]
46. Statystyczny, G.U. *Dochody i Warunki Życia Ludności Polski–Raport z Badania EU-SILC 2018*; GUS: Warszawa, Poland, 2019.
47. Spitzer, R.L.; Kroenke, K.; Williams, J.B.; Löwe, B. A brief measure for assessing generalized anxiety disorder: The GAD-7. *Arch. Intern. Med.* **2006**, *166*, 1092–1097. [CrossRef] [PubMed]
48. Kroenke, K.; Spitzer, R.L.; Williams, J.B. The PHQ-9: Validity of a brief depression severity measure. *J. Gen. Intern. Med.* **2001**, *16*, 606–613. [CrossRef] [PubMed]
49. Richins, M.L. The Material Values Scale: Measurement Properties and Development of a Short Form. *J. Consum. Res.* **2004**, *31*, 209–219. [CrossRef]
50. Blais, A.-R.; Weber, E.U. A Domain-Specific Risk-Taking (DOSPERT) scale for adult populations. *Judgm. Decis. Mak.* **2006**, *1*, 33–47.
51. Bendau, A.; Plag, J.; Kunas, S.; Wyka, S.; Ströhle, A.; Petzold, M.B. Longitudinal changes in anxiety and psychological distress, and associated risk and protective factors during the first three months of the COVID-19 pandemic in Germany. *Brain Behav.* **2021**, *11*, e01964. [CrossRef]
52. Bell, V.; Wade, D. Mental health of clinical staff working in high-risk epidemic and pandemic health emergencies a rapid review of the evidence and living meta-analysis. *Soc. Psychiatry Psychiatr. Epidemiol.* **2021**, *56*, 1–11. [CrossRef]
53. Ritchie, H.; Ortiz-Ospina, E.; Beltekian, D.; Mathieu, E.; Hasell, J.; Macdonald, B.; Giattino, C.; Appel, C.; Rodés-Guirao, L.; Roser, M. Coronavirus Pandemic (COVID-19). Available online: https://ourworldindata.org/coronavirus (accessed on 10 March 2021).
54. Xie, X.-F.; Stone, E.; Zheng, R.; Zhang, R.-G. The 'Typhoon Eye Effect': Determinants of Distress during the SARS Epidemic. *J. Risk Res.* **2011**, *14*, 1091–1107. [CrossRef]
55. Statystyczny, G.U. *Rocznik Statystyczny Rzeczypospolitej Polskiej*; GUS: Warszawa, Poland, 2021.
56. Hofstede, G. *Culture's Consequences: International Differences in Work-Related Values*; Sage: Beverly Hills, CA, USA, 1980.
57. Ibrahim, S. A binary model of broken home: Parental death-divorce hypothesis of male juvenile delinquency in nigeria and ghana. In *Contemporary Perspectives in Family Research*; Maxwell, S.R., Blair, S.L., Eds.; Emerald Group Publishing Limited: New York, NY, USA, 2015; Volume 9, pp. 311–340.
58. International Labour Office. *World Social Protection Report 2020–22: Social Protection at the Crossroads-in Pursuit of a Better Future*; ILO: Geneva, Switzerland, 2021.
59. Kasser, T. Materialistic values and goals. *Annu. Rev. Psychol.* **2016**, *67*, 489–514. [CrossRef] [PubMed]

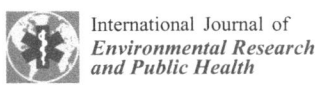

Article

ESG Performance and Stock Price Volatility in Public Health Crisis: Evidence from COVID-19 Pandemic

Dongyi Zhou and Rui Zhou *

School of Economics, Fudan University, Shanghai 200433, China; 17300680139@fudan.edu.cn
* Correspondence: zhourui@sina.cn

Abstract: Unlike traditional financial crises, COVID-19 is a global public health crisis with a significant negative impact on the global economy. Meanwhile, the stock market has been hit hard, and corporate share prices have become more volatile. However, the stock prices of some enterprises with good performance of ESG (Environment, Social, and Governance) are relatively stable in the epidemic. This paper selects ESG rating data from MSCI (Morgan Stanley Capital International) with better differentiation, adopts multiple regression and dummy variables, and adopts the Differences-in-Differences (DID)model with the help of COVID-19, an exogenous event. Empirical test the impact of ESG performance on the company's stock price fluctuations. The results show that the stock price volatility of companies with good ESG performance is lower than that of companies with poor performance. Second, COVID-19 exacerbates volatility in company stock prices, but the increase in stock price volatility of companies with good ESG performance is small. That is, good ESG performance helps reduce the increase in stock price volatility due to COVID-19 shock, and plays a role in enhancing "resilience" and stabilizing stock prices. This paper provides new empirical evidence for the study of ESG performance and corporate stock price volatility, and puts forward relevant policy recommendations for enterprises and government departments.

Keywords: public health crisis; ESG; stock price volatility; avoid risk; COVID-19

Citation: Zhou, D.; Zhou, R. ESG Performance and Stock Price Volatility in Public Health Crisis: Evidence from COVID-19 Pandemic. *Int. J. Environ. Res. Public Health* **2022**, *19*, 202. https://doi.org/10.3390/ijerph19010202

Academic Editors: Dirga Kumar Lamichhane and Dean G. Smith

Received: 20 October 2021
Accepted: 23 December 2021
Published: 25 December 2021

Publisher's Note: MDPI stays neutral with regard to jurisdictional claims in published maps and institutional affiliations.

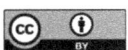

Copyright: © 2021 by the authors. Licensee MDPI, Basel, Switzerland. This article is an open access article distributed under the terms and conditions of the Creative Commons Attribution (CC BY) license (https://creativecommons.org/licenses/by/4.0/).

1. Introduction

In the course of the financial crisis, investors and scholars have paid extensive attention to what type of company's stock price performed better or alleviated the systemic risk. Many scholars have carried out in-depth discussions. The research found that companies with good ESG performance had a strong slow-release effect on systemic risk [1–8]. Especially during the COVID-19 pandemic, relevant studies have reached a new climax. Most studies show that ESG has obvious "resilience" and good avoid risk effect in crisis, thus effectively reducing systemic risk [9–11].

The sudden outbreak of COVID-19 made the world suffer a public health crisis as well as a heavy economic blow. After a short break during the Spring Festival in 2020, China's stock market experienced a "1000 share limit drop", with the CSI 300 index plummeting from 4200 to 3700 points, and the fluctuation of enterprise stock prices increased under the impact of the epidemic. This raises new questions about what types of stocks perform better in a crisis and are more resistant to systemic financial risk. What role does ESG performance play in stabilizing stock prices and reducing volatility? Can the improvement of ESG's performance become a "cushion" for enterprises in a crisis? What will be the effect on investors? These questions are worthy of our study.

The purpose of this study is to explore the relationship between ESG performance and stock price volatility under COVID-19. The research is divided into three levels: first, linear regression is used to test the effect of ESG performance on corporate volatility during COVID-19; Then, referring to the research ideas of Diaz et al. [12], the samples were stratified according to ESG score, and the groups of companies with better ESG performance and those with poor ESG performance were selected. Dummy variables were set to explore the volatility difference between the groups, so as to verify whether the volatility of companies with better ESG performance was significantly lower than that of companies with poor ESG performance. Finally, considering the impact of the COVID-19 outbreak and using the research ideas of Hoepner and Oikonomou [13] for reference, difference-in-differences (DID for short) are used to explore the impact of the COVID-19 outbreak. Does ESG performance enhance the company's "resilience"?

The innovation of this paper lies in: (1) the research perspective is novel. From the perspective of COVID-19, this paper studies the relationship between ESG performance and stock price volatility of enterprises under the impact of COVID-19. Most existing studies focus on the relationship between ESG performance, corporate performance and enterprise value, while this paper focuses on the effect of ESG performance on stock price volatility of enterprises. (2) High data quality. Existing literature is mostly used at present in China "picture of melt green" institutions such as disclosure of ESG rating data. However, these data are the enterprise of ESG performance roughly divided into several levels, A+ to D and for companies at the same level of ESG, the marking and no difference, so this method is divided into A rough, poor differentiation. The data used in this paper are MSCI ESG rating scores disclosed by Bloomberg data terminal, which quantifies enterprise ESG performance into floating point numbers with higher accuracy and better differentiation. (3) Use of new econometric methods. Most of the literature related to ESG used the multivariate linear regression method. This paper treats the outbreak of COVID-19 pandemic as a quasi-natural experiment and studies the effect of ESG performance on the share price volatility in the public health crisis using the difference-in-difference method (DID).

The following structure of this paper is as follows: The second part is a literature review, which reviews the concept and development of CSR and ESG, and summarizes the impact of COVID-19 on the stock market and the avoiding risk role of ESG. The third part is research design, including data source, variable selection and econometric model construction. The fourth part is the analysis of test results, including descriptive statistics, baseline regression, robustness test; The fifth part is the conclusion and enlightenment.

2. Literature Review

2.1. Corporate Social Responsibility (CSR) and Environmental Social Governance (ESG)

Corporate social responsibility (CSR) refers to the responsibility of industrial and commercial enterprises to not only be responsible to shareholders but also meet the expectations of different stakeholders in society when carrying out business activities [14]. ESG is an acronym developed by 20 financial institutions in response to the appeal of UN Secretary-General Kofi Anon in a 2004 report, which represents three different dimensions of Environment, Social responsibility and corporate Governance. It is the main evaluation method to inspect whether the enterprise operation conforms to sustainable development, and it is also the extension of the concept of green finance. Generally speaking, CSR refers to the activities of a company in promoting social responsibility and becoming a better corporate citizen. ESG refers to how companies and investors integrate environmental, social and governance issues into their business models. The difference between the two terms is that ESG explicitly encompasses governance, while CSR indirectly encompasses governance issues, as both involve environmental and social factors. Therefore, ESG is a broader concept than CSR [15].

North America and Europe are world leaders in CSR practices. After years of practice, a number of sustainable development frameworks and related standards have been put forward. At present, the mainstream enterprise sustainable development frameworks and related standards include SA8000, UNGC, G4-GRI and ISO 26000. Meanwhile, ESG related investment strategies develop rapidly and have gradually evolved into one of the mainstream investment strategies. In contrast, China's practice and related theoretical research started late and is limited in scale. The research of Chandan and Das [16] shows that the state-centric corporate social responsibility (CSR) model is different from the market model in the United States and the relationship model in the European Union. Hou and Li [17] believe that the differences in the development of CSR in China, Europe and the United States are caused by history, economy and enterprise development. ESG's domestic development in China is still not fully mature. In developed countries, institutional investors play a very important role in ESG investment practice. Institutional investors continually monitor ESG performance as they build their portfolios. In China, institutional investors exist but are not mainstream, and most investors are still retail investors. Accordingly, the demand for ESG products is still relatively small, and investors are more inclined to consider the factor of ESG performance on a psychological level, rather than systematically including it into the scope of investigation when allocating asset portfolios in a quantitative form [9].

2.2. The Impact of COVID-19 on China's Stock Market

In January 2020, COVID-19 was detected in Wuhan, China. Within a month, the number of cases in Wuhan soared to 60,000, leading to a total "lockdown" in the city and much of China. The virus brought about an unprecedented global public health crisis, followed by a global market-wide financial crisis. At 10 am on 23 January, Wuhan was locked down and the stock market was closed for the Lunar New Year. China's stock markets reacted to the public health crisis shortly after the lockdown of Wuhan. On 3 February 2020, the market reopened and the CSI 300 index fell sharply from 4200 to 3700. In general, the epidemic has brought a great negative impact on the stock market. To be specific, the study by Baker et al. [18] shows that in the 22 trading days from 24 February to 24 March 2020, 18 markets had a fluctuation of 2.5% or more every day. COVID-19 has affected policymakers, investors and companies across the globe. Dayong et al. [19] found that COVID-19 has caused markets to become highly volatile and unpredictable. Duan et al. [20] discovered that stock returns and turnover rates were positively predicted by the COVID-19 sentiments during the period from 17 December 2019 to 13 March 2020, which illustrated how the effects of the pandemic crisis were amplified by the sentiments. Further research found that COVID-19 had an unprecedented negative impact on stock market volatility compared to the impact of other epidemics. Duan et al. [21] develop two COVID-19 sentiment indices that capture the moods related to COVID-19. Our sentiment indices are real-time and forward-looking indices in the stock market. We discover that stock returns and turnover rates were positively predicted by the COVID-19 sentiments during the period from December 17, 2019 to March 13, 2020. Hanif et al. [22] studied the spillover effect of the stock market and found that COVID-19 increased the risk spillover effect of the market between March 2020 and April 2020. Huang et al. [23] found that the stock price crash risk of energy firms significantly decreases in the post-COVID-19 period and the effect of COVID-19 on stock price crash risk is less severe for state-owned enterprises (SOEs) than for non-SOEs in the post-COVID-19 period.

2.3. Avoid Risk Role of ESG
2.3.1. ESG and Risk

There is a view that the risk exposure of a company is related to ESG status. Heinkel et al. [1] established a model and divided the capital market according to investors' preferences. The study believed that companies with high ESG scores were given higher valuations and suffered lower systemic risks. Chen et al. [2] verified the inhibitory effect of CSR/ESG performance on the downside risk of stock price by describing the asymmetry of stock return distribution. Mishra and Modi [3] use empirical analysis to verify that good corporate social responsibility can help reduce non-systemic risks. The empirical study of Diemont, et al. [4] shows that tail risk measurement is closely related to ESG risk. The research results of Sassen [24] confirm that the improvement of ESG performance has a prominent effect on reducing stock price volatility and eliminating the overall risk of the company. Garcia et al. [5] measured the relationship between ESG performance and systemic risk by analyzing the performance of 365 companies from 2010 to 2012, and verified that the relationship between ESG performance and systemic risk was in an inverted "U" shape. The study of Jagannathan and Ravikumar [6] found that ESG-related risks may be rare, huge and non-diversified, especially related to the downside risks of enterprises. According to the research results of Albuquerque and Koskinen [8], when a company increases product differentiation through social responsibility investment, the higher the social responsibility investment, the lower the systemic risk of the company and the higher the value of the company. Lueg and Krastev [7] studied the two-way influence of ESG disclosure and corporate risk, and the results show that high-quality disclosure of sustainable development performance is conducive to corporate risk reduction. Ilhan et al. [25] found that companies with poorer ESG performance had higher tail risks. The research of Hoepner et al. [13] shows that companies that take an active role in ESG/CSR, especially those that attach importance to the environment, can reduce their downward risks in a crisis. Shakil [26] finds a significant adverse influence of ESG on stock price volatility. However, firm size portrays a non-significant moderating effect on ESG-stock price volatility nexus. And portfolio managers may invest in high achieving ESG firms to leverage the market volatility of their portfolio. Sabbaghi [27] using the Morgan Stanley Capital International (MSCI) indices as proxies for ESG test assets, this study investigates volatility risk for the highest ESG-rated firms through an empirical analysis in assessing how good news and bad news impact the risk of ESG firms. The analysis provides empirical evidence in support of the hypothesis that the impact of news on the volatility of ESG firms is larger for bad news, compared to good news. Employing an EGARCH framework, the analysis also finds that, in response to bad news, the observed volatility increases for small size ESG firms is lower compared to large and mid-cap ESG firms. James [28] also found that stocks with low ESG risk ratings (green stocks) not only have higher realized returns but also provide better tail-risk protection than stocks with high ESG risk ratings (brown stocks), especially during the COVID-19 crisis. The tail-risk protection provided by green stocks is robust within sectors and styles. Green funds and exchange-traded funds (ETFs) that hold green stocks have attracted significantly more fund flow than their counterparts, which is associated with the outperformance for both green funds and stocks.

2.3.2. The Avoid Risk Role of ESG in Crisis

Benabou and Tirole [29] found that companies with different ESG and CSR performance may face different systemic risk exposures, because they are resilient and have the ability to recover faster from crises. Oikonomou et al. [30] used downside risk as a measurement index. The author conducted an empirical study based on the S&P 500 index from 1992 to 2009, and the results showed that corporate social responsibility was negatively correlated with financial risk. Krueger [31] believes that companies with better ESG performance can be more "resilient" and recover from shocks more quickly in the face of negative events unique to the company. Lins et al. [32] found that companies with high ESG scores outperformed those with low ESG scores during the 2008–2009 financial crisis. According to Zhang [19], strong ESG/CSR companies face relatively small price elasticity demand due to product differentiation strategy, thus reducing system risk. Broadstock, et al. [9] explored that the performance of companies with high ESG score was better than that of companies with low ESG score in the context of COVID-19, and the event study method was used to prove that ESG played a avoid risk role to a certain extent in the crisis period compared with the normal period. Albuquerque et al. [10] used differential difference method to measure the mitigation effect of ESG input on corporate downside risk during the crisis, and the results showed that the downside risk of companies with excellent ESG performance was significantly lower than that of companies with poor ESG performance. The research of Diaz et al. [12] shows that environment and society are the main dimensions that can reflect the role of avoiding risk during the COVID-19 crisis. Takahashi and Yamada [11] Identify factors affecting the Japanese Stock market during the COVID-19 pandemic period. Studies have shown that governance (ESG) engagement, there is no evidence that firms that have highly rated ESG scores have higher abnormal returns, but firms with ESG funds outperform those without.

Albuquerque et al. [10] selected data during the COVID-19 epidemic to verify that companies with high ES scores in the ESG scoring system showed lower stock price volatility in the first quarter of 2020. However, it should be noted that this paper is significantly different from Albuquerque et al. [10] Albuquerque et al. [10] focuses on the impact of ES (environmental and social responsibility) performance on company stock price performance. This paper focuses on the "buffer" effect of ESG performance on company stock price volatility under the impact of the epidemic. Albuquerque et al. [10] used the main index ES is environment (E) and social responsibility (S), ignoring corporate governance (G). The data in this paper are the MSCI ESG rating score disclosed by Bloomberg data terminal, which quantifies the ESG performance of enterprises into floating point numbers. Other advantages are higher accuracy and better differentiation. In addition, China's ESG investment concept was formed late. A-shares were officially included in the MSCI index in 2018. A-share listed companies were selected as samples in this paper, which contributed Chinese experience to ESG related research.

To sum up, ESG related research is a relatively emerging research topic in recent years, and since performance and income related data are easier to obtain and more frequent, most research focuses on the effect of ESG on corporate performance. In recent years, due to the improvement of ESG information disclosure system, the improvement of data availability and the occurrence of several financial crises, people began to discuss the relationship between ESG and risk under the impact of financial crises. Most of the existing literature on ESG performance and corporate risk in the academic world is to explore the relationship between ESG performance and stock price fluctuations of a company. However, these studies mainly focus on the period of stable economic operation, and seldom consider the "impact" of economic crisis. However, in the few literature that consider the effect of ESG performance on corporate risk under crisis, most of them only focus on ESG performance during the financial crisis, without comparison before and after the crisis. In addition, there is little literature on the impact of financial crises resulting from public health events on financial markets. Therefore, it is of great theoretical and practical significance to further study the avoided risk effect of ESG before and after the impact of the crisis, especially the mitigation effect of ESG on systemic risk under the impact of COVID-19, a public health crisis different from the financial crisis.

3. Study Design

3.1. Data Source

At present, MSCI, FTSE, Thomson Reuters, Morningstar and Sustainalytics are the major ESG rating agencies and systems in the world. In China, there are different ESG scoring matrices given by rating systems such as China Securities Index, Shangdao Ronggreen and Social Investment Alliance. Currently, the available data is mainly based on rough grade classification, while THE MSCI ESG index further discloses the specific score of each dimension of E, S and G on the basis of grade classification, ranging from the minimum 0.1 to the maximum 100, thus providing a complete ESG measure. In combination with the availability of data, this paper quantifies ESG performance in the MSCI index disclosed in Bloomberg database to measure different corporate governance, environmental and social performance of A-share listed companies.

This paper selects listed companies in the A-share market as samples, and the sample range is all trading days from 1 December 2019 to 31 March 2020. At the same time, the following three samples of ST companies, data missing and MCSI's ESG rating system are excluded. The ESG performance score is derived from the MSCI ESG index of Bloomberg Data Terminal. Tobin's Q value came from CSMAR database. Volatility, high price, low price, average price and other corporate financial indicators come from the Wind financial terminal. Finally, valid data for 1021 companies were obtained.

The ESG performance score is derived from the MSCI ESG index of Bloomberg Data Terminal. Tobin's Q value came from CSMAR database. Volatility, high price, low price, average price and other corporate financial indicators come from the Wind financial terminal.

The cleaning, screening and organization of the original data were completed by Microsoft Excel software, and the regression was completed by Stata software.

3.2. Variables Selection

3.2.1. Explained Variable: Volatility

Volatility in this paper is divided into window volatility and intraday volatility. Window period volatility refers to the day after Wuhan was closed down, namely 24 January 2020, as the base date. Different days are set before and after the base date to form window periods covering different time ranges. The calculation formula of window yield is as follows:

$$VOL_i = \sqrt{\frac{\sum_{t=1}^{N}\left[\left(R_{it} - \frac{\sum_{t=1}^{N} R_{it}}{N}\right)^2\right]}{N-1}}$$

$$R_{it} = \frac{P_{it}}{P_{i,t-1}} - 1$$

where, P_{it} is the closing price of stock I on day t, and N is the window period.

Daily stock prices within the window period are selected to calculate the volatility within this range, which is recorded as window period volatility. The window periods selected in this paper include 5 trading days before and after the base date, 10 trading days before and after the base date, and the first quarter of 2020. Intraday volatility is the intraday high, low and average price of all trading days between 1 November 2019 and 31 March 2020. The results calculated by using these three groups of data can approximately replace intraday volatility, and the interest calculation formula is as follows:

$$vol_{it} = (High_{it} - Low_{it})/Avg_{it} \tag{1}$$

In Formula (1), vol_{it} is the intra-day volatility of company i on date t, $High_{it}$ is the intra-day high price of company i on date t, Low_{it} is the intra-day low price of company i on date t, Avg_{it} is the intra-day average price of company i on date t. The calculation reflects the maximum daily volatility of a company's stock. We refer to Parkinson [33], Garman and Klass [34], Rogers and Satchell [35], and Yang and Zhang [36]. But we try to study this problem from another angle. This paper pays more attention to the protection and buffer role of ESG performance when the company's stock price fluctuates violently under the impact of the epidemic. In view of the fact that COVID-19 is rapid and has a wide range of impact and is exogenous to enterprises, ESG performance can be divided into processing group and control group based on company characteristics. Therefore, the double difference method is very suitable for this study, and it can identify COVID-19's impact on stock price volatility and the difference of price fluctuation between companies with different ESG performance.

The higher the volatility, the more severe the volatility of financial asset prices, the higher the uncertainty of asset returns. On the contrary, the smaller the volatility, the gentler the price change of financial assets. Volatility in this paper is mainly used to measure risk.

3.2.2. Core Explanatory Variable: ESG

In China, ESG score data is mainly measured by MSCI ESG Index, FTSE Russell ESG Index, China Securities Index, Business Green Index, Social Value Investment Alliance Index and other rating systems.

In the three dimensions of ESG, Governance (G), also known as corporate governance, is the most important, because corporate Governance risks are common and critical to all companies. Compared with corporate governance, Environment (E) and Social (S), namely, Environment and society, are endowed with different degrees of importance in different industries. In the two dimensions of the environment and society, due to the rise of the concept of "climate assistance" in recent years, the discussion on the environmental dimension has become more intense.

The ESG rating system is designed to measure a company's resilience to significant environmental, social and governance risks to the industry over the long term. Taking the MSCI ESG rating used in this paper as an example, the establishment method of ESG scoring matrix is as follows: The first step is to select 35 indicators of different dimensions from the three levels of environment, society and corporate governance. The second step is to look at how companies perform on each of the 35 different indicators and give them a score for their performance. The third step is to calculate the weighted average of the 35 scores according to MSCI's weighting method as the total score of ESG. The last step is to adjust the ESG score of the enterprise into seven grades from "AAA" to "CCC". Among them, AAA and AA mark the leading companies in the industry, A, BBB and BB mark the average company in the industry, and B and CCC mark the backward company in the industry. Other ESG rating systems work in a similar way, assigning certain points to different companies' performance in environmental, social and corporate governance aspects, and quantifying them into an overall score through weighted average. The difference between different systems mostly lies in the selection of indicators of different dimensions and different weights.

As most of the available ESG data are roughly classified, the MSCI ESG index disclosed by Bloomberg platform further discloses the specific scores of E, S and G on the basis of the classification, ranging from the minimum 0.1 to the maximum 100, thus providing a complete ESG measure. Therefore, this paper selects the TOTAL ESG score data of more than 1000 A-share listed companies covered by THE MSCI ESG rating system, and the higher the ESG score, the better the company's performance in CSR.

3.2.3. Control Variables

In this paper, specific characteristics of enterprises and industries are controlled. Referring to the research of Broadstock et al. [9], enterprise Size (Size), financial leverage (Lev), TobinQ and Cash holding ratio (Cash) are selected as enterprise characteristic variables to control. On this basis, Fixed effects of control industry. Sabbaghi [27] found that when negative news occurs, the volatility of stock prices of large-sized enterprises also increases significantly. However, Shakil [26] found in his study that enterprise size had no significant moderating effect on the relationship between ESG and stock price volatility. Therefore, enterprise Size may also affect stock price fluctuations, so we add enterprise Size into the control variable. The size of the enterprise is expressed in this paper by the natural logarithm of the total market value of the company, which is the data disclosed in the 2019 annual report of the company. Industry division is based on the CSRC industry code disclosed by Wind terminal. Variable selection and definition are shown in Table 1.

Table 1. Variable selection and definition.

Variable Types	Variable Name	Variable Code	Variable Definitions
Explained variable	5 days before and after the fluctuations	VOL5	Five (10) days of stock price volatility before and after the window period
	10 days before and after the fluctuation	VOL10	Stock price volatility of 10 days before and after the window period (20 days in total)
	Seasonal fluctuations	VOLQ	Stock price volatility for all trading days in the first quarter of 2020
	Intraday volatility	vol	(Intraday high price—intraday low price)/daytime average price
Explanatory variables	ESG performance	ESG	Quantitative scores given by the MSCI ESG index
Control variables	The enterprise scale	Size	The natural log of a company's total annual market value
	Financial leverage	Lev	Average annual total liabilities/Average annual Total assets × 100
	Tobin Q value	TobinQ	Company market capitalization/total assets
	Cash holding ratio	Cash	The company holds cash/total assets

3.3. Econometric Model

The empirical test in this paper will be divided into three levels, and three models will be used to verify them respectively.

First, establish the regression equation between ESG performance and the company's volatility during COVID-19:

$$VOL_i = \alpha_0 + \alpha_1 ESG_i + \alpha_2 Size_i + \alpha_3 Lev_i + \alpha_4 TobinQ_i + \alpha_5 Cash_i + \varepsilon_i \quad (2)$$

In Formula (2), VOL represents volatility in the window period: 5 trading days before and after the base date, 10 trading days, and the first quarter of 2020 are successively selected, and the volatility in these three window periods are respectively denoted as $VOL5$, $VOL10$ and $VOLQ$. α_0 is a constant term, ε_{it} is a residual term, and α_1 represents the degree of effect of ESG performance on volatility. If α_1 is significantly negative, it verifies that good ESG performance is conducive to reducing the volatility of asset prices, making asset prices more stable and thus reducing risks.

Secondly, on the basis of Formula (2), if the company is divided into the group with better ESG performance and the group with poor ESG performance, whether the volatility of the former group will be significantly lower in the same period compared with the latter group. This paper introduces a dummy variable as an ESG factor to distinguish different groups. Therefore, the regression model for the comparison of volatility between companies with excellent ESG performance and those with poor ESG performance during COVID-19 is constructed:

$$VOL_i = \alpha_0 + \alpha_1 ESGf_i + \alpha_2 Size_i + \alpha_3 Lev_i + \alpha_4 TobinQ_i + \alpha_5 Cash_i + \varepsilon_i \quad (3)$$

In Formula (3), $ESGf$ is the dummy variable. The processing of this variable is to sort the ESG scores of all companies from large to small and divide them into four equal parts, extract the top 25% and the bottom 25% of companies, assign the value of the top 25% to 1, and the $ESGf$ value of the bottom 25% to 0. Thus, companies with excellent ESG performance can be distinguished from those with poor ESG performance. The other assumptions are the same. The dependent variable is volatility in the window period, VOL.

Finally, by comparing the difference between the control group and the experimental group before and after the implementation of quasi-natural experiment, the method constructs the difference statistics reflecting the implementation effect of quasi-natural experiment. At the same time, this statistic can also reflect the enhancement or alleviation of experimental implementation effect by dividing treatment groups and the basis of illumination. Because the impact of COVID-19 is global, all businesses are affected almost simultaneously. Therefore, the control group and the treatment group were constructed from the perspective of enterprise characteristics by referring to many literatures [37]. In this paper, the treatment group and the control group were divided according to the ESG score of enterprises. That is, the virtual variable ESGf in Model (2) was directly used as the grouped virtual variable.

The DID method was used to study whether companies with excellent ESG performance had stronger "resilience" after the outbreak compared with those with poor ESG performance before the outbreak, that is, whether they could recover from the shock more quickly. Therefore, in order to characterize the effect of ESG performance on corporate volatility before and after COVID-19, the following regression equation is constructed in this paper:

$$vol_{it} = \beta_0 + \beta_1 ESGf_{it} + \beta_2 Post_{it} + \beta_3 ESGf_{it} \times Post_{it} + \beta_4 Size_{it} \\ + \beta_5 Lev_{it} + \beta_6 TobinQ_{it} + \beta_7 Cash_{it} + \varepsilon_{it} \quad (4)$$

In Formula (4), the time span is selected from trading days between 8 January 2020 and 19 February 2020. The dependent variable is intraday volatility, vol. The sample companies also select the 25% with the highest ESG score and the 25% with the lowest ESG score, a total of 531 companies. Set $ESGf$ and $Post$ dummy variables and their interaction item $ESG*Post$. The meaning and treatment of $ESGf$ are the same as above; $Post$ is a time dummy variable used to distinguish between before and after the epidemic impact. The division is based on the closing day of Wuhan, China on 23 January 2020. This variable in the data of subsequent trading days is assigned as 1, and the previous data is assigned as 0.

4. Analysis of Inspection Results

4.1. Descriptive Statistics

Table 2 lists the sample size, mean, standard value, minimum value and maximum value of each variable. As the intraday volatility covers multiple dates and is panel data, there are many observed values.

Table 2. Descriptive Statistics.

Variable Name	Variable Code	Sample Size	Mean Value	Standard Deviation	Min	Max
5-Day Fluctuation	VOL5	1021	2.020	0.222	1.079	2.807
Fluctuation In the Last 10 Days	VOL10	1021	1.818	0.219	1.002	2.714
Quarterly Fluctuation	VOLQ	1021	1.743	0.241	1.029	2.534
Intraday Fluctuation	vol	38,690	0.2294	0.4204	0	1
Esg Performance	ESG	1021	24.80	7.650	11.21	61.72
Tobin Q Value	TobinQ	1021	1.693	1.313	0.730	14.09
Enterprise Scale	Size	1021	23.54	1.159	20.62	28.09
Cash Ratio	Cash	1021	0.0018	0.0282	0	0.876
Financial Leverage	Lev	1021	51.51	21.72	0.836	229.0

4.2. Benchmark Regression

4.2.1. Volatility between ESG and COVID-19

As can be seen from the regression results in Table 3, excellent ESG performance of listed companies contributes to the stability of the company's stock price. Since the coefficient α_1 before ESG is significantly negative, it can be inferred that, for a firm, the higher the ESG score, the lower its volatility over time. As window volatility is selected for 5 trading days before and after the base date, 10 trading days, and the volatility for the whole first quarter of 2020, ESG coefficients α_1 in columns (1), (3) and (5) of Table 3 are all significantly negative, so this conclusion is robust. In addition, Table 3 (2), (4) and (6) are listed as the results of the fixed effect model regression. Controlling the industry fixed effect can solve the endogeneity problem caused by the missing variables to a certain extent. The ESG coefficient α_1 is significantly negative, being -0.127, -0.145 and -0.132 respectively, indicating that when the ESG score increases by 1, stock price volatility decreases by 0.127, 0.145 and 0.132 over 5 trading days, 10 trading days, and the first quarter of 2020.

Table 3. Regression results of ESG and corporate volatility during COVID-19.

	(1)	(2)	(3)	(4)	(5)	(6)
	VOL5	VOL5	VOL10	VOL10	VOLQ	VOLQ
ESG	−0.099 **	−0.127 **	−0.121 ***	−0.145 ***	−0.126 **	−0.132 **
	(0.047)	(0.051)	(0.046)	(0.050)	(0.051)	(0.054)
Size	−0.001	−0.018 ***	0.007	−0.009 *	0.032 ***	0.012 **
	(0.006)	(0.006)	(0.006)	(0.005)	(0.006)	(0.006)
Lev	−0.002 ***	−0.001 ***	−0.001 ***	−0.000	−0.000	0.001
	(0.000)	(0.000)	(0.000)	(0.000)	(0.000)	(0.000)
TobinQ	−0.031 ***	−0.017 ***	−0.034 ***	−0.020 ***	−0.040***	−0.027 ***
	(0.006)	(0.007)	(0.006)	(0.006)	(0.007)	(0.007)
Cash	−0.598 **	−0.493 **	−0.624 ***	−0.541 **	−0.790 ***	−0.698 ***
	(0.237)	(0.224)	(0.235)	(0.221)	(0.258)	(0.238)
Constant term	2.901 ***	2.574 ***	2.725 ***	2.406 ***	2.696 ***	2.383 ***
	(0.141)	(0.144)	(0.140)	(0.142)	(0.153)	(0.153)
Sample size	1021	1021	1021	1021	1021	1021
R^2	0.100	0.233	0.091	0.238	0.095	0.265
Fixed effects		YES		YES		YES

Note: *, ** and *** represent significant at the level of 10%, 5% and 1% respectively.

4.2.2. Comparison of Volatility of ESG Performance during COVID-19

Further, we analyze and compare the COVID-19 volatility between high performing and low performing ESG companies. As can be seen from the regression results in Table 4, companies with excellent ESG performance have higher avoid risk ability compared with companies with poor ESG performance, and their volatility is significantly lower than that of companies with poor ESG performance. As the coefficient before ESG is significantly negative, which is −0.044, −0.046 and −0.047 respectively, that is, the stock price volatility of companies with good ESG performance is 0.044, 0.046 and 0.067 lower than that of companies with average ESG performance in the 5 trading days and 10 trading days before and after the base date of the company and in the first quarter of 2020. This shows that companies with good ESG performance have a strong ability to resist risks.

Table 4. Regression results of the volatility of companies with high and low ESG performance during COVID-19.

	(1) VOL5	(2) VOL10	(3) VOLQ
ESGf	−0.044 **	−0.046 **	−0.067 ***
	(0.021)	(0.020)	(0.022)
Size	−0.030 ***	−0.033 ***	−0.027 ***
	(0.009)	(0.009)	(0.009)
Lev	−0.001 *	−0.000	0.001
	(0.001)	(0.001)	(0.001)
TobinQ	−0.007	0.000	0.012
	(0.008)	(0.008)	(0.009)
Constant term	2.810 ***	2.628 ***	2.349 ***
	(0.199)	(0.197)	(0.208)
Sample size	526	526	526
R^2	0.248	0.257	0.292
Fixed effects	YES	YES	YES

Note: *, ** and *** represent significant at the level of 10%, 5% and 1% respectively.

4.2.3. The Effect of ESG on Corporate Volatility before and after COVID-19

(1) Parallel trend test

Figure 1 shows the intra-group mean changes of intraday volatility in the experimental group (companies with high ESG performance) and the control group (companies with low ESG performance) before and after the outbreak. The results showed that the variation trend of intraday volatility of the experimental group and the control group before the epidemic impact was basically the same, meeting the parallel trend test, and the intraday volatility of the experimental group was always lower than the control group, which was consistent with the above analysis.

(2) Regression analysis

The regression results of the impact of ESG on the company's stock price volatility before and after COVID-19 are shown in Table 5. As can be seen from Table 5, since the time dummy variable represents the time limit of the impact of COVID-19, and the former coefficient is significantly positive, this shows that under the impact of COVID-19, the stock price volatility of enterprises has increased and the degree of instability has increased. The coefficient β_1 before the policy dummy variable $ESGf$ is significantly negative, this indicates that the stock price volatility of companies with excellent ESG performance is lower than that of companies with poor ESG performance. The coefficient β_3 before interaction term is significantly negative, indicating that after excluding other impacts of COVID-19, the increase of volatility of companies with excellent ESG performance is 0.002 lower than that of companies with poor ESG performance. This phenomenon can be seen as an illustration of the "weakening" of ESG performance against shocks. In the crisis,

ESG performance becomes the "cushion" of the company, enabling the company to have stronger "resilience" and recover from shocks faster.

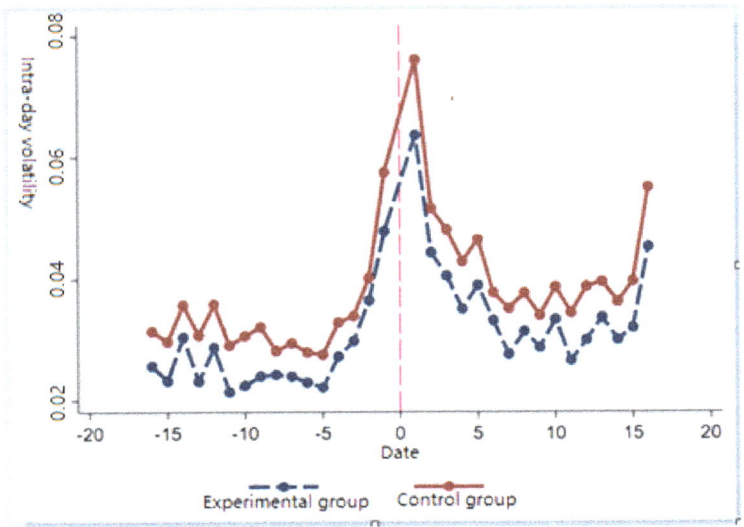

Figure 1. Intra-day volatility trend of the experimental and control groups before and after COVID-19 outbreak.

Table 5. Regression results of ESG's effect on corporate volatility before and after COVID-19.

	(1) VOL	(2) VOL
Post	0.011 ***	0.011 ***
	(0.001)	(0.001)
ESGf	−0.005 ***	−0.002 ***
	(0.001)	(0.001)
ESGf*Post	−0.002 ***	−0.002 ***
	(0.001)	(0.001)
Size		−0.001 ***
		(0.000)
Lev		−0.000 ***
		(0.000)
TobinQ		0.002 ***
		(0.000)
Cash		−0.025 ***
		(0.005)
Constant term	0.033 ***	0.063 ***
	(0.000)	(0.004)
N	13,247	13,247
R^2	0.059	0.085

Note: *, ** and *** represent significant at the level of 10%, 5% and 1% respectively.

In general, we consider ESG investment as a kind of good deed to society and a cost investment made by enterprises at the expense of economic resources. However, the research results of this paper have obvious economic significance. The research results reveal the negative correlation between ESG performance and stock price volatility, thus helping enterprises and investors to understand the benefits of ESG input more comprehensively. On the one hand, ESG performance can help companies achieve more robust stock price performance. On the other hand, it also helps investors better manage risks and build portfolios based on ESG factors.

4.3. Robustness Test

4.3.1. Change the Subsample Selection Method

As for the second regression model Formula (3) above, the classification of ESG factor is based on the 25% companies with the highest ESG score and the 25% with the lowest ESG score. As the two groups of companies with the best performance and the worst performance are selected as sub-samples, the regression results may be affected by this selection method. Therefore, we changed the selected sub-sample, adjusted the combination of the highest 25% and the lowest 25% ESG score to the highest 25% and 50–75% ESG score companies, and assigned the value $ESGf$ of the top 25% companies to 1, and the value $ESGf$ of the 50–75% companies to 0, and then regression. The regression results are shown in Table 6.

Table 6. Change the subsample selection method.

	(1) VOL5	(2) VOL10	(3) VOLQ
ESGf	−0.028	−0.040 **	−0.048 **
	(0.020)	(0.020)	(0.021)
Size	−0.029 ***	−0.030 ***	−0.032 ***
	(0.009)	(0.008)	(0.009)
Lev	−0.000	0.001	0.002 **
	(0.001)	(0.001)	(0.001)
TobinQ	−0.009	0.001	0.018 *
	(0.009)	(0.009)	(0.009)
Cash	−0.445 *	−0.494 **	−0.609 **
	(0.237)	(0.230)	(0.244)
Constant term	2.737 ***	2.503 ***	2.388 ***
	(0.197)	(0.191)	(0.203)
Sample size	526	526	526
R^2	0.257	0.277	0.315
Fixed effects	YES	YES	YES

Note: *, ** and *** represent significant at the level of 10%, 5% and 1% respectively.

As can be seen from Table 6, when the volatility in the window period is selected for 10 trading days before and after the base day and the first quarter of 2020, the regression result is still significantly negative; while when the volatility in the window period is selected for 5 days before and after the base day, the regression effect is no longer significant. The reason for this result may be that it takes a period of time for ESG performance to show its weakening effect on volatility. Compared with the short term, the weakening effect will be more obvious after a period of time. Therefore, on the whole, the model is robust.

4.3.2. Change the Time Span

As the third econometric model Formula (4) mentioned above may be affected by the number of periods included in the time span before and after COVID-19 impact when it is tested by DID method. Therefore, this paper adjusts the time span, extending the trading daytime span from 8 January 2020 to 19 February 2020 to 2 December 2019 to 31 March 2020, and then makes a regression according to the model ideas mentioned above. The test results are shown in Table 7, which shows that the results are still robust.

Table 7. Change the time span.

	(1) VOL	(2) VOL
Post	0.015 ***	0.015 ***
	(0.000)	(0.000)
ESGf	−0.005 ***	−0.003 ***
	(0.000)	(0.000)
ESGf*Post	−0.002 ***	−0.002 ***
	(0.000)	(0.000)
Size		−0.001 ***
		(0.000)
Lev		−0.000
		(0.000)
TobinQ		0.002 ***
		(0.000)
Cash		−0.027 ***
		(0.003)
Constant term	0.030 ***	0.052 ***
	(0.000)	(0.002)
N	38,638	38,638
R^2	0.122	0.142

Note: *, ** and *** represent significant at the level of 10%, 5% and 1% respectively.

5. Conclusions

From the perspective of COVID-19 shock, this paper selects THE MSCI ESG data disclosed by Bloomberg data terminal and uses the difference in difference (DID) method to test the relationship between ESG performance and stock price volatility of enterprises under COVID-19 shock. The results show that: (1) excellent ESG performance of single listed companies is conducive to reducing stock price volatility under the impact of crisis and stabilizing stock price; (2) Compared with companies with poor ESG performance, companies with excellent ESG performance had lower volatility and more stable stock prices in the same period of time; (3) Volatility of listed companies generally rose before and after the impact of the epidemic. In this process, companies with excellent ESG performance saw a lower increase in volatility than those with poor ESG performance, showing stronger "resilience" and the ability to recover faster from the impact of the crisis. As a result, ESG performance can act as a "cushion" for a company and serve as a good hedge in a crisis.

At the same time, the research of this paper also gives us the following enlightenment: From an investor's perspective, investors should factor ESG into their asset allocation considerations and avoid companies with low ESG scores, thereby avoiding costly risks. From the perspective of enterprises, companies with good ESG performance have relatively low stock price volatility. Therefore, enterprises should take an active role in ESG, integrate the concept of corporate social responsibility into the operation system, and create "ESG reputation" for enterprises. From the perspective of policy makers, since ESG performance can reduce the systemic risk of enterprises, relevant policy departments should strengthen support for green enterprises and related projects and encourage participation in the construction of green projects. The government can adopt top-down measures to escort companies with good CSR performance.

Author Contributions: Conceptualization, D.Z.; methodology, D.Z. and R.Z.; analysis, D.Z. and R.Z.; data source, D.Z. and R.Z.; writing—original draft, D.Z.; writing—review and editing, R.Z.; supervision, R.Z.; project administration, D.Z. and R.Z. All authors have read and agreed to the published version of the manuscript.

Funding: This research was supported by the Major Program of the National Social Science Foundation of China (Grant No. 21&ZD117).

Institutional Review Board Statement: Not applicable.

Informed Consent Statement: Not applicable.

Conflicts of Interest: The authors declare no conflict of interest.

References

1. Heinkel, R.; Kraus, A.; Zechner, J. The Effect of Green Investing on Corporate Behavior. *J. Financ. Quant. Anal.* **2001**, *36*, 431–449. [CrossRef]
2. Chen, J.; Hong, H.; Stein, J.C. Forecasting Crashes: Trading Volume, Past Returns, and Conditional Skewness in Stock Prices. *J. Financ. Econ.* **2001**, *61*, 345–381. [CrossRef]
3. Mishra, S.; Modi, S.B. Positive and Negative Corporate Social Responsibility, Financial Leverage, and Idiosyncratic Risk. *J. Bus. Ethics* **2013**, *117*, 431–448. [CrossRef]
4. Diemont, D.; Moore, K.; Soppe, A. The Downside of Being Responsible: Corporate Social Responsibility and Tail Risk. *J. Bus. Ethics* **2016**, *137*, 213–229. [CrossRef]
5. Garcia, A.S.; Mendes, W.; Orsato, R.J. Sensitive Industries Produce Better ESG Performance: Evidence from Emerging Markets. *J. Clean. Prod.* **2017**, *150*, 135–147. [CrossRef]
6. Jagannathan, R.; Ravikumar, A.; Sammon, M. Environmental, Social, and Governance Criteria: Why Investors Should Care. *J. Invest. Manag.* **2018**, *16*, 18–31.
7. Lueg, K.; Krastev, B.; Lueg, R. Bidirectional Effects between Organizational Sustainability Disclosure and Risk. *J. Clean. Prod.* **2019**, *229*, 268–277. [CrossRef]
8. Albuquerque, R.; Koskinen, Y.; Zhang, C. Corporate Social Responsibility and Firm Risk: Theory and Empirical Evidence. *Manag. Sci.* **2019**, *65*, 4451–4469. [CrossRef]
9. Broadstock, D.C.; Chan, K.; Cheng, L.T.; Wang, X. The Role of ESG Performance during Times of Financial Crisis: Evidence from COVID-19 in China. *Financ. Res. Lett.* **2021**, *38*, 1–11. [CrossRef]
10. Albuquerque, R.; Koskinen, Y.; Yang, S.; Zhang, C. Resiliency of Environmental and Social Stocks: An Analysis of the Exogenous COVID-19 Market Crash. *Rev. Corp. Financ. Stud.* **2020**, *9*, 593–621. [CrossRef]
11. Takahashi, H.; Yamada, K. When the Japanese stock market meets COVID-19: Impact of ownership, China and US exposure, and ESG channels. *Int. Rev. Financ. Anal.* **2021**, *74*, 101670. [CrossRef]
12. Díaz, V.; Ibrushi, D.; Zhao, J. Reconsidering Systematic Factors during the COVID-19 Pandemic—The Rising Importance of ESG. *Financ. Res. Lett.* **2021**, *38*, 1–6. [CrossRef]
13. Cojoianu, T.F.; Ascui, F.; Clark, G.L.; Hoepner, A.G.; Wójcik, D. Does the Fossil Fuel Divestment Movement Impact New Oil & Hoepner Gas Fundraising. *J. Econ. Geogr.* **2020**, *21*, 1–33.
14. Bowen, H.R. Graduate education in economics. *Am. Econ. Rev.* **1953**, *43*, iv-223.
15. Gillan, S.L.; Koch, A.; Starks, L.T. Firms and Social Responsibility: A Review of ESG and CSR Research in Corporate Finance. *J. Corp. Financ.* **2021**, *66*, 1–16. [CrossRef]
16. Chandan, H.C.; Das, R. Evolution of Responsible and Sustainable Corporate Identity for Chinese Firms. In *The China Business Model*; Chandos Publishing: Cambridge, UK, 2017; pp. 71–96.
17. Hou, S.; Li, L. Reasoning and Differences Between CSR Theory and Practice in China, the United States and Europe. *J. Int. Bus. Ethics* **2014**, *7*, 19–30.
18. Baker, S.R.; Bloom, N.; Davis, S.J.; Terry, S.J. COVID-Induced Economic Uncertainty, National Bureau of Economic Research. NBER Working Papers. 2020. No. w26983. Available online: https://www.nber.org/papers/w26983 (accessed on 19 October 2021).
19. Zhang, D.; Hu, M.; Ji, Q. Financial markets under the global pandemic of COVID-19. *Financ. Res. Lett.* **2021**, *36*, 101528. [CrossRef]
20. Duan, Y.; Liu, L.; Wang, Z. COVID-19 Sentiment and the Chinese Stock Market: Evidence from the Official News Media and Sina Weibo. *Res. Int. Bus. Financ.* **2021**, *58*, 101432. [CrossRef]
21. Liu, Z.; Huynh, T.L.D.; Dai, P.-F. The Impact of COVID-19 on the Stock Market Crash Risk in China. *Res. Int. Bus. Financ.* **2021**, *57*, 1–10. [CrossRef] [PubMed]
22. Hanif, W.; Mensi, W.; Vo, X.V. Impacts of COVID-19 Outbreak on the Spillovers between US and Chinese Stock Sectors. *Financ. Res. Lett.* **2021**, *7*, 1–18. [CrossRef]
23. Huang, S.; Liu, H. Impact of COVID-19 on stock price crash risk: Evidence from Chinese energy firms. *Energy Econ.* **2021**, *101*, 105431. [CrossRef]
24. Sassen, R.; Hinze, A.K.; Hardeck, I. Impact of ESG Factors on Firm Risk in Europe. *J. Bus. Econ.* **2016**, *86*, 867–904. [CrossRef]
25. Ilhan, E.; Sautner, Z.; Vilkov, G. Carbon Tail Risk. *Rev. Financ. Stud.* **2019**, *34*, 1540–1571. [CrossRef]
26. Shakil, M.H. Environmental, social and governance performance and stock price volatility: A moderating role of firm size. *J. Public Aff.* **2020**, *10*, e2574. [CrossRef]
27. Sabbaghi, O. The impact of news on the volatility of ESG firms. *Glob. Financ. J.* **2020**, *4*, 100570. [CrossRef]
28. James, X.X. The Impact of ESG Risk on Stocks. *J. Impact ESG Invest.* **2021**, *2*, 22–42.
29. Benabou, R.; Tirole, J. Individual and Corporate Social Responsibility. *Economica* **2010**, *77*, 1–19. [CrossRef]
30. Oikonomou, I.; Brooks, C.; Pavelin, S. The Impact of Corporate Social Performance on Financial Risk and Utility: A Longitudinal Analysis. *Financ. Manag.* **2012**, *41*, 483–515. [CrossRef]

31. Krueger, P.; Zacharias, S.; Tang, D.Y.; Rui, Z. The Effects of Mandatory ESG Disclosure Around the World (30 November 2021). European Corporate Governance Institute—Finance Working Paper No. 754/2021, Swiss Finance Institute Research Paper No. 21–44. Available online: http://dx.doi.org/10.2139/ssrn.3832745 (accessed on 19 October 2021).
32. Lins, K.V.; Servaes, H.; Tamayo, A. Social Capital, Trust, and Firm Performance: The value of corporate social responsibility during the financial crisis. *J. Financ.* **2017**, *72*, 1785–1824. [CrossRef]
33. Parkinson, M. The Extreme Value Method for Estimating the Variance of the Rate of Return. *J. Bus.* **1980**, *53*, 61–65. [CrossRef]
34. Garman, M.B.; Klass, M.J. On the Estimation of Security Price Volatilities from Historical Data. *J. Bus.* **1980**, *53*, 67–78. [CrossRef]
35. Rogers, L.C.G.; Satchell, S.E. Estimating Variance from High, Low and Closing Prices. *Ann. Appl. Probab.* **1991**, *1*, 504–512. [CrossRef]
36. Yang, D.; Zhang, Q. Drift Independent Volatility Estimation Based on High, Low, Open, and Close Prices. *J. Bus.* **2000**, *73*, 477–492. [CrossRef]
37. Campello, M.; Larrain, M. Enlarging the contracting space: Collateral menus, access to credit, and economic activity. *Rev. Financ. Stud.* **2016**, *29*, 349–383.

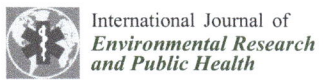

Article

The Impacts of COVID-19 on China's Economy and Energy in the Context of Trade Protectionism

Feng Wang and Min Wu *

School of Economics and Finance, Xi'an Jiaotong University, Xi'an 710061, China; wangfeng123@xjtu.edu.cn
* Correspondence: wumin2019@stu.xjtu.edu.cn

Abstract: In the current context of rising trade protectionism, deeply understanding the impacts of COVID-19 on economy and energy has important practical significance for China to cope with external shocks in an uncertain environment and enhance economic resilience. By constructing an integrated economic and energy input-output model including the COVID-19 shock, this paper assesses the impacts of COVID-19 on China's macro-economy and energy consumption in the context of trade protectionism. The results are shown as follows. First, in the context of protectionism, the outbreak of COVID-19 in China would cause a 2.2–3.09% drop in China's GDP and a 1.56–2.48% drop in energy consumption, while adverse spillovers from global spread of COVID-19 would reduce its GDP by 2.27–3.28% and energy consumption by 2.48–3.49%. Second, the negative impacts of domestic outbreak on China's construction, non-metallic mineral products, and services would be on average 1.29% higher than those on other industries, while the impacts of global spread of COVID-19 on export-oriented industries such as textiles and wearing apparel would be on average 1.23% higher than other industries. Third, the effects of two wave of the pandemic on China's fossil energy consumption would be on average 1.44% and 0.93% higher than non-fossil energy consumption, respectively.

Keywords: COVID-19; trade protectionism; economy; energy; input-output model

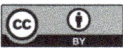

1. Introduction

Since the outbreak of the 2008 financial crisis, trade protectionism has gradually risen in the international market [1,2]. According to Global Trade Alert (GTA), China has experienced the highest number of protectionist measures. The coronavirus disease (COVID-19) outbreak was discovered in Wuhan, China, in December 2019 and then spread rapidly to multiple countries around the world in early 2020, which was characterized as a pandemic by the World Health Organization (WHO). The COVID-19 pandemic not only has a direct impact on China's economy, but also entails disruptions of global value chains and recessions in major economies, thus exposing China to adverse global spillovers. Meanwhile, the panic caused by the pandemic may further exacerbate global trade protectionism [3,4]. This shows that the COVID-19 pandemic poses a huge challenge to China's economy in the context of trade protectionism. In addition, some scholars found that the pandemic may also affect energy consumption, which may be due to a bidirectional causality between energy consumption and economic growth [5,6]. For example, Smith et al. [7] argued that the pandemic would cause a decline in energy consumption in major carbon-emitting countries. Norouzi et al. [8] found that the pandemic has delivered a shock to electricity and oil demand in China. Similarly, Wang and Su [9] suggested that the reductions in economic activity and the restrictions on transport caused by COVID-19 has significantly decreased China's energy consumption, especially coal consumption. The above evidence indicates that the COVID-19 pandemic will not only bring substantial challenges to China's economy but also affect its energy consumption.

Much of the current literature on the pandemic analyzes its social and economic impacts, such as its impact on output [10], industry volatility [11] and interest rates [12]. Other literature focuses on the effects of the pandemic on energy and environment, such as its impact on energy consumption [13] and air pollution [14,15]. However, most researchers focusing on the economic impacts of COVID-19 ignored the effects of the pandemic on the flow of energy products [10–12], while those examining the impacts of the pandemic on energy consumption rarely considered the relationship between energy and economy [13–15]. In addition, no studies have been found in the searchable literature that analyze the impact of the pandemic on China in the current context of rising trade protectionism. Currently, China is experiencing the shock of COVID-19 in the context of rising trade protectionism. Combined with the international context that China is facing, deeply understanding the effects of the pandemic on China's economy and energy in this context is of great significance for China to respond to external shocks in an uncertain environment, enhance economic resilience, safeguard national security, and promote high-quality development. Therefore, this paper will evaluate the impacts of the COVID-19 shock on China's economy and energy in the context of trade protectionism. Specifically, this paper will first construct an integrated economic and energy input-output (IEEIO) model including the COVID-19 shock based on the characteristics of such shock. This model can capture the changes in the global economic supply chain and energy conversion chain under the pandemic shock. Then, according to the development of the pandemic, we will set scenarios to simulate the shock of the COVID-19 outbreak in China and the shock of the COVID-19 global spread. Finally, based on the IEEIO model, including the COVID-19 shock and related scenarios, this paper will simulate and evaluate the impacts of the outbreak and spread of the pandemic on China's macro-economy, industry outputs, and energy consumption in the context of trade protectionism.

This paper makes three contributions to the literature. First, this paper is the first to assess the impacts of the COVID-19 shock on China's economic development, industry outputs, and energy flows from the perspective of economic–energy interactions. Although some researchers have evaluated the effects of the COVID-19 pandemic on the economy or on energy [10–15], most of them focus on a single dimension, and there is a lack of studies that comprehensively examine the impacts of the pandemic on the macro-economic level and on energy flows from the perspective of economic–energy interactions. Second, fully considering the nature and characteristics of the shock of COVID-19, we introduce the pandemic's impact on supply-side and demand-side in different forms into the IEEIO model, thus constructing the IEEIO model including the COVID-19 shock. This model can capture the changes from the shock of COVID-19 in global supply chains and energy conversion chains. Third, given the characteristics of the outbreak and spread of the pandemic and its uncertainty, this paper innovatively sets up 11 scenarios to simulate and extrapolate the impacts of the pandemic on China's economy and energy in the context of trade protectionism.

The structure of this paper is as follows: Section 2 reviews the relevant literature; Section 3 constructs an IEEIO model including the COVID-19 shock; Section 4 introduces the design of scenarios and data sources; Section 5 presents the results and discussion; and the last section provides the conclusions and policy implications.

2. Literature Review

From the existing literature, there are three main types of literature germane to this paper: the first is the literature that assesses the effects of COVID-19; the second is the literature that examines the economic and energy impacts of COVID-19 on China; the third is the literature analyzing the impacts of COVID-19 on the world and other countries.

A variety of methods have been used in the literature to assess the impacts of COVID-19, methods which could be broadly classified into three categories. One of the common methods is the computable general equilibrium (CGE) model. This model can be used to evaluate the effects of the pandemic from a macro and comprehensive perspective [16]. Based on global hybrid dynamic stochastic general equilibrium (DSGE)–computable general equilibrium (CGE) general equilibrium model, McKibbin and Fernando [17] and Jawad et al. [18] predicted the possible progress of COVID-19 in seven scenarios and assessed the macroeconomic impacts of the pandemic under each scenario. Madai Boukar et al. [19] used the CGE model to evaluate the effects of COVID-19 on employment in Cameroon's different sectors. The CGE model can identify all economic activities in a consistent way, in theory, reflecting the interdependence of economic sectors [20]. However, the modeling of the CGE model is complex, and the sensitivity of CGE outputs to shocks, model types, and closure rules may hinder the applicability of this paper to impact assessments of structural changes caused by shocks [21]. The input-output model is another common method for evaluating the impacts of the pandemic on economy and energy. Based on the input-output model, Sayan and Alkan [22] and Bonet-Morón et al. [23] assessed the economic costs of the pandemic control measures, while Huang and Tian [24] analyzed the impacts of the pandemic on inequality in carbon emissions. The input-output model has been simplified to the easily constructed inter-industry-based tables [25], which is suitable for capturing the impacts of sudden shocks on the economy [20]. However, this model has the limitations that the technical coefficient is assumed to be constant, the production function is assumed to be linear, and it is only applicable to static analysis. The third type of common methods for assessing the impact of the pandemic is the econometric model. Using econometric models, Aruga et al. [26] examined the impacts of COVID-19 on energy consumption in India, Shaikh [27] revealed the effects of the COVID-19 on energy markets, and Iqbal et al. [28] assessed the impacts of the pandemic on energy consumption and carbon emissions. The econometric model can reflect the historical trend of the economy and the schedule of economic impact, but it is constrained by the nature of past economic relations and cannot predict possible changes in economic events or activities. In conclusion, since the COVID-19 shock is a sudden short-term shock, the input-output model that is relatively simple and more suitable for assessing shock bursts is more appropriate for this study.

From the emergence of COVID-19 in China, many researchers have begun to examine the domestic impact of the pandemic. Relevant studies mainly focus on the social and economic impacts of the pandemic on China, as well as the energy and environmental impacts. In terms of the social and economic impacts, Zhou et al. [29] and Hu et al. [10] evaluated the macroeconomic effects of COVID-19 on China using the CGE model, and found that the pandemic had heterogeneous impacts on industrial outputs, and the impact on the secondary industry was significantly greater than that on the tertiary industry. Taking a different approach, Duan et al. [30] adopted a quarterly CGE model to assess the economic impacts of COVID-19 on China at the national and industrial levels, and suggested that the service sector was most affected by the pandemic; Tan et al. [31] also found that firms and activities related to the service sector were most affected. Regarding the impacts of COVID-19 on energy and environment in China, related studies found that the pandemic is reducing energy consumption and pollutant emissions [9,32]. Specifically, the electricity demand [8,33] and oil demand [8] in China were found to be severely affected by the pandemic. However, Wang and Su [9] suggested that energy consumption and greenhouse gas emissions might exceed the prepandemic levels when China resumes large-scale industrial production. Furthermore, some scholars also focused on the changes in China's economy, energy and environment during the pandemic. For example, Xu et al. [34] examined the causal relationship between economic development and environmental quality during this public health crisis. Their results indicated that economic activities mainly caused environmental pollution and energy use through the COVID-19 shock in China. Jia et al. [35] also suggested that the decline of global carbon emissions caused by the pandemic was only due to economic recession.

As COVID-19 rapidly spread internationally, many scholars have also studied the impacts of the pandemic on the world, as a whole, and in other countries individually. Research on the global level focuses on the pandemic's impacts on the macroeconomic and microeconomic levels [17,36] as well as on the social economy [37], environment [38], and energy [39,40]. Related studies found that the pandemic hit the global economy significantly [17], caused huge losses of economic well-being and social capital [37], and also severely impacted energy and environmental sectors [39,40]. Some scholars have also examined the economic impacts of COVID-19 on a range of countries around the world. Salisu et al. [41] and Chudik et al. [42] found that the pandemic had negative effects on the economies of many countries to varying degrees, with more profound and lasting effects on developed economies than emerging economies. In addition, some scholars have conducted studies on some countries where the pandemic was more serious, and assessed the economic shocks of the pandemic on the United States [43,44], Britain [45], India [46,47], Australia [48], Italy [45] and Canada [49] as well as its impacts on energy demand and energy consumption in the United States [50], India [26] and Canada [51].

In summary, the methods for evaluating the pandemic's impacts used by most of the literature fail to describe in detail the changes in energy conversion chain under the shock, and fail to incorporate the interaction between energy and economy. Moreover, studies on the effects of COVID-19 on China usually examine only its economic or energy impacts. There remains a paucity of research on assessing comprehensively the impacts of the pandemic on economic growth, industry development, and energy flows. Therefore, we will construct an IEEIO model including the COVID-19 shock, and evaluate the impacts of the shock on China's economic growth and energy flows in the context of trade protectionism.

3. Methods

The IEEIO model was constructed by our research group [52]; it can be used to assess the impacts of external shocks on China's economy and energy. Due to space limitations, this paper will briefly introduce the basic IEEIO model and explain how to construct the IEEIO model including the COVID-19 shock.

3.1. Basic IEEIO Model

The IEEIO model is constructed by integrating the global multi-regional input-output (GMRIO) model and the global energy multi-regional supply and use (GEMRSU) model. The introduction of the GMRIO model and the GEMRSU model is shown in Appendix A. Then, we will introduce the IEEIO model.

The link between the GMRIO model and the GEMRSU model is established by the energy products use intensity matrix T of non-energy industries. By collation, the total outputs of energy products E can be expressed as:

$$E = L_E T L_n Y \cdot e + L_E H_E \cdot e \quad (1)$$

where L_E is the energy product total requirements matrix of energy industries. T refers to the energy products use intensity matrix of non-energy industries. L_n denotes the submatrix of Leontief inverse matrix L, $L = (I - A)^{-1}$, representing the total requirements matrix for non-energy products in each industry. Y is the final demand matrix. H_E denotes the final demand matrix of energy products for households and e refers to the summation vector consisting entirely of ones.

3.2. The IEEIO Model including the COVID-19 Shock

This paper constructs an IEEIO model including the COVID-19 shock to assess the pandemic's impacts on China's economy and energy in the context of trade protectionism. First, this paper incorporates the context of protectionism into models by changing the trade relations among regions. This is done by changing the data associated with trade, as described in more detail in Wang and Wu [52]. Then, as the pandemic weighs on both demand and supply, we incorporate the COVID-19 shock into economic model by changing the final demand structure and adding supply constraints in the optimization problem. The pandemic shock will be further transmitted from economic system to energy system through the IEEIO model.

The procedure for introducing the COVID-19 shock into models is as follows.

(1) Add supply constraints in the optimization problem to introduce the supply shock arising from COVID-19, change final demand structure s to introduce the demand shock, and solve the optimization problem including the impacts on obtaining the final demand Y (in monetary units) and the value added V (in monetary units) in the optimal solution;
(2) Estimate the total outputs of energy products E (in energy units) using the IEEIO model including the COVID-19 shock;
(3) Compare the value added V (in monetary units) and the total outputs of energy products E (in energy units) estimated in this scenario with those in the baseline scenarios including trade protectionism to obtain the pandemic's economic and energy impacts in the context of trade protectionism.

It is worth noting that since the IEEIO model is constructed based on the input-output model, it also suffers from that model's same limitations, which mainly include three aspects: first, the technical coefficient is assumed to be a constant; second, the production function is assumed to be linear; and third, this model is only applicable to static analysis. Next, we will describe the effects of these limitations on interpreting results. First, the assumption of the constant technical coefficient is relatively reasonable for the study in this paper. Since this paper aims to analyze the short-term effects of COVID-19 on China's economy and energy, technology could be assumed to be constant in the short term. Second, the assumption of the linear model does have a certain impact on the research of this paper. In fact, the pandemic's impacts on China's economy and energy might be nonlinear. However, it is difficult to capture these nonlinear impacts and to characterize them accurately. Therefore, to simplify the analysis, this paper simulates the shock of the pandemic based on the linear assumption, which is relatively reasonable and could provide a good benchmark for the evaluation of this shock. Finally, although the input-output model is only suitable for static analysis, it is feasible to use this model to evaluate the effects of the pandemic on China's economy and energy because the pandemic shock simulated in this paper is a sudden short-term shock.

4. Scenarios and Data

Based on the IEEIO model including the COVID-19 shock, this paper defines various scenarios to simulate and assess the pandemic's economic and energy impacts on China in the context of trade protectionism. In addition, the data for the COVID-19 pandemic is introduced in this section, while the data for the GMRIO table and GEMRSU table is shown in Appendix B. According to the number published by GTA of discriminatory trade restrictions implemented by countries against China, this paper divides countries covered by the World Input-Output Table (WIOT) into three trade regions: China; countries with many discriminatory trade restrictions against China (simply CTR hereafter, including the United States, India, Germany, Brazil, and Canada); and rest of the World (simply ROW hereafter).

4.1. Detailed Information about Incorporating the COVID-19 Pandemic into Models

The COVID-19 pandemic could be roughly divided into two waves based on its emergence and spread. The initial wave of the pandemic refers to the outbreak of COVID-19 in China (mainly in the first quarter of 2020), and the second wave is the global spread of COVID-19.

(1) The initial wave of the pandemic

The initial wave of the pandemic delivered a shock to China's economy. This paper introduces this shock into the economic model of supply and demand. On the supply side, the pandemic control measures reduce labor supply and disrupt transportation, thus lowering productivity. Therefore, we add supply constraints in the optimization problem shown in Appendix A.1 to introduce the supply shock arising from the domestic outbreak:

$$X_i^{CHN} \leq (1 - \alpha_i^{CHN}) X_i^{CHN,0} \qquad (2)$$

where X_i^{CHN} is the element of total outputs vector X, representing the output of industry i in China. $X_i^{CHN,0}$ refers to the baseline value of the output of industry i in China. α_i^{CHN} represents the productivity loss rate of industry i in China under domestic outbreak.

On the demand side, the pandemic not only decreases consumption of wholesale and retail, accommodation and food service, travel and other services, but also negatively affects investment. Since the pandemic shock on consumption and investment in China will cause changes in final demand structure, we introduce the demand shock arising from domestic outbreak by changing final demand structure in the optimization problem. The specific steps are as follows. First, estimate the decline rate of China's final demand for products of each trade region. Second, estimate final demand of each trade region. Finally, recalculate the final demand structure s under domestic outbreak.

(2) The second wave of the pandemic

The pandemic continues to spread across the world although the pandemic in China has been brought under control. CTR and ROW economies have been hit by the second wave of the pandemic; therefore, this paper introduces the impacts of the global spread of COVID-19 on these economies into the economic model through supply- and demand-side. On the supply side, the spread of the pandemic would have a direct negative impact on production activities in these two regions. We incorporate the supply shock arising from global spread of the pandemic on these regions by adding supply constraints in the optimization problem:

$$X_j^{CTR} \leq (1 - \alpha_j^{CTR})X_j^{CTR,0},\ X_k^{ROW} \leq (1 - \alpha_k^{ROW})X_k^{ROW,0} \quad (3)$$

where X_j^{CTR} and X_k^{ROW} refer to the elements of total outputs vector X, which represent the outputs of industry j in CTR and industry k in ROW, respectively. $X_j^{CTR,0}$ and $X_k^{ROW,0}$ are the baseline values of X_j^{CTR} and X_k^{ROW}. α_j^{CTR} and α_k^{ROW} represent the productivity loss rates of industry j in CTR and industry k in ROW, respectively.

On the demand side, global spread of the pandemic delivers a negative shock to consumption and investment in CTR and ROW. This is reflected in the optimization problem as the changes in final demand structure. Thus, we reestimate the final demand structure to introduce the demand shock arising from the spread of the pandemic on CTR and ROW into the economic model. The estimation steps of final demand structure under the spread of the outbreak are basically consistent with that under domestic outbreak.

4.2. Design of Scenarios

Since the purpose of this paper is to simulate and assess the impact of COVID-19 on China's economy and energy in the context of trade protectionism, we set the baseline scenarios to include the context of trade protectionism. In order to cope with the uncertainty of trade policies across regions, this paper sets up five baseline scenarios (baseline scenarios 1–5 in Figure 1) based on the extreme trade relations among regions that may be caused by trade protectionism.

Baseline scenarios

Baseline scenario 1		Demanders			Baseline scenario 2		Demanders			Baseline scenario 3		Demanders			Baseline scenario 4		Demanders			Baseline scenario 5		Demanders		
		CHN	CTR	ROW			CHN	CTR	ROW			CHN	CTR	ROW			CHN	CTR	ROW			CHN	CTR	ROW
Suppliers	CHN	=	−	−	Suppliers	CHN	=	−	=	Suppliers	CHN	+	−	=	Suppliers	CHN	+	−	=	Suppliers	CHN	=	−	=
	CTR	−	+	=		CTR	=	=	=		CTR	−	+	=		CTR	−	=	=		CTR	−	+	=
	ROW	=	=	=		ROW	=	+	=		ROW	=	=	=		ROW	=	+	=		ROW	+	=	=

The first stage

Scenario 1		Demanders			Scenario 2		Demanders			Scenario 3		Demanders			Scenario 4		Demanders			Scenario 5		Demanders		
		CHN	CTR	ROW			CHN	CTR	ROW			CHN	CTR	ROW			CHN	CTR	ROW			CHN	CTR	ROW
Suppliers	CHN	=	−	−	Suppliers	CHN	=	−	=	Suppliers	CHN	+	−	=	Suppliers	CHN	+	−	=	Suppliers	CHN	=	−	=
	CTR	−	+	=		CTR	=	=	=		CTR	−	+	=		CTR	−	=	=		CTR	−	+	=
	ROW	=	=	=		ROW	=	+	=		ROW	=	=	=		ROW	=	+	=		ROW	+	=	=
Note: The shock of the initial wave of the pandemic is introduced.					Note: The shock of the initial wave of the pandemic is introduced.					Note: The shock of the initial wave of the pandemic is introduced.					Note: The shock of the initial wave of the pandemic is introduced.					Note: The shock of the initial wave of the pandemic is introduced.				

Figure 1. Cont.

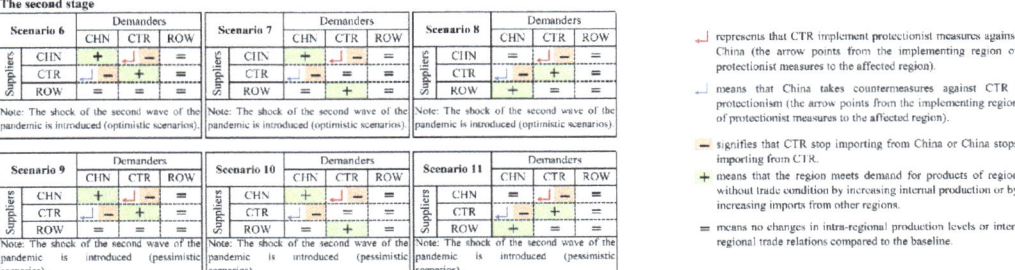

Figure 1. Design of baseline scenarios and scenarios for COVID-19.

Next, to facilitate the scenario analysis, we divide the shock of COVID-19 into two stages according to the development of the pandemic: the first stage is assumed to be the stage with the outbreak of COVID-19 in China, and the second stage is assumed to be the stage in which COVID-19 is controlled in China, but spreads globally. Then, we will introduce baseline scenarios and the scenarios designed at these two stages, as shown in Figure 1.

In terms of baseline scenarios, as shown in Figure 1, baseline scenarios 1 and 2 assume that CTR do not import from China and meet demand for China's products by increasing internal production (baseline scenario 1) or imports from ROW (baseline scenario 2). Baseline scenarios 3–5 assume that CTR do not import from China, while China does not import from CTR. Specifically, baseline scenario 3 assumes that CTR demand for China's products and China's demand for CTR products could be met by their own products; baseline scenario 4 assumes that CTR demand is met by ROW products and China's demand is met by domestic products; and baseline scenario 5 assumes that CTR demand is met by their own products and China's demand is met by ROW products.

At the first stage, China's domestic outbreak may exacerbate trade protectionism. This means that the actual trade relations among regions at this stage may be closer to the extreme trade relations in the baseline scenarios. Therefore, this paper introduces the shock of the initial wave of the pandemic into the five baseline scenarios and defines them as scenarios 1–5, as shown in Figure 1. The trade relations in scenarios 1–5 correspond to those in baseline scenarios 1–5, respectively. At the second stage, the global spread of COVID-19 may further aggravate global trade protectionism. This paper introduces the shock of the second wave of the pandemic into baseline scenarios 3–5, and sets optimistic scenarios (scenarios 6–8) and pessimistic scenarios (scenarios 9–11) considering the uncertainty of the spread of the pandemic, as presented in Figure 1. The trade relations in scenarios 6–8 and scenarios 9–11 correspond to those in baseline scenarios 3–5, respectively.

Overall, we set 11 scenarios to simulate the shock of COVID-19 in the context of trade protectionism. Scenarios 1–5 at the first stage and scenarios 6–11 at the second stage are used to simulate the impacts of the pandemic in China and the global spread of COVID-19 in the context of trade protectionism, respectively.

4.3. Data for the COVID-19 Pandemic

To introduce the demand and supply shocks arising from COVID-19 into the optimization problem, we calculated the productivity loss rates and the decline rates of final demand in China under the initial and second waves of the pandemic.

(1) Data for the initial wave of the pandemic

Due to the lack of information on the productivity loss of China's industries during the domestic outbreak of COVID-19, the productivity loss rates caused by the initial wave of the pandemic were estimated using the decline rates of value added of China's industries in the first quarter of 2020. Following Zhou et al. [29], this paper converted the productivity loss rates in the first quarter of 2020 to those in the full year based on the annual shares of industrial value added in the first quarter of 2019.

Furthermore, due to the paucity of data for final demand change of China's industries during the outbreak, the impacts of domestic outbreak on consumption in services and fixed asset investment were estimated by two indicators, i.e., the decline rates of total retail sales of consumer goods and fixed asset investment in the first quarter of 2020. First, using the annual shares of these two indicators in the first quarter of 2019, this paper converted the decline rates of consumption in services and fixed asset investment in the first quarter of 2020 to those in the full year. Then, based on these data for the full year, the decline rates of China's final demand caused by the initial wave of the pandemic were estimated using the weight of the shares of final consumption expenditure by households and gross fixed capital formation in final demand. The basic data can be obtained from the National Bureau of Statistics of China.

(2) Data for the second wave of the pandemic

The Global Economic Prospects (GEP) released by the World Bank Group in January 2021 and the World Economic Outlook (WEO) released by the International Monetary Fund in October 2020 reported the GDP growth rates of countries in 2020. This paper used these data to estimate the range of the productivity loss rates in CTR and ROW caused by the second wave of the pandemic. First, based on the GDP growth rates of countries in 2020 reported by GEP and WEO, the weighted GDP decline rates of CTR and ROW were calculated using the GDP of countries in 2019 as weights. Then, due to the lack of information on the impacts of the global spread of COVID-19 on specific industries in regions, the GDP decline rates of CTR and ROW were appropriately adjusted to represent the productivity loss rates of various industries in these regions, according to the industry characteristics and the different effects of the initial wave of the pandemic on China's industries. Finally, this paper sets optimistic scenarios and pessimistic scenarios under the second wave of the pandemic based on the range of the productivity loss rates of industries in CTR and ROW.

Moreover, due to the lack of data for final demand change of CTR and ROW during the spread of COVID-19, the growth rates of private consumption and fixed investment in emerging markets in 2020 reported by GEP were used to estimate the decline rates of final demand in CTR and ROW under the second wave of the pandemic. This paper used different data sources to calculate the decline rates of final demand in CTR and ROW because of the differences in countries covered by these two regions. Given the geographical location and the severity of outbreaks in countries covered by CTR, data for South Asia Region, Latin America and the Caribbean, Europe and Central Asia reported by GEP were used to estimate the impact of global spread of COVID-19 on CTR final demand. ROW consist of countries and regions in the world except for China and CTR. It should be noted that China, the main economy in East Asia and Pacific (EAP), has brought domestic outbreak under control while the pandemic continues to spread across the world, and China's investment and consumption are recovering gradually. Therefore, to avoid a disruption in China's demand recovery, this paper adopted data for emerging markets, except EAP, to estimate the impact of the global spread of COVID-19 on ROW demand.

5. Results and Discussion

Based on the scenarios and stages defined in the previous section, this paper analyzes the impacts of COVID-19 on China's economy and energy in the context of trade protectionism. The simulation results of scenarios 1–5 at the first stage are presented in Figures 2–5, showing the impacts of the COVID-19 outbreak in China in the context of trade protectionism. The results of scenarios 6–11 at the second stage are reported in Figures 6–9, which reflect the effects of global spread of COVID-19 in the same context.

5.1. The Impacts of the COVID-19 Outbreak in China on China's Economy and Energy in the Context of Trade Protectionism

At the first stage, the COVID-19 outbreak in China not only had a direct impact on China's economy and trade, but may also have prompted some countries to implement more trade restrictions. This paper sets scenarios 1–5 by introducing the shock of domestic outbreak into five baseline scenarios to assess the impacts of the outbreak on China's economic development and energy consumption in the context of trade protectionism.

5.1.1. The Impact of the COVID-19 Outbreak in China on GDP

Figure 2 presents the impact of the COVID-19 outbreak on China's economy in the context of trade protectionism. Overall, the simulation result indicates that domestic outbreak will involve a 2.20–3.09% decline in China's GDP relative to prepandemic levels. This finding is basically in line with those of previous studies such as Zhou et al. [29], who evaluated the macroeconomic effects of COVID-19 based on the CGE model and found that the pandemic would lead to a 1.43% drop in China's GDP. In a similar study, Hu et al. [10] suggested that China's GDP would fall by 1.27% under the optimistic scenario and by 2.07% under the pessimistic scenario during the pandemic. By contrast, the decline in GDP under the pandemic estimated in this paper is slightly higher than that estimated by Zhou et al. [29]. The main reason for this might be that the different settings of coefficients in the CGE model may lead to differences in the simulation results. For example, there are obvious differences in the estimates of impacts of the pandemic under the optimistic scenario and pessimistic scenario estimated by Hu et al. [10], and our estimates are much closer to their estimates in the pessimistic scenario. In short, the estimation results of these studies could, to some extent, support the credibility of the results of this study.

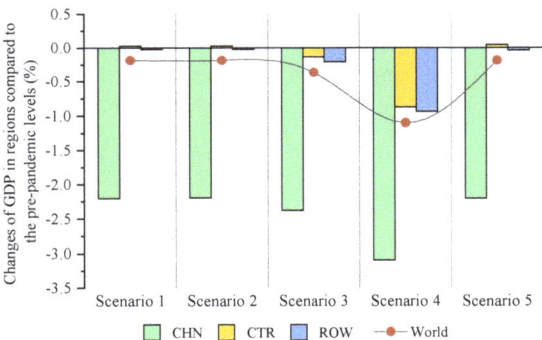

Figure 2. The impact of the COVID-19 outbreak in China on GDP in trade regions in the context of trade protectionism.

Furthermore, the COVID-19 outbreak in China may also affect the economic development in CTR and ROW in the context of trade protectionism. As shown in Figure 2, under scenarios 1, 2 and 5, economic growth in these two regions will be less affected by the outbreak, with GDP changing by less than 0.1%. In contrast, the outbreak in China will deliver a relatively large economic shock to CTR and ROW in scenarios 3 and 4. Under these scenarios, the channel of the outbreak's economic impact ROW might be that the pandemic would cause severe economic losses in China, resulting in a contraction in its import demand for ROW. This would further negatively affect ROW economies. The negative shock of the outbreak to CTR may be due to the fact that ROW economic losses would indirectly affect CTR through trade between these two regions. Based on the above analysis, the possible explanations for the phenomenon that economic growth in CTR and ROW will be less affected by the outbreak under scenarios 1, 2 and 5 are as follows: Since ROW economies would be impacted by the pandemic through the trade between China and ROW, the magnitude of ROW economic losses depends largely on the magnitude of China's economic losses. Under scenarios 1, 2 and 5, China's economic losses were significantly less than those under scenarios 3 and 4, which might explain the smaller economic losses in ROW under these scenarios. Similarly, the impact of the pandemic on CTR is realized by affecting the trade between CTR and ROW. Under scenarios 1, 2 and 5, ROW will be less affected by the pandemic, meaning that trade between CTR and ROW is relatively stable under these scenarios. This is the reason why the outbreak in China would have a smaller impact on CTR under these three scenarios. Globally, the COVID-19 outbreak in China will lead to a decline in global GDP under scenarios 1–5. This suggests that in the context of the integration of the global economy, the outbreak in China would not only negatively affect China's economy, but also generate adverse spillovers for other economies and the world.

5.1.2. The Impact of the COVID-19 Outbreak in China on Industrial Value Added

As can be seen from Figure 3, in the context of trade protectionism, China's industries will be negatively affected by this domestic outbreak, albeit in varying degrees. Of these industries, construction, non-metallic mineral products, wood and wood products, and services will suffer greater output losses, the decline rate in value added relative to them will average 1.29% higher than that of other industries. More concretely, in a scenario with the largest impact from COVID-19 on China's economy (scenario 4), the value added of these four industries will fall by 4.77%, 4.15%, 3.63%, and 3.30%, respectively, relative to prepandemic levels; in a scenario with smaller impact from COVID-19 (scenario 2), the value added relative to them will decline by 3.89%, 3.28%, 2.75%, and 2.41%, respectively, compared to prepandemic levels. The reasons why these four industries would be greatly affected by the outbreak are as follows. First, as a labor-intensive industry, construction is vulnerable to production shutdowns, production delays, and labor shortages, together with the shortage of inputs and with transportation difficulties, making it the severely affected industry during the domestic outbreak. Second, non-metallic mineral products and wood and wood products, the upstream industries of construction and other industries, would be not only directly impacted by the pandemic, but also negatively affected by the output declines and investment weakness in their downstream industries. Third, the outbreak would sharply curb consumption of traditional services such as accommodation, food service, and tourism, but have little influence on emerging services such as financial services, and even drive the development of online services. The overall effect of the outbreak on services is negative as traditional services accounted for a larger proportion.

Figure 3 also shows the impacts of the COVID-19 outbreak in China on industry development in CTR and ROW. Since industry outputs in these two regions will be less affected by the COVID-19 outbreak under scenarios 1, 2, and 5, this paper analyses and discusses the impacts of the outbreak on industries based on the simulation results of scenarios 3 and 4. As can be seen from the graph above, mining and quarrying and manufacture of metals in ROW will be more negatively impacted by the outbreak. According to the WIOT 2014, ROW exports of these two industries accounted for 17.18% and 13.72% of the corresponding industry outputs, and their exports to China accounted for 44.84% and 42.42% of total exports of corresponding industries, respectively. It means that mining and quarrying and manufacture of metals are the main export industries in ROW, and China is the main export destination for these two industries. The COVID-19 outbreak in China would cause output losses in China's industries, resulting in a contraction in its import demand for ROW products. This might be the main reason why these two industries in ROW would be greatly affected by the outbreak. In addition, the value added of CTR industries will decline to varying degrees in scenarios 3 and 4. This phenomenon indicates that even though these scenarios assume that trade between CTR and China stops, and CTR are not directly impacted by the outbreak in China, they would be indirectly affected through trade with ROW.

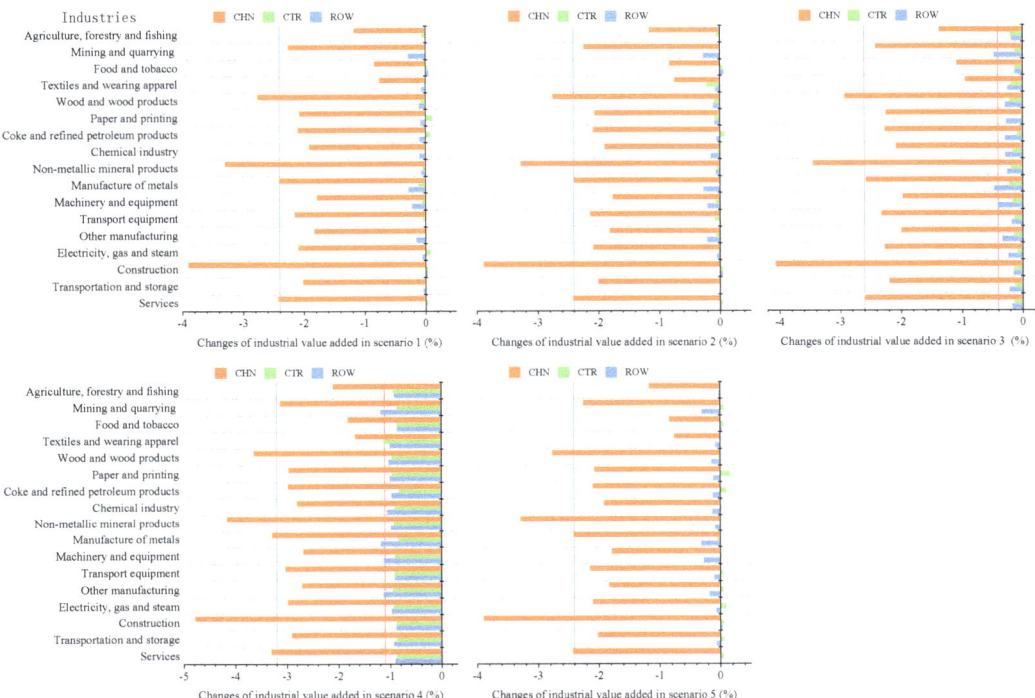

Figure 3. The impact of the COVID-19 outbreak in China on industrial value added in trade regions in the context of trade protectionism.

5.1.3. The Impact of the COVID-19 Outbreak in China on Total Energy Consumption

Figure 4 shows that under scenarios 1–5, the domestic COVID-19 outbreak will cause a 1.56–2.48% drop in China's total energy consumption in the context of trade protectionism, relative to prepandemic levels. This result may be explained by the fact that the COVID-19 shock could be transmitted from economic system to energy system through the interaction between economy and energy. After the pandemic hit, China adopted control measures such as shutdowns or delays of production and restrictions on transport. These measures delivered a significantly negative shock to economic activities, thus resulting in a substantial decline in domestic demand for energy products. The outbreak impact under scenario 4 would have the most severely adverse effect on China's total energy consumption. This scenario's simulation results, in Section 5.1.1, suggest that the outbreak would lead to large economic losses in China. This is the reason why there is a big drop in China's total energy consumption under this scenario. Furthermore, the simulation results show that the decline in China's GDP caused by domestic outbreak is slightly higher than that in its total energy consumption. The possible explanations for this are as follows: The production in some energy-intensive industries is related to the stability of people's livelihood and the control and prevention of the pandemic. Furthermore, since energy demand in these industries is less affected by the outbreak, and human life has a rigid demand for energy products, the drop in energy consumption is less than that in GDP.

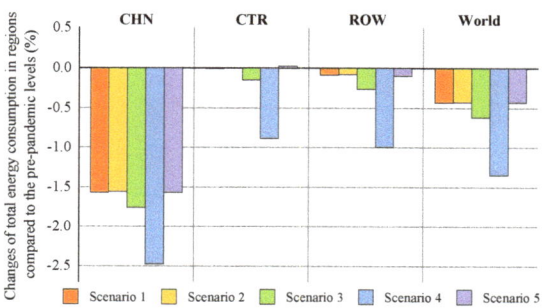

Figure 4. The impact of the COVID-19 outbreak in China on total energy consumption in trade regions in the context of trade protectionism.

As illustrated in Figure 4, the changes of total energy consumption in CTR and ROW are less than 0.1% under scenarios 1, 2, and 5. Thus, this paper analyses the impact of the COVID-19 outbreak in China on their energy consumption based on the simulation results of scenarios 3 and 4. The results show that relative to prepandemic levels, the total energy consumption in CTR will fall by 0.15% and 0.89% in scenarios 3 and 4, respectively, and will decline, in ROW, by 0.27% and 1% under these two scenarios, respectively. There are two main reasons for the decline in ROW total energy consumption caused by China's domestic outbreak. First, industry outputs in ROW would shrink due to the negative spillovers from the outbreak, which reduces their energy consumption as well. Second, the pandemic would cause a decline in China's energy demand, with a contraction in its import demand for ROW energy products such as coal, oil, and natural gas. This would further steepen the drop in ROW energy consumption. Moreover, a major reason for the decline in CTR energy consumption is that industry outputs in CTR would be indirectly affected by the outbreak in China, thus resulting in a reduction in their energy demand. For the world, the simulation results suggest that the outbreak in China will involve a 0.43–1.35% decline in global energy consumption relative to prepandemic levels.

5.1.4. The Impact of the COVID-19 Outbreak in China on Consumption of Energy Products

The simulation result of the domestic impact of the COVID-19 outbreak on China's fossil energy and non-fossil energy consumption in the context of trade protectionism is presented in Figure 5. As can be seen from this figure, the COVID-19 outbreak will deliver a significantly negative shock to China's fossil energy consumption, reducing it by 1.69–2.6% relative to prepandemic levels. In contrast, non-fossil energy consumption would be less impacted by the outbreak, with a 0.26–1.18% decline compared to prepandemic levels, a decline rate 1.44% lower than fossil energy consumption on average. There may be two reasons for this phenomenon. Firstly, the outbreak would affect China's energy consumption mainly by hitting energy demand in energy-intensive industries such as the chemical industry, non-metallic mineral products, and manufacture of metals. Energy consumption of these energy-intensive industries is dominated by fossil fuels such as coal. Therefore, fossil energy consumption is more sensitive to the COVID-19 shock than non-fossil energy consumption. Secondly, China has provided a series of support policies for power generation from renewables to promote its development. These policies could offset to some extent the adverse effects from the pandemic on non-fossil energy demand. In addition, the finding that fossil energy consumption would be more affected by the outbreak is basically consistent with that of the Annual Report on China's Energy Development 2019. The report shows that the pandemic would lead to a decline in China's fossil energy consumption such as coal and oil, while non-fossil energy consumption would continue to grow, with a drop in growth rate. However, the result in this paper indicates that the outbreak would also hit China's non-fossil energy consumption, which differs from the estimates in the report. Non-fossil energy is mainly used for power generation, heating, and biofuel production. It could be inferred that there are two reasons for the decline in non-fossil energy consumption: first, the outbreak would cause a fall in China's electricity demand, thereby reducing the consumption of non-fossil fuels used for power generation; second, transportation would be hard hit by the pandemic, thus lowering the demand for biofuels.

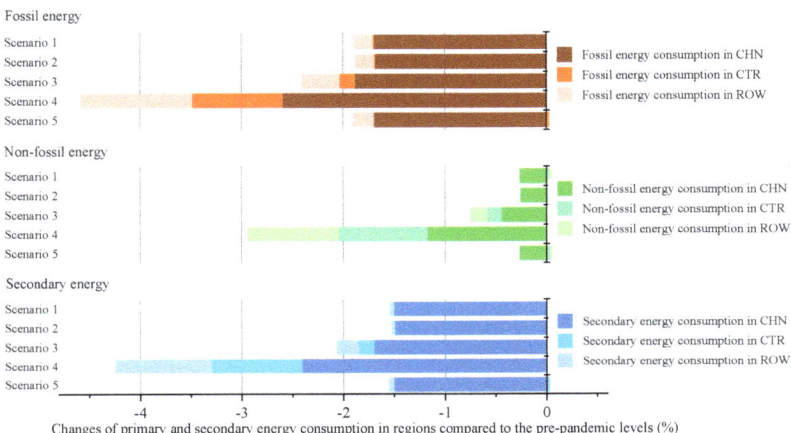

Figure 5. The impact of the COVID-19 outbreak in China on primary and secondary energy consumption in trade regions in the context of trade protectionism.

Figure 5 also shows the impacts of the COVID-19 outbreak in China on fossil energy and non-fossil energy consumption in CTR and ROW in the context of trade protectionism. The simulation results show that under scenario 3, fossil energy and non-fossil energy consumption in CTR will decline by 0.15% and 0.14%, respectively, relative to prepandemic levels, and those in ROW will drop by 0.36% and 0.16%, respectively. Under scenario 4, those in CTR will fall by 0.89% and 0.87%, respectively, and those in ROW will decline by 1.09% and 0.90%, respectively. These results suggest that fossil energy consumption in both CTR and ROW would be slightly more impacted by the outbreak in China than non-fossil energy consumption, which is in agreement with the simulation result for China's energy consumption. According to the WIOT, the shares of fossil energy in primary energy consumption in CTR and ROW were 92% and 89% in 2014, respectively. BP's Statistical Review of World Energy 2020 reports that fossil energy still accounted for 84 % of global primary energy consumption in 2019. This could explain the phenomenon that fossil energy consumption in these regions would be greatly affected by the outbreak in China.

5.2. The Impacts of Global Spread of COVID-19 on China's Economy and Energy in the Context of Trade Protectionism

At the second stage, COVID-19 continues to spread across the world, although in China the spread has been brought under control. This may aggravate global trade protectionism. With the deepening of China's embedding in global value chains, the global spread of COVID-19 (simply global pandemic spread hereafter) and increased trade protectionism would have direct or indirect impacts on China's economy and energy. By introducing the shock of the pandemic on CTR and ROW into baseline scenarios 3–5, this paper sets optimistic scenarios (scenarios 6–8) and pessimistic scenarios (scenarios 9–11) to evaluate the impacts of the global pandemic spread on China's economic development and energy consumption in the context of trade protectionism.

5.2.1. The Impact of Global Pandemic Spread on GDP

Figure 6 shows the impact of global pandemic spread on China's economy in the context of trade protectionism. As can be seen from this figure, global pandemic spread will reduce China's GDP by 2.27–3.18% under the optimistic scenarios (scenarios 6–8) and by 2.46–3.28% under the pessimistic scenarios (scenarios 9–11), compared with prepandemic levels. This means that although China has effectively brought domestic outbreak under control, the global pandemic spread would also generate adverse spillovers for China's economy. The possible explanations for this phenomenon are as follows: Data from the National Bureau of Statistics of China show a high degree of China's dependence on foreign trade, which was close to 32% in 2019. This implies that China is highly dependent on international markets and its growth is vulnerable to economic fluctuations in other economies. It could be inferred that global pandemic spread would cause cross-border spillovers to China through a negative impact on demand and supply in other economies. Concretely, first, the degree of export dependence in China is generally higher than that of import dependence, meaning that the negative spillover impacts of the pandemic on China come mainly from the demand side. Global pandemic spread would cause economic contractions in many countries, resulting in a decline in their demand for China's products. This demand shock, together with disruptions to trade and transportation caused by pandemic-control measures, would deal a significant blow to China's exports. Second, global pandemic spread would also negatively affect China's economy through supply channels. In fact, some raw materials and crucial components needed by China's manufacturing industry are highly dependent on imports. The pandemic spread would disrupt the production and supply of these products, thus leading to further output losses in the manufacturing industry. Moreover, it is found that the impact of global pandemic spread on China's economy is slightly larger than that of the outbreak in China. COVID-19 rapidly struck the world in early 2020, the outbreaks in many countries were worse than that in China, which would lead to the economic recession in China's major trading partners and in turn hit China significantly. This might be the main reason why global pandemic spread would deliver a larger economic shock to China than domestic outbreak.

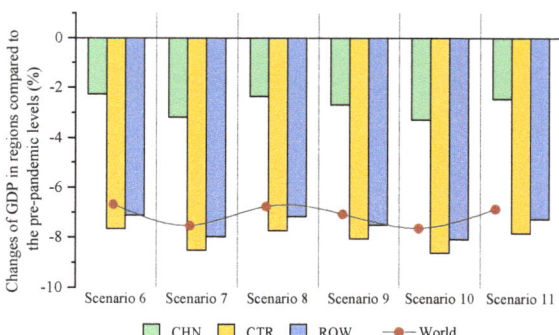

Figure 6. The impact of global pandemic spread on GDP in trade regions in the context of trade protectionism.

Figure 6 indicates that global pandemic spread will reduce CTR GDP by 7.66–8.61% and ROW GDP by 7.13–8.08%, relative to prepandemic levels. By contrast, the declines in GDP of these two regions at this stage are roughly three times as steep as that of China's GDP at the first stage. This implies that the adverse economic impacts of global pandemic spread on CTR and ROW are much larger than that of the domestic outbreak in China. This might be related to the severity of the outbreaks in different regions. In addition, the simulation results show that economic growth in CTR would be slightly more affected by global pandemic spread than that in ROW. The possible explanation for this is that CTR contain some countries with larger outbreaks, such as the United States, India, and Brazil, which were the three countries with the largest cumulative confirmed cases of COVID-19 as of 15 December 2020, according to real-time data of COVID-19. For the world, relative to prepandemic levels, global pandemic spread will involve a 6.66–7.62% decline in global GDP in the context of trade protectionism. This suggests that the pandemic would cause a deep global recession.

5.2.2. The Impact of Global Pandemic Spread on Industrial Value Added

As shown in Figure 7, China's industries will be negatively impacted by global pandemic spread in varying degrees in the context of trade protectionism. Of these industries, textiles and wearing apparel, machinery and equipment, and other manufacturing will suffer greater output losses, the decline rate in value added of them would be on average 1.23% higher than that of other industries. According to the analysis in Section 5.2.1, global pandemic spread would impact China's economy mainly by hitting export demand. Therefore, China's export-oriented industries such as textiles and wearing apparel, machinery and equipment, and other manufacturing will be significantly affected by the pandemic spread. Specifically, in the optimistic scenarios (scenarios 6–8), the value added of textiles and wearing apparel will fall by 3.82–4.75% relative to prepandemic levels, that of machinery and equipment by 3.30–4.21%, and that of other manufacturing by 3.48–4.39%; in the pessimistic scenarios (scenarios 9–11), the value added of these three industries will decline by 3.93–4.85%, 3.56–4.32%, and 3.66–4.49%, respectively, compared with prepandemic levels. The simulation results in Section 5.1.2 suggest that the COVID-19 outbreak in China will have the most severely negative impact on its construction, non-metallic mineral products, wood and wood products, and services. It is observed that industries more affected by global pandemic spread differ from those more affected by the domestic outbreak. This phenomenon might be explained as follows: At the first stage, domestic outbreak hit China's economy through the supply and demand side. Thus, construction and manufacturing that are vulnerable to shutdowns and restricted labor supply, together with services that are vulnerable to consumption reduction, would suffer greater output losses caused by the outbreak. While at the second stage, the pandemic spread would generate negative spillovers for China's economy mainly through demand-side channels, which delivers a significantly negative shock to its exports. This is the reason why export-oriented industries such as textiles and wearing apparel, and machinery and equipment would be more impacted by global pandemic spread.

Figure 7 shows that there are also differences in the impacts of global pandemic spread on various industries in CTR and ROW. In terms of CTR, construction, non-metallic mineral products, and services will be more negatively impacted by global pandemic spread, and the value added of them will fall by 7.71–8.65%, 7.75–8.70%, and 7.69–8.63%, respectively, relative to prepandemic levels. While for ROW, construction, textiles and wearing apparel, and services will be more affected by global pandemic spread, their value added will drop by 7.26–8.20%, 7.23–8.22%, and 7.19–8.15% compared to prepandemic levels, respectively. As can be seen, industries more affected by global pandemic spread in these regions are construction, manufacturing, and services, which are basically in line with industries in China more affected by domestic outbreak. This result may be explained by the fact that the basic characteristics of industries could determine to some extent the degree of the pandemic's impacts on them. For example, construction, a labor-intensive industry, is vulnerable to shutdown and labor shortages, so construction in these three regions would be subject to severely adverse impacts; lockdowns and quarantines to slow the spread of the pandemic would dampen consumption of offline services such as accommodation and food service, making it the directly affected industry during the pandemic.

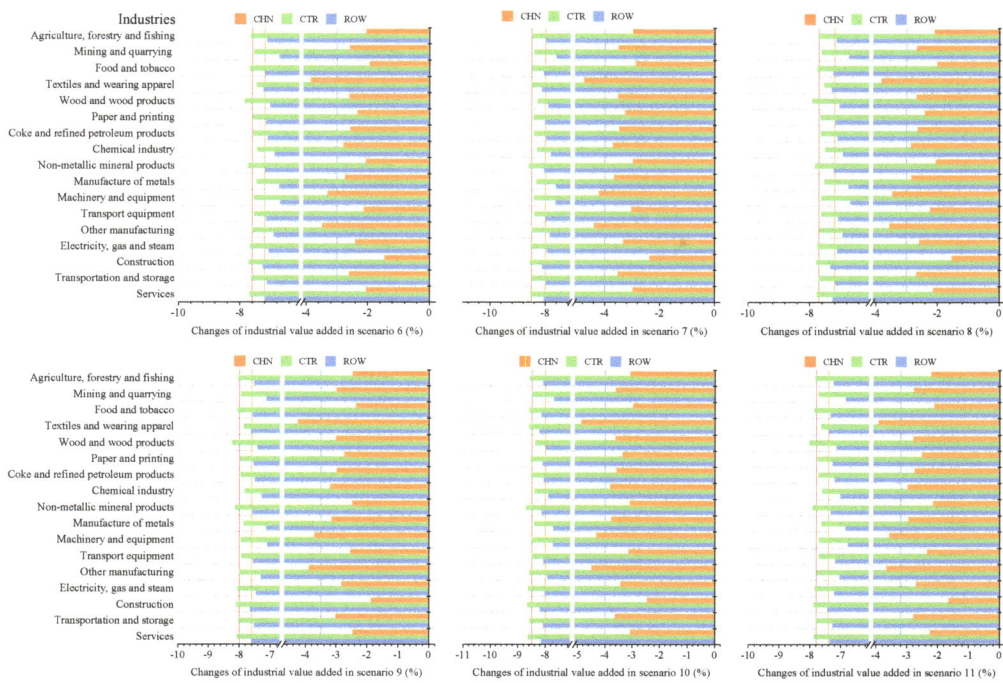

Figure 7. The impact of global pandemic spread on industrial value added in trade regions in the context of trade protectionism.

5.2.3. The Impact of Global Pandemic Spread on Total Energy Consumption

The simulation result of the impact of global pandemic spread on China's total energy consumption in the context of trade protectionism is presented in Figure 8. From this figure we can see that global pandemic spread will reduce total energy consumption in China by 2.48–3.39% under the optimistic scenarios (scenarios 6–8) and by 2.68–3.49% under the pessimistic scenarios (scenarios 9–11), relative to pre-pandemic levels. These results indicate that global pandemic spread would deliver a significantly negative shock to China's energy consumption. There may be two reasons for this. In the first place, the negative spillover impacts of the pandemic spread will lead to a decline in export demand for China's manufacturing industries, such as textiles and wearing apparel, and machinery and equipment. This would have a significant negative impact on manufacturing industries, resulting in a reduction in their energy demand. Secondly, according to the World Economic Survey (WES) database in 2014 and the China Statistical Yearbook in 2018, China exported energy products such as coke, kerosene, gasoline and diesel to some countries covered by ROW. ROW would suffer large economic losses from global pandemic spread. This would cause a contraction in ROW energy demand, thereby reducing their import demand for China's energy products as well. To some degree, the above analysis could be supported by data from the CCS, which shows a decline in China's exports of some energy products during the pandemic. For example, the cumulative amount of China's exports of coke fell by 57% in 2020.

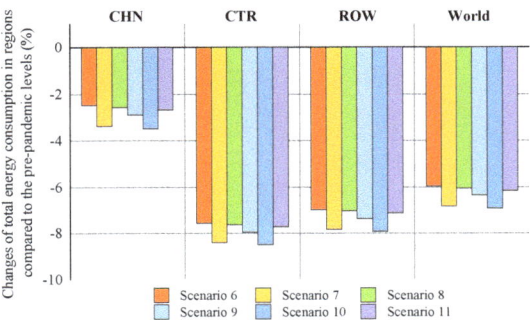

Figure 8. The impact of global pandemic spread on total energy consumption in trade regions in the context of trade protectionism.

Figure 8 also presents the impact of global pandemic spread on energy consumption in CTR and ROW. Under scenarios 6–11, CTR total energy consumption will fall by 7.56–8.5% relative to pre-pandemic levels, and ROW by 6.98–7.93%. Global pandemic spread may affect ROW' energy consumption through multiple channels. First, the pandemic spread would have a direct negative impact on outputs in ROW, resulting in a large drop in their energy consumption. Second, CTR would be also directly affected by the pandemic, with a decline in outputs, thereby leading to a severe contraction in their import demand for ROW energy products such as coal, oil, and natural gas. Third, China's energy demand would shrink due to the negative spillovers of the pandemic spread, which reduces its demand for ROW energy products. Unlike ROW, there may be two channels for the pandemic's impact on CTR energy consumption. The first is that the direct impact of the pandemic on CTR would cause a sharp decline in their energy demand, thus reducing the total energy consumption. On the other hand, energy demand contraction in ROW caused by global pandemic spread would reduce their import demand for CTR energy products such as oil and biofuels. For the world, relative to prepandemic levels, global pandemic spread will lead to a 5.96–6.93% reduction in global energy consumption in the context of trade protectionism.

5.2.4. The Impact of Global Pandemic Spread on Consumption of Energy Products

As can be seen from Figure 9, in the context of trade protectionism, China's fossil energy and non-fossil energy consumption will be affected by the global pandemic spread in varying degrees. The simulation result shows that relative to prepandemic levels, fossil energy consumption in China will decline by 2.49–3.4% under the optimistic scenarios (scenarios 6–8) and by 2.69–3.51% under the pessimistic scenarios (scenarios 9–11), while non-fossil energy consumption will drop by 1.56–2.47% under the optimistic scenarios and by 1.75–2.57% under the pessimistic scenarios. It implies that China's fossil energy consumption is more sensitive to the shock of the pandemic spread; its decline rate would be 0.93% higher than non-fossil energy consumption on average. Three reasons might account for this. First, the energy consumption structure dominated by fossil energy could explain to some extent why fossil energy consumption would be more affected by the pandemic. Second, China's support policies for renewables could help offset the negative impact of the pandemic on non-fossil energy demand. These two reasons are the same as the reasons why fossil energy consumption would be more impacted by domestic outbreak at the first stage. In addition, the third reason is that the pandemic spread would cause a contraction in ROW import demand for China's energy products. The WES database in 2014 shows that China exported coke, natural gas and other fossil fuels to some countries covered by ROW. This means that weak external demand may lead to a decline in fossil energy consumption in China, but may not hit non-fossil energy consumption. In addition, this phenomenon is basically consistent with the characteristics of the impact of the outbreak in China on China's primary energy consumption.

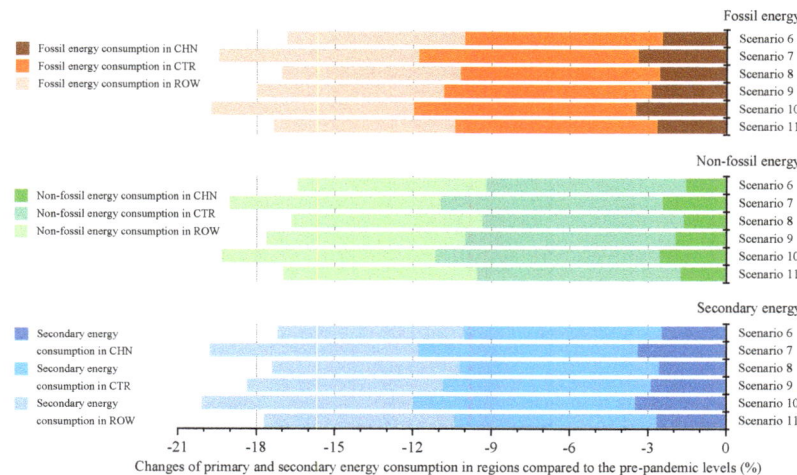

Figure 9. The impact of global pandemic spread on primary and secondary energy consumption in trade regions in the context of trade protectionism.

The simulation results show that global pandemic spread will affect fossil energy and non-fossil energy consumption in CTR and ROW. Overall, CTR fossil energy consumption will fall by 7.55–8.5% and ROW by 6.76–7.73%, while CTR non-fossil energy consumption will drop by 7.65–8.59% and ROW by 7.19–8.15%, compared with prepandemic levels. The World Energy Outlook 2020 released by the IEA suggests that global oil consumption was expected to decline by 8% and coal consumption by 7% in 2020. This could, to some degree, support the credibility of the declines, in these two regions, of fossil energy consumption estimated in this paper. Furthermore, the possible explanations for the phenomenon that non-fossil energy consumption in CTR and ROW would be more affected by the pandemic are as follows. On the one hand, according to the WES database in 2014, biomass accounted for more than 90% of renewable energy consumption in CTR and ROW. On the other hand, global pandemic spread may lead to a drop in biomass use for two reasons. First, the pandemic would cause interruptions or delivery delays of biomass power projects, resulting in a reduction in biomass use. Second, lower transport fuel demand caused by the pandemic, together with weaker competitiveness of biofuels due to a lowering of fossil fuel prices [53], would reduce the demand for transport biofuels, thereby leading to a decline in biomass use. Put differently, a high share of biomass in non-fossil energy consumption and a large impact of the pandemic on biomass use could explain the drop in non-fossil energy consumption in these two regions.

6. Conclusions and Policy Implications

This paper constructs an integrated economic and energy input-output model that includes the COVID-19 shock, and simulates and assesses the impacts of the pandemic on China's economy and energy in the context of trade protectionism. The principal conclusions of this paper are as follows: Overall, the simulation results indicate that in the context of trade protectionism, domestic outbreak will lead to a 2.20–3.09% decline in China's GDP, while global pandemic spread will cause a 2.27–3.28% drop in its GDP, compared to prepandemic levels. China's industries will be negatively affected by two waves of the pandemic in varying degrees. Domestic outbreak would deliver a relatively large shock to construction, non-metallic mineral products, wood and wood products, and services, while global pandemic spread would have a larger negative impact on China's textiles and wearing apparel, machinery and equipment, and other manufacturing.

Meanwhile, relative to prepandemic levels, the outbreak in China will reduce China's total energy consumption by 1.56–2.48%, while global pandemic spread will cut that by

2.48–3.49%. For primary energy, these two waves of the pandemic would have a larger negative effect on China's fossil energy consumption and a smaller effect on non-fossil energy consumption, with the effect on the former averaging 1.44% and 0.93% higher than the latter, respectively.

Based on these findings, the following policy implications can be obtained in this paper.

Firstly, China should pay more attention to problems in industry development exposed during the pandemic to promote the transformation and upgrading of traditional industries, and achieve high-quality development. The simulation results show that China's industries with a low degree of digitalization, such as construction, traditional manufacturing, and services, will suffer greater output losses from the domestic COVID-19 outbreak. In contrast, industries with a high degree of digitalization such as e-commerce may be less affected by the outbreak. This reveals the problem of the lower degree of digitalization in some traditional industries. Hence, the outbreak should be considered as an opportunity to promote the transformation of traditional industries and accelerate the realization of high-quality development. One is to further increase the application of digital technology and intelligent construction technology in the construction industry, and propel the transformation of this industry in the direction of digital and intelligent aspects. The second is to comprehensively facilitate the deep integration of the internet, big data and artificial intelligence with the real economy, and promote the high-quality development of traditional manufacturing and services with automation, digitalization and intelligence.

Secondly, export-oriented industries in China should enhance their risk resistance and economic resilience to cope with the possible external demand shocks brought by the pandemic. This paper finds that since the global pandemic spread would impact China's economy mainly by hitting export demand, export-oriented industries such as textiles and wearing apparel, machinery and equipment, and other manufacturing will suffer greater output losses. Therefore, China's export-oriented industries should take active measures to cope with the external demand shock. On the one hand, export-oriented industries should increase R&D investment in high-end industries, improve industrial chain structure, and enhance China's position in the global industrial chain. On the one hand, export-oriented industries could enhance their anti-risk capability by developing diversified export markets.

Thirdly, China should attach great importance to energy challenges posed by the pandemic, prevent risks relating to energy security, and ensure the stability and security of energy systems. The simulation results indicate that the pandemic would have a significant negative impact on fossil energy consumption, which might trigger a fall in global oil prices. As the second-largest oil consumer and the largest oil importer in the world, China would face challenges of energy security arising from the pandemic spread and the fall in global oil prices. In the first place, although lower oil prices would reduce China's oil import costs and operating costs of the economy, they might lead to a drop in investment in the oil sector and weaken the competitiveness of renewable energy, which is detrimental to oil production, development of renewable energy and energy security. In the second place, the oil market outlook is subject to significant uncertainty as the duration of the pandemic remains unknown. This may even cause shortfalls in oil supply, threatening the security of energy supply in China. Against this background, China can take the following measures to ensure energy security. First, the country should further increase strategic oil reserves to enhance its ability to address emergency risks in global oil markets. Second, it is important to expand domestic oil and gas demand and develop strong policy support for oil and gas companies. These measures could alleviate the adverse impact of the pandemic on China's oil sector and promote the secure and sustainable development of this sector. Third, vigorously developing renewables and reducing import dependence on fossil fuels could help to ensure energy security.

This study has the following limitations. Since the World Input-Output Table (WIOT) is only updated to 2014, this paper constructs the GMRIO model based on the WIOT

2014, and accordingly constructs the GEMRSU model based on the World Energy Statistics database in 2014. If the input-output data closer to the year of the COVID-19 outbreak can be used, the GMRIO model and the GEMRSU model could more precisely reflect the reality, which will more accurately describe the economic linkages and flow of energy products among various sectors in regions. This will better assess the impacts of the pandemic on China's economy and energy in the context of trade protectionism. With the continuous updating of data, the data closer to the year of the outbreak of COVID-19 should be used in further research.

Author Contributions: Conceptualization, F.W.; methodology, M.W.; software, M.W.; data curation, M.W.; writing—original draft preparation, M.W.; writing—review and editing, F.W.; visualization, M.W.; supervision, F.W.; project administration, F.W.; funding acquisition, F.W. All authors have read and agreed to the published version of the manuscript.

Funding: This research was funded by the National Natural Science Foundation of China [grant number 71673217] and the Research Project of Humanities and Social Sciences of the Ministry of Education of People's Republic of China in 2021: Research on the forced mechanism and economic impact of China's "carbon neutralization" target [grant number 21XJA790004].

Data Availability Statement: The data presented in this study are available on request from the corresponding author. The data are not publicly available due to some restrictions, and they are available on reasonable request.

Conflicts of Interest: The authors declare no conflict of interest.

Appendix A. The GMRIO Model and the GEMRSU Model

Appendix A.1. The GMRIO Model

The GMRIO model is constructed based on the World Input-Output Tables (WIOT), and the structure diagram of the GMRIO table is depicted in Figure A1.

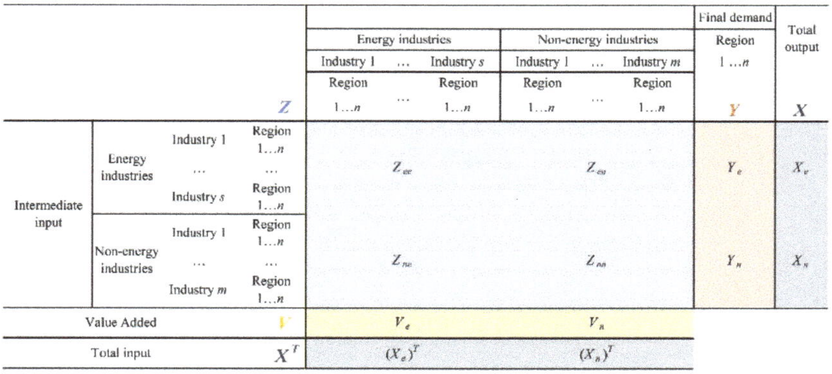

				Energy industries		Non-energy industries		Final demand	Total output
				Industry 1 ...	Industry s	Industry 1 ...	Industry m	Region 1...n	
				Region 1...n	Region 1...n	Region 1...n	Region 1...n		
			Z					Y	X
Intermediate input	Energy industries	Industry 1	Region 1...n	Z_{ee}		Z_{en}		Y_e	X_e
		Industry s	Region 1...n						
	Non-energy industries	Industry 1	Region 1...n	Z_{ne}		Z_{nn}		Y_n	X_n
		Industry m	Region 1...n						
Value Added			V	V_e		V_n			
Total input			X^T	$(X_e)^T$		$(X_n)^T$			

Figure A1. Structure diagram of the GMRIO table.

In Figure A1, matrix Z is the multiregional interindustry flows matrix, matrix V denotes the multiregional value added matrix, matrix Y refers to the multiregional final demand matrix, and column vector X is the total outputs vector. Next, we adopt the Leontief–Kantorovich model to find an optimal resource allocation. This could provide the basis for simulating the impacts of external shocks on China's economy and energy. The optimization problem could be described as follows: find an optimal resource allocation that could maximize final demand for a given level of primary resources, which can be expressed as

$$\begin{aligned} \text{Max } & y = e' \cdot Y \cdot e \\ s.t. \ & (I - A) \cdot X \geq y \cdot s \cdot e \\ & v \cdot X \leq V \cdot e \\ & X \geq 0 \\ & y \geq 0 \end{aligned} \quad (A1)$$

where, y represents the global final demand. Matrix A is the direct input coefficients matrix. Matrix s refers to the final demand structure matrix, $s = Y \cdot y^{-1}$. Matrix v denotes the input coefficients matrix of factors, $v = V \cdot (\hat{X})^{-1}$. e and e' refer to the summation vectors of appropriate dimension. The total outputs X under the conditions of optimal resource allocation could be obtained by solving the optimization problem. Then, the changes in the value added matrix V can be calculated by the equation $\Delta V = \Delta(v \cdot \hat{X})$ based on the changes in the total outputs X. Furthermore, this optimization problem only contains the primal resource allocation constraints. We will introduce other constraints according to the possible shock of COVID-19 to evaluate the pandemic's impacts. A more detailed description of this is provided in Section 4.

Appendix A.2. The GEMRSU Model

The physical GEMRSU table can be used to portray the energy conversion chain, and its structure diagram is shown in Figure A2.

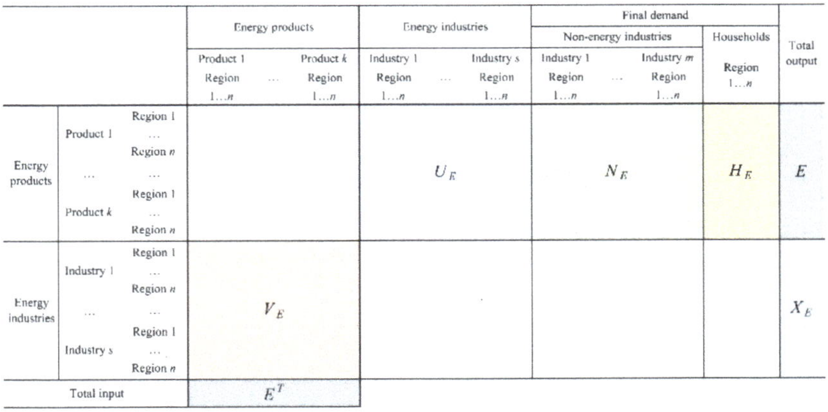

Figure A2. Structure diagram of the GEMRSU table.

In Figure A2, matrix U_E refers to the use matrix of energy products, matrix V_E denotes the make matrix of energy products, matrix N_E and H_E are the final demand matrices of energy products for non-energy industries and households, respectively. Column vector X_E is the total outputs vector of energy industries. Column vector E refers to the total outputs vector of energy products. By defining the total requirements matrix of energy products in energy industries L_E, the total outputs of energy products E can be written as:

$$E = L_E(N_E \cdot e + H_E \cdot e) \quad (A2)$$

where e is the summation vector of appropriate dimension.

Appendix B. Data for GMRIO Table and GEMRSU Table

GMRIO table is constructed using WIOT 2014, while GEMRSU table is constructed based on the World Energy Statistics (WES) database in 2014 released by the International

Energy Agency (IEA). The concrete data processing and model construction are described in Wang and Wu [52].

References

1. Wang, K.; Tong, J. The dynamic effect of trade protection barriers on export trade: Evidence from China's HS-6 ex-port products to the US. *Nankai Econ. Stud.* **2020**, *4*, 163–178. (In Chinese) [CrossRef]
2. Xu, H.; Chen, Y.X.; Ruan, C.Y. Quantitative analysis method on international market segmentation based on fuzzy clustering model. In Proceedings of the 2019 IEEE 4th International Conference on Cloud Computing and Big Data Analysis (ICCCBDA), Chengdu, China, 12–15 April 2019; IEEE: Piscataway, NJ, USA, 2019; pp. 327–332.
3. Evenett, S.; Fiorini, M.; Fritz, J.; Hoekman, B.; Lukaszuk, P.; Rocha, N.; Ruta, M.; Santi, F.; Shingal, A. Trade policy responses to the COVID-19 pandemic crisis: Evidence from a new data set. *World Econ.* **2021**, 1–23. [CrossRef]
4. Pinna, A.M.; Lodi, L. Trade and global value chains at the time of COVID-19. *Int. Spect.* **2021**, *56*, 92–110. [CrossRef]
5. Ouyang, Y.; Li, P. On the nexus of financial development, economic growth, and energy consumption in China: New perspective from a GMM panel VAR approach. *Energy Econ.* **2018**, *71*, 238–252. [CrossRef]
6. Shahbaz, M.; Zakaria, M.; Shahzad, S.J.H.; Mahalik, M.K. The energy consumption and economic growth nexus in top ten energy-consuming countries: Fresh evidence from using the quantile-on-quantile approach. *Energy Econ.* **2018**, *71*, 282–301. [CrossRef]
7. Smith, L.V.; Tarui, N.; Yamagata, T. Assessing the impact of COVID-19 on global fossil fuel consumption and CO_2 emissions. *Energy Econ.* **2021**, *97*, 105170. [CrossRef] [PubMed]
8. Norouzi, N.; Zarazua de Rubens, G.; Choupanpiesheh, S.; Enevoldsen, P. When pandemics impact economies and climate change: Exploring the impacts of COVID-19 on oil and electricity demand in China. *Energy Res. Soc. Sci* **2020**, *68*, 101654. [CrossRef]
9. Wang, Q.; Su, M. A preliminary assessment of the impact of COVID-19 on environment—A case study of China. *Sci. Total Environ.* **2020**, *728*, 138915. [CrossRef] [PubMed]
10. Hu, B.; Fan, Y.; Zheng, L. COVID-19, economic shock and government intervention. *J. Quant. Tech. Econ.* **2020**, *37*, 42–61. (In Chinese) [CrossRef]
11. Choi, S.Y. Industry volatility and economic uncertainty due to the COVID-19 pandemic: Evidence from wavelet coherence analysis. *Financ. Res. Lett.* **2020**, *37*, 101783. [CrossRef]
12. Janus, J. The COVID-19 shock and long-term interest rates in emerging market economies. *Financ. Res. Lett.* **2021**, *43*, 101976. [CrossRef] [PubMed]
13. Jiang, P.; Fan, Y.V.; Klemes, J.J. Impacts of COVID-19 on energy demand and consumption: Challenges, lessons and emerging opportunities. *Appl. Energy* **2021**, *285*, 116441. [CrossRef] [PubMed]
14. Brodeur, A.; Cook, N.; Wright, T. On the effects of COVID-19 safer-at-home policies on social distancing, car crashes and pollution. *J. Environ. Econ. Manag.* **2021**, *106*, 102427. [CrossRef] [PubMed]
15. Dang, H.-A.H.; Trinh, T.-A. Does the COVID-19 lockdown improve global air quality? New cross-national evidence on its unintended consequences. *J. Environ. Econ. Manag.* **2021**, *105*, 102401. [CrossRef]
16. Zhang, L.; Li, H.; Lee, W.-J.; Liao, H. COVID-19 and energy: Influence mechanisms and research methodologies. *Sustain. Prod. Consum.* **2021**, *27*, 2134–2152. [CrossRef]
17. McKibbin, W.; Fernando, R. The Global Macroeconomic Impacts of COVID-19: Seven Scenarios. *CAMA Cent. Appl. Macroecon. Anal.* **2021**, *20*, 1–30. [CrossRef]
18. Jawad, M.; Maroof, Z.; Naz, M. Impact of pandemic COVID-19 on global economies (a seven-scenario analysis). *MDE Manag. Decis. Econ.* **2021**, *42*, 1897–1908. [CrossRef]
19. Madai Boukar, A.; Mbock, O.; Kilolo, J.M.M. The impacts of the COVID-19 pandemic on employment in Cameroon: A general equilibrium analysis. *Afr. Dev. Rev.* **2021**, *33*, S88–S101. [CrossRef]
20. Shan, Y.; Ou, J.; Wang, D.; Zeng, Z.; Zhang, S.; Guan, D.; Hubacek, K. Impacts of COVID-19 and fiscal stimuli on global emissions and the Paris Agreement. *Nat. Clim. Chang.* **2021**, *11*, 200–206. [CrossRef]
21. Zhou, L.; Chen, Z. Are CGE models reliable for disaster impact analyses? *Econ. Syst. Res.* **2020**, *33*, 20–46. [CrossRef]
22. Sayan, S.; Alkan, A. A novel approach for measurement and decomposition of the economywide costs of shutting down tourism and related service sectors against COVID-19. *Tour. Econ.* **2021**, 1–18. [CrossRef]
23. Bonet-Morón, J.; Ricciulli-Marín, D.; Pérez-Valbuena, G.J.; Galvis-Aponte, L.A.; Haddad, E.A.; Araújo, I.F.; Perobelli, F.S. Regional economic impact of COVID-19 in Colombia: An input–output approach. *Reg. Sci. Policy Pract.* **2020**, *12*, 1123–1150. [CrossRef]
24. Huang, R.; Tian, L. CO_2 emissions inequality through the lens of developing countries. *Appl. Energy* **2021**, *281*, 116043. [CrossRef]
25. Munn, I.A.; Hussain, A.; Spurlock, S.; Henderson, J.E. Economic impact of fishing, hunting, and wildlife-Associated recreation expenditures on the Southeast U.S. regional economy: An input–output analysis. *Hum. Dimens. Wildl.* **2010**, *15*, 433–449. [CrossRef]
26. Aruga, K.; Islam, M.M.; Jannat, A. Effects of COVID-19 on Indian Energy Consumption. *Sustainability* **2020**, *12*, 5616. [CrossRef]
27. Shaikh, I. Impact of COVID-19 pandemic on the energy markets. *Econ. Chang. Restruct.* **2021**. [CrossRef]
28. Iqbal, S.; Bilal, A.R.; Nurunnabi, M.; Iqbal, W.; Alfakhri, Y.; Iqbal, N. It is time to control the worst: Testing COVID-19 outbreak, energy consumption and CO_2 emission. *Environ. Sci. Pollut. Res. Int.* **2021**, *28*, 19008–19020. [CrossRef]

29. Zhou, M.; Liu, Y.; Zhang, J.; Cui, Q. COVID-19 and its macroeconomic countermeasures in China: Impact and effectiveness. *J. Quant. Tech. Econ.* **2020**, *37*, 24–41. (In Chinese) [CrossRef]
30. Duan, H.; Bao, Q.; Tian, K.; Wang, S.; Yang, C.; Cai, Z. The hit of the novel coronavirus outbreak to China's economy. *China Econ. Rev.* **2021**, *67*, 101606. [CrossRef]
31. Tan, L.; Wu, X.; Guo, J.; Santibanez-Gonzalez, E.D.R. Assessing the Impacts of COVID-19 on the Industrial Sectors and Economy of China. *Risk Anal.* **2021**. [CrossRef] [PubMed]
32. Wang, K.; Wang, Y.W.; Chang, C.P. The impacts of COVID-19 pandemic on air pollution from energy consumption: Diverse evidence from China. *Int. J. Green Energy* **2021**. [CrossRef]
33. Wang, Q.; Li, S.; Jiang, F. Uncovering the impact of the COVID-19 pandemic on energy consumption: New insight from difference between pandemic-free scenario and actual electricity consumption in China. *J. Clean. Prod.* **2021**, *313*, 127897. [CrossRef]
34. Xu, S.; Liu, Q.; Lu, X. Shock effect of COVID-19 infection on environmental quality and economic development in China: Causal linkages (Health Economic Evaluation). *Environ. Dev. Sustain.* **2021**, 1–16. [CrossRef]
35. Jia, Z.; Wen, S.; Lin, B. The effects and reacts of COVID-19 pandemic and international oil price on energy, economy, and environment in China. *Appl. Energy* **2021**, *302*, 117612. [CrossRef]
36. Dube, K.; Nhamo, G.; Chikodzi, D. COVID-19 cripples global restaurant and hospitality industry. *Curr. Issues Tour.* **2021**, *24*, 1487–1490. [CrossRef]
37. Wei, X.L.; Li, L.J.; Zhang, F. The impact of the COVID-19 pandemic on socio-economic and sustainability. *Environ. Sci. Pollut. Res.* **2021**. [CrossRef] [PubMed]
38. Bherwani, H.; Nair, M.; Musugu, K.; Gautam, S.; Gupta, A.; Kapley, A.; Kumar, R. Valuation of air pollution externalities: Comparative assessment of economic damage and emission reduction under COVID-19 lockdown. *Air Qual. Atmos. Health* **2020**, *13*, 683–694. [CrossRef]
39. Mofijur, M.; Fattah, I.M.R.; Alam, M.A.; Islam, A.; Ong, H.C.; Rahman, S.M.A.; Najafi, G.; Ahmed, S.F.; Uddin, M.A.; Mahlia, T.M.I. Impact of COVID-19 on the social, economic, environmental and energy domains: Lessons learnt from a global pandemic. *Sustain. Prod. Consum.* **2021**, *26*, 343–359. [CrossRef]
40. Priya, S.S.; Cuce, E.; Sudhakar, K. A perspective of COVID 19 impact on global economy, energy and environment. *Int. J. Sustain. Eng.* **2021**, 1–16. [CrossRef]
41. Salisu, A.A.; Adediran, I.A.; Gupta, R. A note on the COVID-19 shock and real GDP in emerging economies. *Emerg. Mark. Financ. Trade* **2021**, 1–9. [CrossRef]
42. Chudik, A.; Mohaddes, K.; Pesaran, M.H.; Raissi, M.; Rebucci, A. A counterfactual economic analysis of COVID-19 using a threshold augmented multi-country model. *J. Int. Money Financ.* **2021**, *119*, 102477. [CrossRef] [PubMed]
43. Li, Z.Y.; Farmanesh, P.; Kirikkaleli, D.; Itani, R. A comparative analysis of COVID-19 and global financial crises: Evidence from US economy. *Econ. Res.-Ekon. Istraz.* **2021**, 1–15. [CrossRef]
44. Yousfi, M.; Ben Zaied, Y.; Ben Cheikh, N.; Ben Lahouel, B.; Bouzgarrou, H. Effects of the COVID-19 pandemic on the US stock market and uncertainty: A comparative assessment between the first and second waves. *Technol. Forecast. Soc. Chang.* **2021**, *167*, 120710. [CrossRef]
45. Su, C.W.; Dai, K.; Ullah, S.; Andlib, Z. COVID-19 pandemic and unemployment dynamics in European economies. *Econ. Res.-Ekon. Istraz.* **2021**, 1–13. [CrossRef]
46. Goswami, B.; Mandal, R.; Nath, H.K. COVID-19 pandemic and economic performances of the states in India. *Econ. Anal. Policy* **2021**, *69*, 461–479. [CrossRef]
47. Ramakumar, R.; Kanitkar, T. Impact of COVID-19 pandemic on the Indian economy: A critical analysis. *Investig. Econ.* **2021**, *80*, 3–32. [CrossRef]
48. Beck, M.J.; Hensher, D.A. Insights into the impact of COVID-19 on household travel and activities in Australia—The early days of easing restrictions. *Transp. Policy* **2020**, *99*, 95–119. [CrossRef] [PubMed]
49. Barichello, R. The COVID-19 pandemic: Anticipating its effects on Canada's agricultural trade. *Can. J. Agric. Econ.-Rev. Can. D Agroecon.* **2020**, *68*, 219–224. [CrossRef]
50. Ou, S.Q.; He, X.; Ji, W.Q.; Chen, W.; Sui, L.; Gan, Y.; Lu, Z.F.; Lin, Z.H.; Deng, S.L.; Przesmitzki, S.; et al. Machine learning model to project the impact of COVID-19 on US motor gasoline demand. *Nat. Energy* **2020**, *5*, 666–673. [CrossRef]
51. Rouleau, J.; Gosselin, L. Impacts of the COVID-19 lockdown on energy consumption in a Canadian social housing building. *Appl. Energy* **2021**, *287*, 116565. [CrossRef] [PubMed]
52. Wang, F.; Wu, M. How does trade policy uncertainty affect China's economy and energy? *Struct. Chang. Econ. Dyn.* under review.
53. IEA. *World Energy Outlook 2020*; IEA: Paris, France, 2020; Available online: https://www.iea.org/reports/world-energy-outlook-2020 (accessed on 25 November 2021).

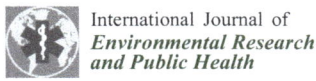

Article

COVID-19 Prevalence among Czech Dentists

Jan Schmidt [1], Vojtech Perina [2,*], Jana Treglerova [2], Nela Pilbauerova [1], Jakub Suchanek [1] and Roman Smucler [3]

1. Department of Dentistry, Charles University, Faculty of Medicine in Hradec Kralove and University Hospital Hradec Kralove, 500 05 Hradec Kralove, Czech Republic; Jan.Schmidt@lfhk.cuni.cz (J.S.); Nela.Pilbauerova@lfhk.cuni.cz (N.P.); SuchanekJ@lfhk.cuni.cz (J.S.)
2. Department of Oral and Maxillofacial Surgery, Masaryk University, Faculty of Medicine and University Hospital Brno, 625 00 Brno, Czech Republic; treglerova.jana@fnbrno.cz
3. Czech Dental Chamber, Slavojova 270/22, 128 00 Prague, Czech Republic; Smucler@dent.cz
* Correspondence: Perina.Vojtech@fnbrno.cz

Abstract: This work evaluates the prevalence of coronavirus disease (COVID-19), a viral infection caused by severe acute respiratory syndrome coronavirus 2 (SARS-CoV-2), among members of the Czech Dental Chamber. The assessment was based on an online questionnaire filled out by 2716 participants, representing 24.3% of all chamber members. Overall, 25.4% of the participants admitted they were diagnosed with COVID-19 by 30 June 2021, with no statistical differences between the sexes. While in the age groups under 50 the reported prevalence was around 30%, with increasing age, it gradually decreased to 15.2% in the group over 70 years. The work environment was identified as a place of contagion by 38.4% of the respondents. The total COVID-19 PCR-verified positivity was 13.9%, revealing a statistically lower prevalence ($p = 0.0180$) compared with the Czech general population, in which the COVID-19 PCR-verified positivity was ~15.6% (fourth highest rank in the world). The total infection–hospitalization ratio (IHR) was 2.8%, and the median age group of hospitalized individuals was 60–70 years. For respondents older than 60 years, the IHR was 8.7%, and for those under 40 years, it was 0%. Of the respondents, 37.7% admitted that another team member was diagnosed with COVID-19, of which the most frequently mentioned profession was a nurse/dental assistant (81.2%). The results indicate that although the dentist profession is associated with a high occupational risk of SARS-CoV-2 infection, well-chosen antiepidemic measures adopted by dental professionals may outweigh it.

Keywords: COVID-19; SARS-CoV-2; prevalence; dentistry; pandemic; dentist; occupational health; infection

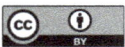

1. Introduction

Coronavirus disease (COVID-19) is a viral infection caused by the newly isolated severe acute respiratory syndrome coronavirus 2 (SARS-CoV-2). The standard clinical features are of a wide flulike spectrum, including fatigue, taste and smell loss, cough, headache, or fever. However, in some patients, it can lead to a more severe form, including breathing difficulties, respiratory failure, or acute inflammatory response, which could be fatal [1,2]. The rapid spread of SARS-CoV-2 is mainly due to the type of its transmission from person to person via respiratory droplets or mucosal contact or less often by contact with fomites [3–5]. The first official case of SARS-CoV-2 was reported in Wuhan City, Hubei Province, China, in December 2019 [6]. Due to its global spread, it soon became a worldwide health threat broadly affecting human society and leading the World Health Organization to classify COVID-19 as a pandemic disease as of 11 March 2020 [7].

The first cases of COVID-19 were recorded in the Czech Republic at the beginning of March 2020. The Czech government quickly issued a number of antiepidemic measures, which made the virus spread very limited. At the end of August 2020, the cumulative numbers of COVID-19 PCR-verified cases and total deaths per 100,000 people were 230 and 4, respectively [8,9]. However, since September 2020, the number of infected patients has risen sharply. During the autumn of 2020 and the spring of 2021, the Czech Republic was one of the countries most affected by COVID-19. As of the reference period of this study (i.e., 30 June 2021), the Czech Republic had 15,546 cumulatively PCR-verified infected per 100,000 people, which was the fourth highest number in the world [10]. On the same date, the number of total deaths related to COVID-19 per 100,000 people was 283, which was the fourth highest number in the world [11].

The transmission of SARS-CoV-2 is mainly via droplets, and in areas where there is a great fluctuation and accumulation of individuals, the spread of the disease is heightened. This also applies to medical facilities, making healthcare professionals vulnerable to COVID-19, with a special risk for those whose work is associated with mucus and saliva droplets. This is especially true for dental professionals. The dentist's work is associated with close contact with many people and producing a large amount of aerosol containing the patient's saliva and mucus droplets. Due to the high speed of dental rotary instruments, the aerosol swirls at a high speed to a distance of several meters from the source. Thus, the work environment of dentists is particularly risky, and dentists are one of the highly vulnerable groups [12].

During the COVID-19 pandemic, general healthcare was suppressed in the Czech Republic. However, a survey performed among members of the Czech Dental Chamber revealed that Czech dentists worked even throughout the pandemic [13]. During the spring of 2020, in the Czech Republic also called the "first wave" of COVID-19, more than 90% of the participating dentists replied that their practices were open. During the period from autumn 2020 to spring 2021, also called the "second wave" of COVID-19, more than 96% of them replied their practices remained open. From those who closed their practices during the period from March 2020 to March 2021, only less than 10% reported that the closure was longer than 4 weeks. The data showed that Czech dentistry remained very operational during the whole pandemic. This approach was rare on a European and global scale [13]. Such conditions make Czech dentists a unique study group to assess the impact of COVID-19 on dental professionals as it minimizes the bias resulting from their workplace.

Based on the combination of these three factors—high national prevalence, a significant risk of infection due to work settings, and high workload during pandemics—Czech dentists form a unique group with a presumption of high COVID-19 prevalence. At the same time, it could be assumed that dentists will be more affected by COVID-19 than the Czech general population due to the work environment. Furthermore, as Czech dentists remained more operative during the pandemic than their counterparts in other countries, it can be assumed that the regional impact of COVID-19 on this professional group was greater. However, these assumptions are hypotheses only and have not yet been addressed in any study.

On the other hand, Czech dentists were aware of these risks, and in order to maintain high operability, they adopted strict antiepidemic measures, such as an anamnestic questionnaire for each patient, regular testing of dental team members, planning a daily schedule to minimize patient accumulation in dental practices, rubber dam use, barrier precautions, minimizing aerosol spread, or establishing dental centers for the treatment of COVID-19-positive patients. These measures were aimed at minimizing the risk of transmission from patients to staff and vice versa, between staff, and between patients. The Czech Dental Chamber was one of the first dental chambers in Europe to issue antiepidemic recommendations for its members, and ordinary members of the chamber were also very proactive in this regard. These thorough measures could significantly reduce the risk of COVID-19 transmission in dental practices. However, so far, there are no data available to confirm this assumption.

To reflect the need to obtain statistically relevant quantifying data, the Czech Dental Chamber decided to conduct a survey among its members, the results of which are presented in this study.

The aim of this work is to assess the impact of COVID-19 on Czech dentists.

2. Materials and Methods

2.1. Design

This ad hoc, self-administered, cross-sectional, online survey was conducted by the Czech Dental Chamber and filled out by chamber members. All participants were informed about the purpose of the study, and none of them had a patient status. The questionnaire was anonymous; reported data did not include any identifying information that could be used to trace the participants and did not allow any association with the person answering. The participants were not rewarded with any direct benefits for participating in the survey. This study was conducted in accordance with the Declaration of Helsinki.

The presented data were obtained from the answers to 9 questions. Out of these questions, 8 were close-ended, and 1 was semi-close-ended (prefilled close-ended answers along with the option to reply in an open form). The whole questionnaire was in the Czech native language and was designed in collaboration with experts from the chamber, the academic community, and general practitioners.

A description of the questions, including the type and number of answers, is given in Table 1.

Table 1. Questions and their classification.

Question Mark	Question	Question Type	Number of Closed-Ended Answer Options	Answer Choice
Q1	Sex	Closed	2	Single
Q2	Age	Closed	6	Single
Q3	Were you diagnosed with COVID-19 by 30 June 2021?	Closed	3	Single
Q4	How was COVID-19 diagnosed?	Closed	8	Multiple
Q5	Where did the treatment take place?	Closed	5	Single
Q6	Do you know where you got infected?	Closed	3	Single
Q7	Where did the transmission of COVID-19 occur?	Semiclosed	6	Single
Q8	Was another member of the team diagnosed with COVID-19?	Closed	2	Single
Q9	Which team member was it?	Closed	5	Multiple

2.2. Sample

To address the members of the Czech Dental Chamber, invitations for participation in the survey were sent to all 9922 officially registered e-mail addresses in the chamber database. Each address represents one chamber member. The addressees were asked to fill out the questionnaire from 23 June to 4 September 2021. According to the Czech Dental Chamber 2020 Annual Report, the chamber had 11,160 members as of 31 December 2021 [14]. Thus, the survey addressed 88.9% of the chamber members. Membership in the Czech Dental Chamber is compulsory for all dentists working in the Czech Republic.

2.3. Sample Size Relevancy

Based on the total number of chamber members, the minimum relevant number of survey participants was set at 372. This quantification was assessed by the online Netquest calculator using Formula (1). For the calculation, a study universe of the members of the Czech Dental Chamber (N = 11,162), a margin of error of 5%, a confidence level of 95%, and a standard heterogeneity of 50% were used. As the sample size of this study (2716 participants) significantly exceeds the minimum required value ($n = 372$), the results are statistically relevant.

$$n = \frac{N \cdot Z^2 \cdot p \cdot (1-p)}{(N-1) \cdot e^2 + Z^2 \cdot p \cdot (1-p)} \quad (1)$$

Formula (1). Relevant sample size calculation. Sample size calculated (*n*), size of the universe (N), deviation from the mean value (Z), maximum margin of error tolerated (e), expected proportion (p).

2.4. Data Collection

The invitation to participate was sent by e-mail to 9922 officially registered e-mail addresses of the chamber members. The e-mail contained a link to an online questionnaire in Google Forms (Google, Mountain View, CA, USA). The compatibility of the questionnaire interface was not limited and included a mobile phone, desktop computer, laptop, or tablet with support for all the most used operating systems. The collected data were stored in the Google Forms cloud database and downloaded after the whole survey was completed.

2.5. Statistical Analysis

After the survey was completed, the results of all the questions were downloaded from the Google Forms cloud database. The results of close-ended questions (Q1–6, Q8, and Q9) were analyzed and presented as the percentage of individual answers within all the answers provided. Blank responses were not included in the total number of responses.

Responses to the semi-close-ended question (Q7) were analyzed individually. Each open-ended answer was evaluated independently by two authors (J.S. (Jan Schmidt), V.P.). Results disagreeing between the authors were resolved by a decision of the third author (J.T.). Open responses that were of similar meaning to closed responses were transferred to the appropriate closed response category. The remaining answers were put into new groups according to their meaning. Newly formed groups that exceeded the specified limit in frequency ($n = 5$) were presented as separate answers within the results. Answers that did not exceed this limit were classified in the "Others" category. Results were analyzed and presented as the percentage of individual answers within all answers provided. Blank responses were not included in the total number of responses.

To compare the COVID-19 prevalence between the Czech Dental Chamber members and the Czech general population, it was necessary to use the same methodology. The available COVID-19 prevalence rate within the Czech general population was based on PCR-confirmed cases and did not include cases diagnosed with clinical symptoms. As of the end of this survey, the COVID-19 cumulative cases among the Czech general population was 15,546 per 100,000 people [10]. In order to compare these values with the results of our study, only PCR-verified diagnoses were used.

The data were analyzed using custom Microsoft Office Excel formulas (version 2106 for Windows, Microsoft Corporation, Redmond, WA, USA) and GraphPad Prism (version 8.0.0 for Windows, GraphPad Software, San Diego, CA, USA). Chi-square with test Yates's correction was used for statistical analysis; * indicates $p < 0.05$.

3. Results

3.1. Response Rate

A total of 2716 respondents took part in the survey. Based on the 9922 e-mails sent, the response rate was 27.4%, representing 24.3% of all the chamber members ($n = 11,162$) (Figure 1).

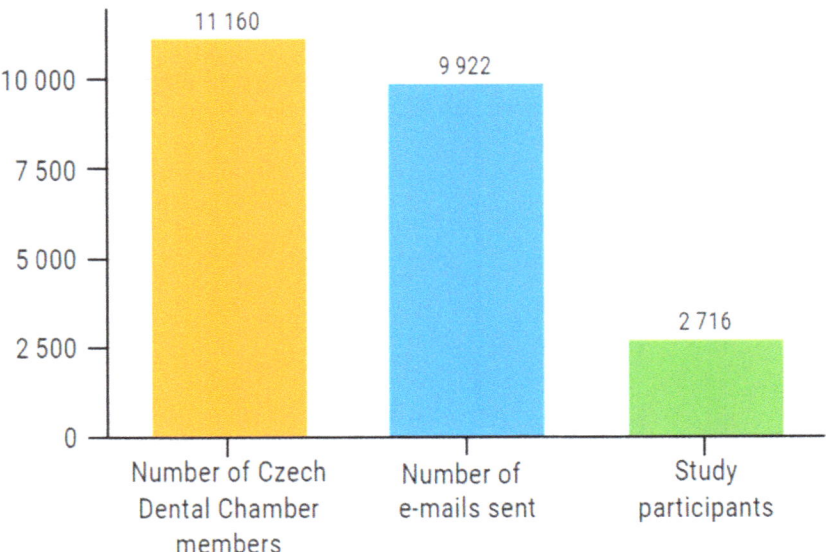

Figure 1. Response rate. The 2716 participants represent 27.4% of all the e-mail addresses included and 24.3% of the Czech Dental Chamber members.

3.2. Sex Distribution

A total of 2708 respondents stated their sex, and 8 skipped this question. A total of 1871 (68.9%) selected the female option, and 837 (30.8%) selected the male option (Figure 2), which also corresponds to the dominant representation of women among Czech dentists (64.9%) [14].

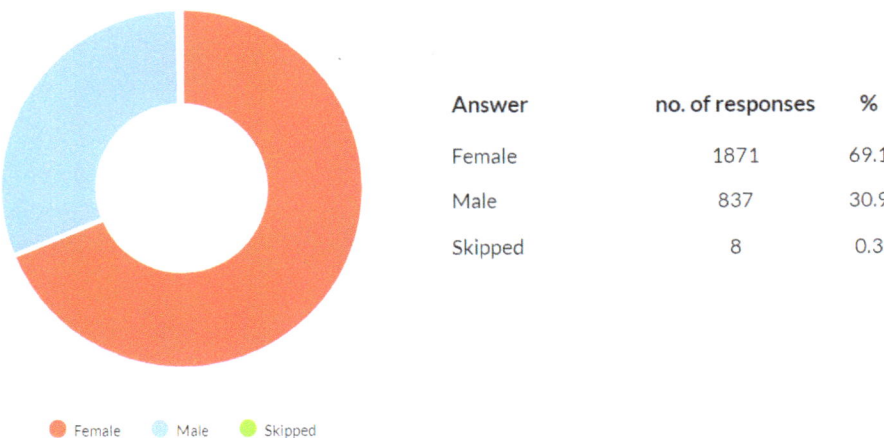

Figure 2. Sex distribution of the study participants.

3.3. Age Distribution

A total of 2712 respondents stated their age, and 4 skipped this question. The distribution is illustrated in Figure 3 and approximately corresponds to the age composition of the chamber members [14]. The median age group is 50–60 years.

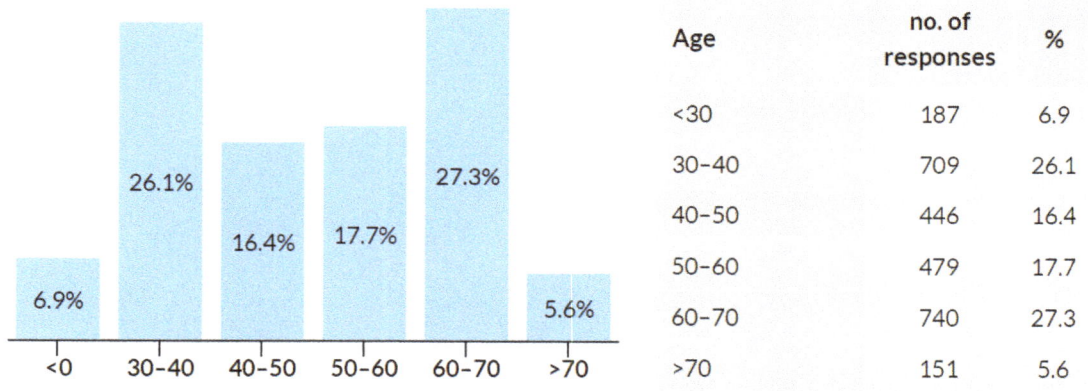

Age	no. of responses	%
<30	187	6.9
30–40	709	26.1
40–50	446	16.4
50–60	479	17.7
60–70	740	27.3
>70	151	5.6

Figure 3. Age distribution of the study participants.

3.4. COVID-19 Prevalence

3.4.1. COVID-19 Prevalence in the Whole Study Population

A total of 2716 respondents replied to this question. No respondent skipped this question. The results are presented in Figure 4. These data reveal that 691 (25.4%) respondents admitted they were diagnosed with COVID-19 by 30 June 2021.

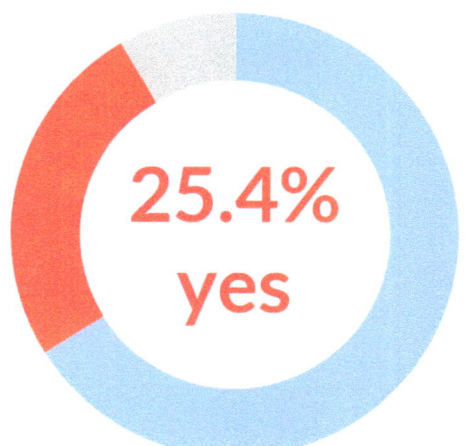

Answer	no. of responses	%
No	1793	66.0
Yes	643	23.7
Yes, only positive test	33	1.2
Yes, repeatedly	15	0.6
Did not know	232	8.5

Figure 4. COVID-19 positivity, the whole study population.

3.4.2. COVID-19 Prevalence Based on Sex

Sex-based COVID-19 prevalence is provided in Figure 5. Detailed data about the answers provided are available in the Supplementary Material.

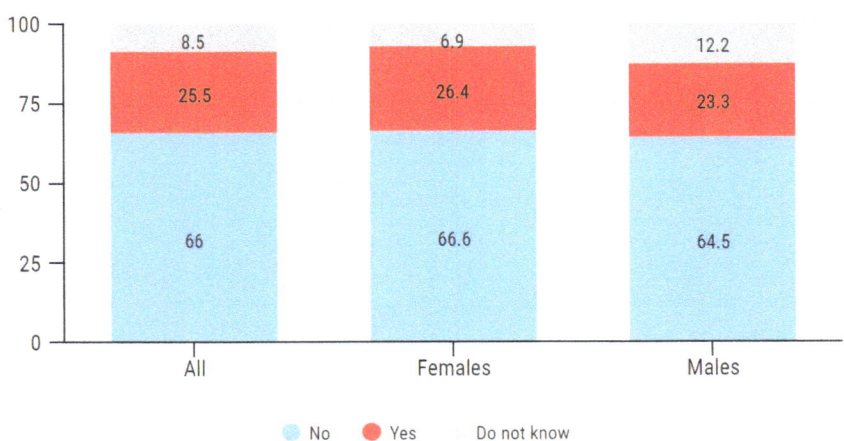

Figure 5. COVID-19 positivity, distribution by sex.

3.4.3. COVID-19 Prevalence Based on Age

Age-based COVID-19 prevalence is illustrated in Figure 6. Age- and sex-based COVID-19 prevalence is shown in Figure 7. Detailed data about the answers provided are available in the Supplementary Material.

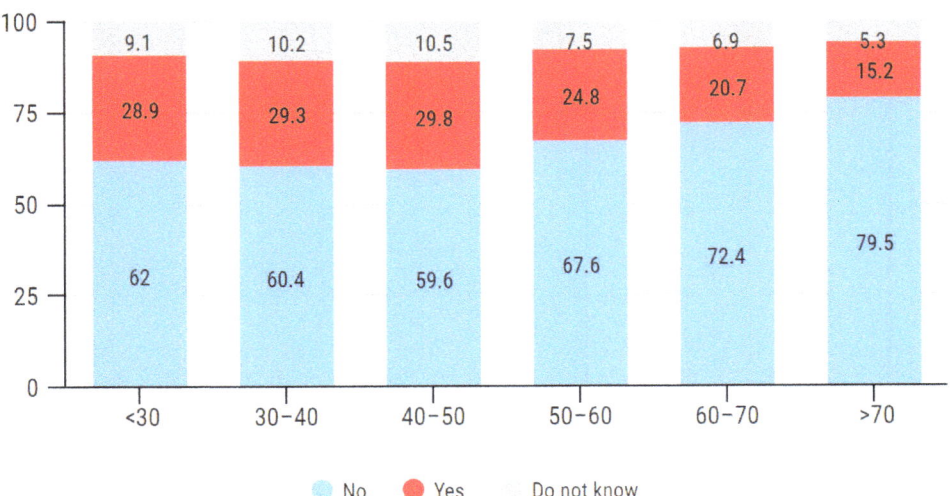

Figure 6. COVID-19 positivity, age distribution.

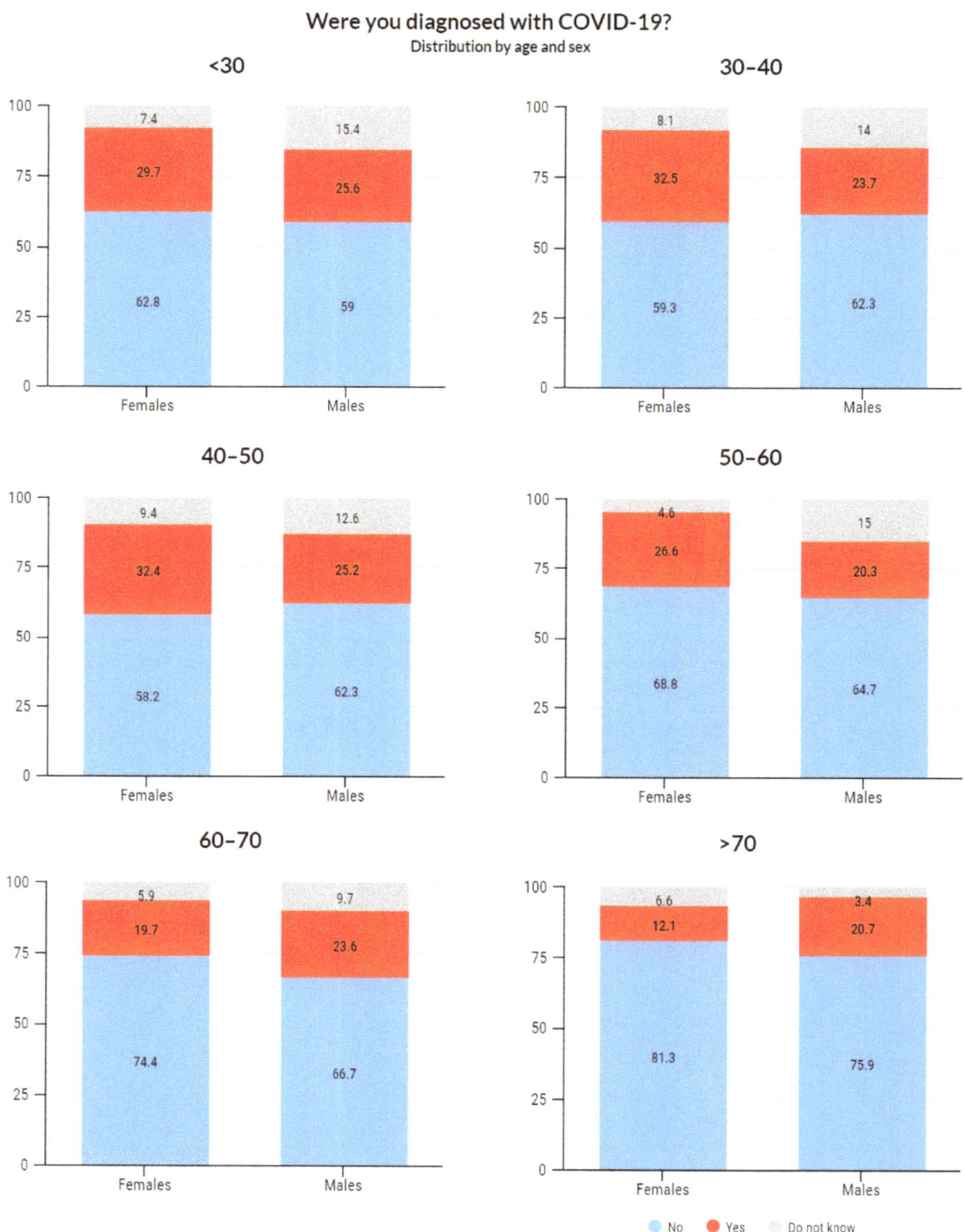

Figure 7. COVID-19 positivity, age and sex distribution.

3.5. COVID-19 Diagnostics

This question was addressed only to the respondents who confirmed they were diagnosed with COVID-19 in Q3 ($n = 691$). A total of 651 (94.2%) respondents reported 1328 answers to this multiple-choice question. The results are presented as a number of answers, percentage of respondents choosing this answer, and frequency of an answer among all answers in Figure 8.

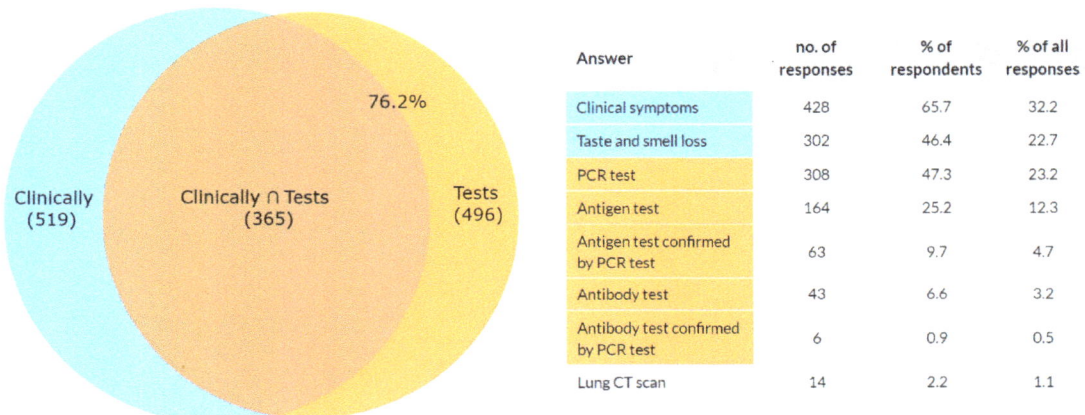

Figure 8. COVID-19 diagnostics.

There were a total of 520 respondents who chose to answer either "clinical symptoms" or "taste and smell loss". An answer containing some type of test was selected by 496 respondents. The intersection of these two groups was 365 respondents. In 76.2% of the respondents, the diagnosis of COVID-19 was confirmed by a test. In 23.7%, it was diagnosed solely on the basis of clinical symptoms. In 57.9%, the diagnosis was confirmed with a PCR test.

3.6. Comparison of COVID-19 Prevalence among the General Population in the Czech Republic

As of the end of this survey, the COVID-19 cumulative cases among the Czech general population was 15,546 per 100,000 people [10]. The PCR-verified prevalence within our study is 13.9%. Compared with the PCR-verified positivity in the general population, the difference is statistically significant ($p = 0.0180$) (Figure 9).

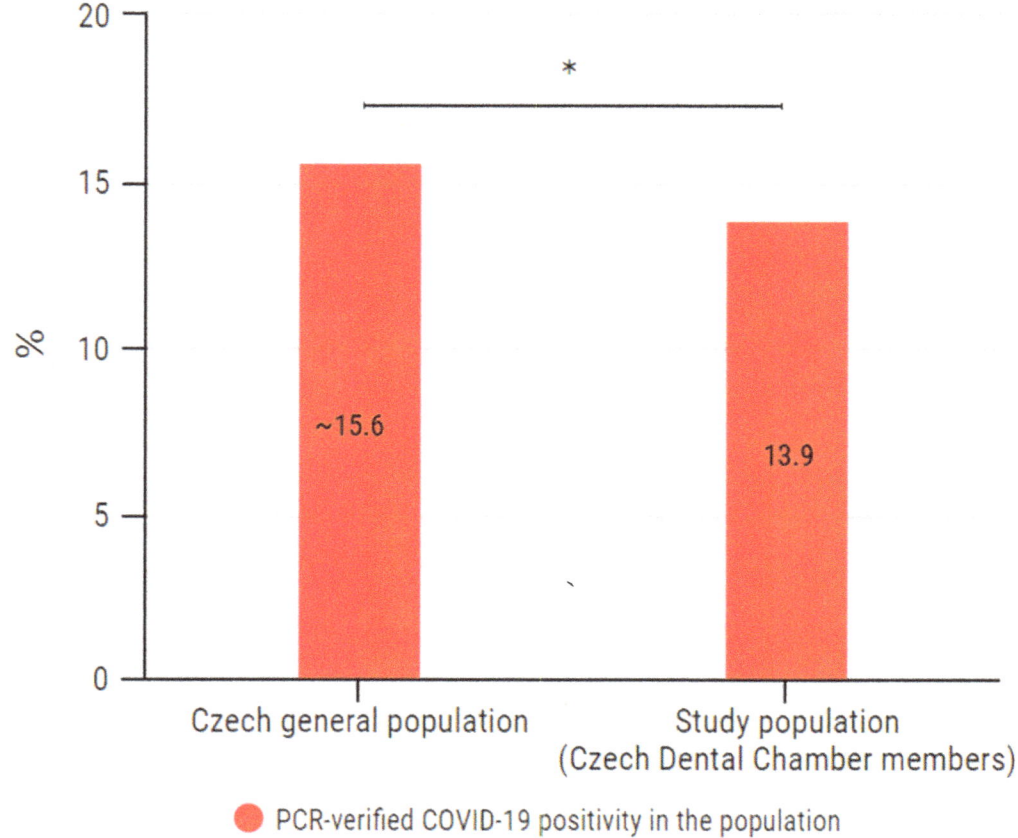

Figure 9. Comparison of COVID-19 prevalence in the Czech general population and its estimation within the population of Czech Dental Chamber members. Chi-square with test Yates's correction was used for statistical analysis; $p = 0.0180$. * indicates $p < 0.05$.

3.7. Place of Treatment

This question was addressed only to the respondents who confirmed they were infected with COVID-19 in Q3 ($n = 691$). A total of 646 (93.5%) respondents answered this question.

The vast majority of the participants (628, 97.2%) answered that they were being treated in the household. Only 2.8% of COVID-19 cases led to hospitalization (Figure 10). The median age group of those hospitalized was 60–70 years. In the group of respondents older than 60 years, the infection–hospitalization ratio (IHR) was 8.7%. On the other hand, none of the hospitalized were under the age of 40; the IHR under the age of 40 was 0%.

Place of treatment

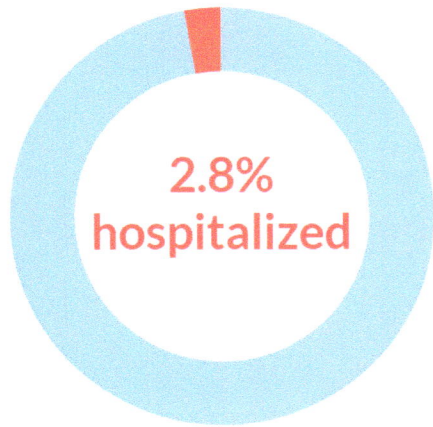

Answer	no. of responses	%
Household	628	97.2
Hospital, standard	5	0.8
Hospital, standard + O2	7	1.1
ICU	4	0.6
Artificial ventilation	2	0.3

Figure 10. Place of treatment.

3.8. Awareness of Where the Infection Occurred

This question was addressed only to the respondents who confirmed they were diagnosed with COVID-19 in Q3 (n = 691). Of them, 650 (94.1%) respondents answered this question. The results are provided in Figure 11.

Awarness of where the infection occurred

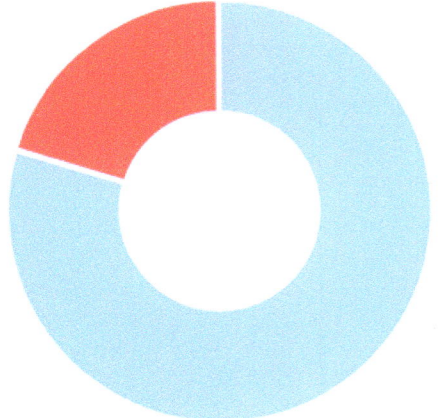

Answer	no. of responses	%
Yes	286	44.0
Probably yes	232	35.7
No	132	20.3

Figure 11. Awareness of where the infection occurred.

3.9. Environment Where the Infection Occurred

This question was addressed only to the respondents who reported that they knew or suspected where they were infected within Q8 (n = 518). Of them, 517 (99.8%) respondents answered this question.

These results show that 199 (38.4%) respondents identified the work environment as a source of infection. Together with the domestic environment (47.0%), these two categories were the dominant source of infection among respondents, jointly responsible for 85.5% of the reported transmission (Figure 12). Detailed data about the answers provided are available in the Supplementary Material.

Environment where the infection occurred

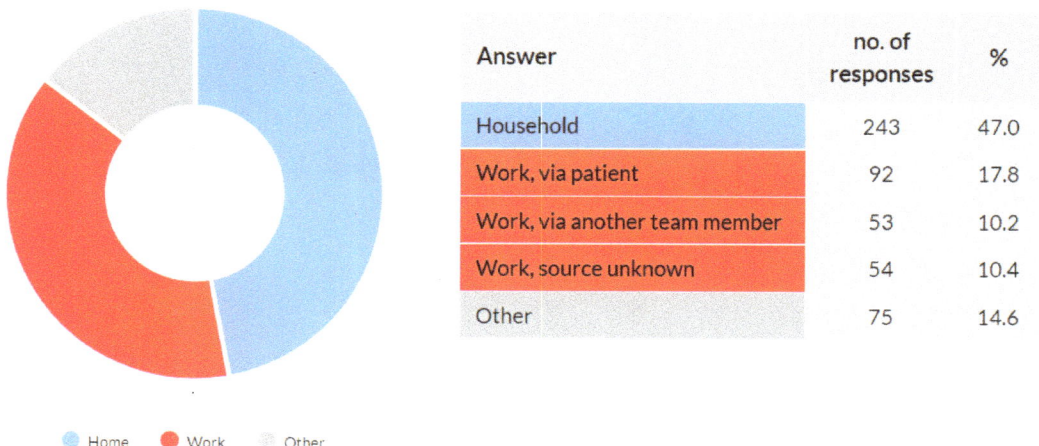

Figure 12. The environment where the infection occurred.

3.10. Prevalence of COVID-19 among Other Team Members

This question was addressed to all survey participants. Of them, 1683 (62.3%) replied that they were not aware of any other team member who was ill with COVID-19. A total of 1018 (37.7%) respondents admitted that another team member was ill with COVID-19.

Of the respondents who admitted they were diagnosed with COVID-19, 43.3% also reported another team member who was diagnosed as well, and 55.6% reported that no additional team member was diagnosed. Among those respondents who replied they were not diagnosed with COVID-19, 34.7% also reported another team member who was diagnosed with COVID-19, while 65% reported that no additional team member was diagnosed with COVID-19.

3.11. Profession Specification among Other Members of the Dental Team Infected with COVID-19

Those who reported an additional team member diagnosed with COVID-19 in the previous question (a total of 1018 participants, 37.7%) were asked to specify the profession of the infected individual. Of them, 990 (97.3%) replied, providing 1124 answers to this multiple-choice question. The results are presented as a number of answers, percentage of respondents choosing this answer, and frequency of an answer among all answers in Figure 13.

Profession specification among other members of the dental team infected with COVID-19

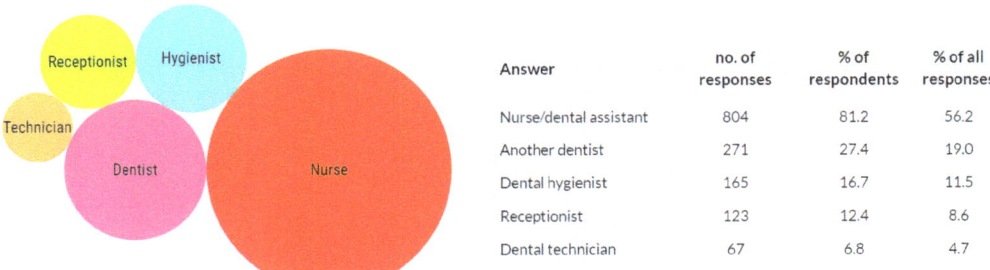

Answer	no. of responses	% of respondents	% of all responses
Nurse/dental assistant	804	81.2	56.2
Another dentist	271	27.4	19.0
Dental hygienist	165	16.7	11.5
Receptionist	123	12.4	8.6
Dental technician	67	6.8	4.7

Figure 13. Profession specification among other members of the dental team infected with COVID-19.

4. Study Limitations

There was one limitation that the authors had to address when planning this study and that they would like to discuss in this section. This limitation was not accidentally identified during the survey but was known to the authors before the research began. This chapter describes the limitation causes, possible approaches, and the approach by which the authors decided to address it.

The aim of the study is to describe the impact of COVID-19 on chamber members. In order to describe the prevalence of this disease among the respondents, it was necessary to establish diagnostic criteria. The authors considered whether these criteria would include only test-verified infections or whether they would be accepted together with diagnosis based on sole clinical symptoms.

Criteria based exclusively on tests would enhance the validity of the data. However, this method would lead to skewed results, as a large part of the Czech population was not tested and passed COVID-19 without test confirmation. At the time of the pandemic, test sites were overloaded due to the massive community-based virus spreading, and testing was unavailable to many patients. It is also important to note that one of the recommendations of the Ministry of Health of the Czech Republic was that people with COVID-19 should stay at home and be treated at home unless their condition is serious. The aim of this measure was to keep people with symptoms of COVID-19 in isolation and not to spread the infection just because of laboratory verification of the infection. Such a measure was medically correct but led to the real prevalence of COVID-19 among the population being significantly higher than the prevalence confirmed by the test.

We had two options to address this fact in determining the prevalence of COVID-19 among the study participants. One of them was to consider infected only those respondents in which positivity for COVID-19 was confirmed by a test. This option would lead to the acquisition of meticulous solid data but would significantly differ from the real prevalence. The second option was to accept the infection status regardless of the diagnostic method (i.e., both test-verified diagnosis and diagnosis based on clinical symptoms). This option would lead to less solid total data gain but would better correspond to the actual situation. In the end, we decided to obtain data combining the benefits of both of the abovementioned options.

In order to avoid skewing the results, we decided to include in the study both the group with the test-confirmed infection and the group diagnosed on the basis of clinical symptoms. To be able to distinguish these two groups in the results, the respondents were asked to indicate how COVID-19 was diagnosed, including sorting by the test used for diagnosis. Thanks to this procedure, the survey was as inclusive as possible, methodologically reflecting the epidemiological situation in the country and at the same time providing meticulous solid data. We consider this procedure to be appropriate, as it offers as much

5. Discussion

As there were no relevant quantitative data on the COVID-19 impact on Czech dentists, the Czech Dental Chamber decided to issue a survey among its members addressing their COVID-19 anamnesis. The data from this survey are presented in this study. Compared with studies with a similar focus and methodology, our work is one with the highest nationwide participation rates [15,16].

As mentioned in the Introduction, it was assumed that the prevalence of this disease would be high in this group. This assumption was confirmed as 25.4% of the respondents stated that they were diagnosed with COVID-19. Of the total reported positive cases among the respondents, the data show that the prevalence was 26.4% among females and 23.3% among males. An interesting phenomenon was observed across age groups. While in the age groups under 50 years, the prevalence was around 30%, with increasing age, it gradually decreased. In the group of 50–60 years, it was 24.8%, in the group of 60–70 years 20.7%, and in the group over 70 years 15.2%. These results may indicate that older members of the chamber acted with more caution. It is likely that they have reduced their workload and protected themselves more. Such behavior is only logical because there is a higher risk of fatal consequences in these age groups. Overall, the highest prevalence was recorded among women aged 30–40 and 40–50 years (32.5% and 32.4%, respectively), and the lowest among women between 60–70 years and above 70 years (19.7% and 12.1%, respectively). Additionally, a significant proportion (38.4%) stated that they were infected in the work environment.

The PCR-confirmed positivity within the population of this study was 13.9%. As of the end of this survey, the COVID-19 prevalence among the Czech general population was 15,546 cumulatively infected per 100,000 people (~15.6%) [10]. This comparison (15.6% and 13.9%) reveals that the prevalence among the respondents of this study was lower than in the general population. The difference is statistically significant ($p = 0.0180$). These outcomes suggest that although the dental profession is associated with a high occupational risk of droplet infection transmission, including SARS-CoV-19, the working conditions of dentists in the Czech Republic have not led to a higher prevalence of COVID-19 among them. Such results demonstrate that properly set working conditions focused on infection control led to a reduction in occupational infection risk.

For the majority of the respondents (97.2%), COVID-19 infection did not lead to hospitalization, and they were treated at home. However, 2.8% of the participants stated that their condition required hospitalization. This result is higher than the usual rate of COVID-19-related hospitalization. However, this may be influenced by the age composition of the respondents, as the condition for entering the chamber is a university degree in dentistry. According to Manochemi et al., the COVID-19 infection–hospitalization ratio (IHR) is 2.1% [17]. However, the IHR varies considerably across age groups, ranging from 0.4% for those younger than 40 years to 9.2% for those older than 60 years. In our study, the median age of the hospitalized individuals was 60–70 years. Among those older than 60 years, the infection–hospitalization ratio (IHR) was 8.7%. On the other hand, none of those hospitalized were under the age of 40; the IHR under the age of 40 was 0%. These findings are in accordance with those of Manochemi et al.

Overall, 37.7% of the respondents admitted that another team member was diagnosed with COVID-19, of which the most frequently mentioned profession was nurse/dental assistant (81.2%), followed by another dentist (27.4%), dental hygienist (16.7%), receptionist (12.4%), and dental technician (6.8%). These data may indicate that the distance from the site of aerosol production decreases the risk of infection. However, these results may be influenced by the uneven staffing of dental teams. Further studies would be needed to confirm this conclusion.

To compare the prevalence of COVID-19 among Czech dentists and their foreign counterparts, it is necessary to find studies of a similar methodology carried out in a similar period of time. However, a literature search revealed a lack of studies that met both of these criteria. In June 2020, a methodologically similar work was performed by the American Dental Association [15]. The questionnaire survey addressed 2195 dentists in the USA. Of them, 355 reported that they had been tested for COVID-19. Testing via respiratory, blood, and salivary samples revealed 3.7%, 2.7%, and 0% COVID-19 positivity. Despite the methodological similarity of this and our research, the data are not comparable, as they are separated by an interval of 1 year. Another online survey of dentists, dental hygienists, and dental assistants from around the world was conducted in August and September 2020 by Gluckman et al. [18]. The respondents were asked about the COVID-19 positivity among their dental practice staff. Of the total number of 1154 participants, 210 (18.2%) admitted COVID-19 infection, of which 186 (16.1%) were confirmed by a test. However, the results of this study were affected by uneven geographical participation as 48.6% of the participants were from South Africa. The COVID-19 positivity reported by the respondents from South Africa was 19%, by others 13%. Comparison with our study is, again, limited by the time difference of the event.

The literature search shows that studies focusing on the prevalence of COVID-19 among dentists are scant. Although many studies have been published focusing on the impact of COVID-19 on the operability of dental practices, current works on the impact of COVID-19 on dental professionals are lacking [13,19,20]. This condition is alarming due to the high occupational risk of dentists and emphasizes the need for further studies on this topic. Our study describing COVID-19 prevalence among members of the Czech Dental Chamber is thus one of the few that describe the impact on this professional group and, at the same time, the only one that describes this topic a year after the beginning of the pandemic.

6. Conclusions

This survey conducted among 2716 members of the Czech Dental Chamber reveals that 25.4% of the participants admitted to being diagnosed with COVID-19 by 30 June 2021. The total COVID-19 PCR-verified positivity was 13.9%, revealing a statistically lower prevalence ($p = 0.0180$) compared with the Czech general population (~15.6%). The results of this study suggest that although the dental profession is associated with a high occupational risk of droplet infection transmission, including SARS-CoV-19, the working conditions of dentists in the Czech Republic have not led to a higher prevalence of COVID-19 infection among them. Such results demonstrate that properly set working conditions focused on infection control were effective and led to a reduction in the occupational infection risk.

Supplementary Materials: The following are available online at https://www.mdpi.com/article/10.3390/ijerph182312488/s1.

Author Contributions: Conceptualization: V.P., J.S. (Jan Schmidt) and R.S.; methodology V.P. and J.T.; software: V.P. and R.S.; validation, N.P. and J.S. (Jakub Suchanek); formal analysis V.P., J.T., and J.S. (Jan Schmidt); investigation, V.P., J.S. (Jan Schmidt), J.T. and N.P.; resources, J.S. (Jakub Suchanek); data curation, V.P. and J.S. (Jan Schmidt); writing—original draft preparation, V.P., J.S. (Jan Schmidt) and J.S. (Jakub Suchanek); writing—review and editing, N.P., J.T. and R.S.; visualization, V.P. and J.S. (Jan Schmidt); supervision, J.S. (Jakub Suchanek) and R.S.; project administration, J.T., N.P. and R.S.; funding acquisition, J.S. (Jakub Suchanek) and N.P. All authors have read and agreed to the published version of the manuscript.

Funding: This work was supported by Charles University's program PROGRES Q40/13.

Institutional Review Board Statement: Not applicable.

Informed Consent Statement: Not applicable.

Data Availability Statement: The dataset is available on demand from the corresponding author.

Acknowledgments: The authors thank Diksha Ghimire for the English language editing.

Conflicts of Interest: The authors declare no conflict of interest.

References

1. Hu, B.; Huang, S.; Yin, L. The cytokine storm and COVID-19. *J. Med. Virol.* **2021**, *93*, 250–256. [CrossRef] [PubMed]
2. Li, X.; Ma, X. Acute respiratory failure in COVID-19: Is it "typical" ARDS? *Crit. Care* **2020**, *24*, 198. [CrossRef] [PubMed]
3. Lotfi, M.; Hamblin, M.R.; Rezaei, N. COVID-19: Transmission, prevention, and potential therapeutic opportunities. *Clin. Chim. Acta* **2020**, *508*, 254–266. [CrossRef] [PubMed]
4. Goldman, E. Exaggerated risk of transmission of COVID-19 by fomites. *Lancet Infect. Dis.* **2020**, *20*, 892–893. [CrossRef]
5. Chin, A.W.H.; Chu, J.T.S.; Perera, M.R.A.; Hui, K.P.Y.; Yen, H.L.; Chan, M.C.W.; Peiris, M.; Poon, L.L.M. Stability of SARS-CoV-2 in different environmental conditions. *Lancet Microbe* **2020**, *1*, e10. [CrossRef]
6. Huang, C.; Wang, Y.; Li, X.; Ren, L.; Zhao, J.; Hu, Y.; Zhang, L.; Fan, G.; Xu, J.; Gu, X.; et al. Clinical features of patients infected with 2019 novel coronavirus in Wuhan, China. *Lancet* **2020**, *395*, 497–506. [CrossRef]
7. World Health Organization. WHO Director-General's Opening Remarks at the Media Briefing on COVID-19—11 March 2020. 2020. Available online: https://www.who.int/director-general/speeches/detail/who-director-general-s-opening-remarks-at-the-media-briefing-on-covid-19---11-march-2020 (accessed on 12 July 2021).
8. Global Change Data Lab. Czechia, Coronavirus Cases per Capita, August 2020. 2021. Available online: https://ourworldindata.org/explorers/coronavirus-data-explorer?tab=map&zoomToSelection=true&time=2020-08-31&facet=none&pickerSort=asc&pickerMetric=location&hideControls=true&Metric=Confirmed+cases&Interval=Cumulative&Relative+to+Population=true&Align+outbreaks=false&country=~{}CZE (accessed on 10 October 2021).
9. Global Change Data Lab. Czechia, Coronavirus Deaths per Capita, August 2020. 2021. Available online: https://ourworldindata.org/grapher/covid-deaths-daily-vs-total-per-million?tab=table&time=2020-01-22..2020-08-31 (accessed on 10 October 2021).
10. Global Change Data Lab. Czechia, Coronavirus Cases per Capita, June 2021. 2021. Available online: https://ourworldindata.org/explorers/coronavirus-data-explorer?tab=table&zoomToSelection=true&time=earliest..2021-06-30&facet=none&pickerSort=asc&pickerMetric=location&hideControls=true&Metric=Confirmed+cases&Interval=Cumulative&Relative+to+Population=true&Align+outbreaks=false&country=~{}CZE (accessed on 10 October 2021).
11. Global Change Data Lab. Czechia, Coronavirus Deaths per Capita, September 2021. 2021. Available online: https://ourworldindata.org/grapher/total-covid-cases-deaths-per-million?tab=table&time=2019-12-31..2021-07-30&country=~{}OWID_WRL (accessed on 10 October 2021).
12. Shields, A.M.; Faustini, S.E.; Kristunas, C.A.; Cook, A.M.; Backhouse, C.; Dunbar, L.; Ebanks, D.; Emmanuel, B.; Crouch, E.; Kröger, A.; et al. COVID-19: Seroprevalence and Vaccine Responses in UK Dental Care Professionals. *J. Dent. Res.* **2021**, *100*, 1220–1227. [CrossRef]
13. Schmidt, J.; Waldova, E.; Balkova, S.; Suchanek, J.; Smucler, R. Impact of COVID-19 on Czech Dentistry: A Nationwide Cross-Sectional Preliminary Study among Dentists in the Czech Republic. *Int. J. Environ. Res. Public Health* **2021**, *18*, 9121. [CrossRef] [PubMed]
14. Czech Dental Chamber. Ročenka ČSK 2020 (Czech Dental Chamber 2020 Annual Report). 2021. Available online: https://www.dent.cz/o-nas/rocenky/ (accessed on 10 July 2021).
15. Estrich, C.G.; Mikkelsen, M.; Morrissey, R.; Geisinger, M.L.; Ioannidou, E.; Vujicic, M.; Araujo, M.W.B. Estimating COVID-19 prevalence and infection control practices among US dentists. *J. Am. Dent. Assoc.* **2020**, *151*, 815–824. [CrossRef] [PubMed]
16. Jungo, S.; Moreau, N.; Mazevet, M.E.; Ejeil, A.-L.; Biosse Duplan, M.; Salmon, B.; Smail-Faugeron, V. Prevalence and risk indicators of first-wave COVID-19 among oral health-care workers: A French epidemiological survey. *PLoS ONE* **2021**, *16*, e0246586. [CrossRef] [PubMed]
17. Menachemi, N.; Dixon, B.E.; Wools-Kaloustian, K.K.; Yiannoutsos, C.T.; Halverson, P.K. How Many SARS-CoV-2-Infected People Require Hospitalization? Using Random Sample Testing to Better Inform Preparedness Efforts. *J. Public Health Manag. Pract.* **2021**, *27*, 246–250. [CrossRef] [PubMed]
18. Gluckman, H.; Pontes, C.; Troelzsch, M.; Scheyer, E. An overview of COVID-19 infection in dental practices—A questionnaire survey. *S. Afr. Dent. J.* **2021**, *76*, 404–408. [CrossRef]
19. Izzetti, R.; Gennai, S.; Nisi, M.; Barone, A.; Giuca, M.R.; Gabriele, M.; Graziani, F. A perspective on dental activity during COVID-19: The Italian survey. *Oral Dis.* **2021**, *27*, 694–702. [CrossRef] [PubMed]
20. Tysiąc-Miśta, M.; Dziedzic, A. The Attitudes and Professional Approaches of Dental Practitioners during the COVID-19 Outbreak in Poland: A Cross-Sectional Survey. *Int. J. Environ. Res. Public Health* **2020**, *17*, 4703. [CrossRef] [PubMed]

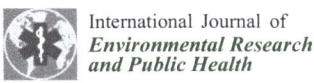

International Journal of Environmental Research and Public Health

Review

The Potential Impact of Smog Spell on Humans' Health Amid COVID-19 Rages

Ammar Javed [1,†], Farheen Aamir [1,†], Umar Farooq Gohar [1], Hamid Mukhtar [1], Muhammad Zia-UI-Haq [2,*], Modhi O. Alotaibi [3], May Nasser Bin-Jumah [3,4], Romina Alina Marc (Vlaic) [5,*] and Oana Lelia Pop [6]

1. Institute of Industrial Biotechnology, Government College University Lahore, Lahore 54000, Pakistan; ammarjaved94@gmail.com (A.J.); farheenaamir15@gmail.com (F.A.); dr.mufgohar@gcu.edu.pk (U.F.G.); hamidmukhtar@gcu.edu.pk (H.M.)
2. Office of Research, Innovation & Commercialization, Lahore College for Women University, Lahore 54000, Pakistan
3. Biology Department, College of Science, Princess Nourah Bint Abdulrahman University, Riyadh 11671, Saudi Arabia; mouotaebe@pnu.edu.sa (M.O.A.); mnbinjumah@pnu.edu.sa (M.N.B.-J.)
4. Environment and Biomaterial Unit, Health Sciences Research Center, Princess Nourah Bint Abdulrahman University, Riyadh 11671, Saudi Arabia
5. Food Engineering Department, Faculty of Food Science and Technology, University of Agricultural Sciences and Veterinary Medicine, 400372 Cluj-Napoca, Romania
6. Department of Food Science, University of Agricultural Science and Veterinary Medicine, 400372 Cluj-Napoca, Romania; oana.pop@usamvcluj.ro
* Correspondence: ahirzia@gmail.com (M.Z.-U.-H.); romina.vlaic@usamvcluj.ro (R.A.M.)
† These authors contributed equally to this paper.

Abstract: Rapid and unchecked industrialization and the combustion of fossil fuels have engendered a state of fear in urban settlements. Smog is a visible form of air pollution that arises due to the over-emissions of some primary pollutants like volatile organic compounds (VOCs), hydrocarbons, SO_2, NO, and NO_2 which further react in the atmosphere and give rise to toxic and carcinogenic secondary smog components. Smog reduces the visibility on roads and results in road accidents and cancellation of flights. Uptake of primary and secondary pollutants of smog is responsible for several deleterious diseases of which respiratory disorders, cardiovascular dysfunction, neurological disorders, and cancer are discussed here. Children and pregnant women are more prone to the hazards of smog. The worsening menace of smog on one hand and occurrence of pandemic i.e., COVID-19 on the other may increase the mortality rate. But the implementation of lockdown during pandemics has favored the atmosphere in some ways, which will be highlighted in the article. On the whole, the focus of this article will be on the dubious relationship between smog and coronavirus.

Keywords: air pollution; COVID-19; photochemical smog; respiratory disorders

1. Introduction

The word smog is an amalgamation of two words, 'smoke' and 'fog'. Fog is reckoned as a visible low lying cloud, made up of small water droplets or ice crystals [1]. In 1905, H. A. Des Voeux used the term 'smog' to define the atmospheric conditions of many towns in Britain. In 1911, this word became famous when H. A. Des Voeux reported 1000 deaths in his paper 'Smoke and Fog' due to 'smoke-fog' in Edinburgh and Glasgow [2]. Nowadays, Lahore, Faisalabad, Delhi, Beijing, Los Angles, Mexico, and London are mostly affected by the smog [3–9].

Currently, various studies have provided knowledge to the general population about the relationship between smog and its adverse effects on human health. Earlier researchers had confirmed that health effects are related to persons' age, health, and socioeconomic status [10]. However, the impact of smog is also influenced by its time of exposure. The risk of long-term exposure is much higher than that of short-term exposure. Both the long-term unceasing exposure and short-term peak do not have the same consequences and they follow different dynamics. The effects range from short-term irritation in the trachea to long-term genetic mutations. However, some recent studies have observed a link between adverse mortality and short-term exposure to smog [11]. These adverse health effects have a broad array from subclinical effects like irritation in the trachea to long-term genetic mutations and premature deaths. Some of the major diseases which are harbored by smog are respiratory diseases (asthma, coughing, and bronchiolitis), cardiovascular disease, neurological disorders, cancer, infant health, low birth weight, and other problems like eye irritation and breathing difficulties [12–15].

On the other hand, the novel coronavirus outbreak has shaken the world. It originated from Wuhan, China, and has engulfed the whole world within a year. The root cause of this pandemic i.e., SARS-CoV-2 (Severe acute respiratory syndrome coronavirus-2) is transmissible from humans to humans. It targets the respiratory tract of humans, attaches with the angiotensin-converting enzyme-2 (ACE2), and down-regulates its production to cause severe respiratory illnesses. Although the mortality rate of coronavirus disease of 2019 (COVID-19) is less than 10% together with smog, the increase in fatality can be observed because both target the respiratory tract of humans [16]. In elderly people, coronavirus invasion is facilitated as immune responses are weakened by age and smog [17]. Together they may worsen the disease and can lead to hospitalization and eventually death occurs [18] as shown in Figure 1. Studies have backed the hypothesis that components of air pollution like nitrogen dioxide (NO_2) and particulate matter (PM) cause the excessive production of the Angiotensin-converting enzyme-2 (ACE2) which is the binding target for SARS-CoV-2 [19–21]. This increased production increases the susceptibility towards COVID-19. Thus the combination of coronavirus and air pollution can exacerbate the situation. The regions like China, India, and the USA a positive correlation is observed between COVID-19 mortality and high air pollution. This aggravates the need to control air pollution to reduce coronavirus cases where they share common hotspots [22,23]. However, there is another aspect of this pandemic. Due to the pandemic, people are locked in their houses to avoid SARS-CoV-2 infection. This reduction in human activities has a positive has brought a positive impact on nature like less water, air, and noise pollution. The lockdown periods have also prevented several deaths due to a reduction in air pollutants [24]. The purpose of the paper is to highlight the negative aspects of the relation of smog with the current coronavirus pandemic. Along with negative aspects, positive aspects of the lockdown on air pollution are also discussed in the paper.

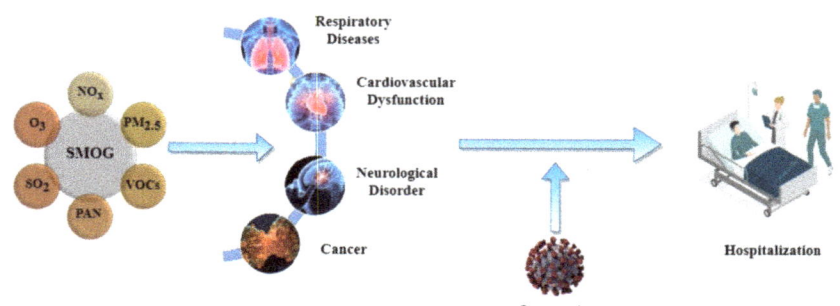

Figure 1. Relationship between COVID-19 and smog.

2. Research Methodology

2.1. Identifying the Research Question

The following questions are established to address the relation of smog with coronavirus disease.

1. What are the components of the smog that are of concern during the pandemic?
2. Does amalgamation of coronavirus and smog increase the health risks?

3. Does the COVID-lockdown bring any positive effects on the air quality?

2.2. Finding and Selecting the Relevant Studies

To draft this review, we have searched PubMed for the articles that discussed the relationship between smog and coronavirus disease and have to obtain the most relevant studies using simple keywords "Smog", "Air pollution", "Coronavirus" and "COVID-19". We have also gone through the references section of these articles to select the pertinent publications.

3. Smog

The 20th century marks some of the disastrous events related to smog. In the 1930s, the areas of Liège and Huy alongside River Meuse were hubs of industries in Continental Europe. After the industrial revolution fertilizer, glass, zinc smelters, steelworks, and explosive manufacturing plants were established in these areas [25]. At the end of the year, these areas were shrouded by a thick fig for five days (1–5 December). Within 3 days hundreds of people contracted the signs and symptoms of respiratory diseases. The government was baffled completely after the death of 63 people. On the 6th of December, smog disappeared completely with improvement in respiratory troubles [26].

On the 28th of November 1939, dwellers of ST. LOUIS faced a thick smog for over a month as they were burning cheap coal to keep themselves warm from cold weather. Kings-highway and neighboring areas were completely covered by darkness during the daytime. That day is attributed as 'Black Tuesday' in history. ST. LOUIS faced smog events later in the next year after which the authorities took proper actions to resolve the pollution issue [27–29].

On October 26, 1948 fog mixed with industrial pollutants engulfed the atmosphere of Donora, Pennsylvania [30]. Donora Zinc Works, part of US Steel was blamed by the authorities as a major contributor to smog. About 5000–7000 residents became ill, 400 were hospitalized and 20 people died. After five days on 31st October 1948, the smog was dispersed by the rain [31]. Donora also faced small smog events on the 4th and 14th of October, 1923 [32]. After the events, the Donora Zinc Works was shut down [31].

In 1952, London (England's capital) was engulfed for five days by the lethal black haze called, Great London Smog of 1952 [33]. In December residents of London burned the high sulfur coal [2] to keep themselves warm. This black smoke escaped from their chimneys and mixed with fog [34]. Then this smog cooled by air covered the atmosphere and blocked the sunlight. This black haze proved to be hazardous when converted into sulfur dioxide and sulfuric acid (i.e., corrosive) and affected the eyes, skin, respiratory and cardiac systems of Londoners [33]. This smog caused an increase in hospitalization (48%), respiratory diseases (163%), and asthma in newborn children (20%) [35].

Historical events are discussed to bring an insight into the occurrence of the smog. It helps to determine the possible season, time, or region in which smog is most prevalent. If one knows the possible time of occurrence of smog during the pandemic, then measures can be taken accordingly.

Different types of smog contribute to air pollution. They are London smog (high content of sulfur oxides), Polish smog (PM_{10}, $PM_{2.5}$, PM_1, and various polycyclic aromatic hydrocarbons such as benzo-pyrene), photochemical smog (nitrogen oxides, ozone, hydrocarbons, and VOCs) as shown in Figure 2, and the natural smog released from volcanoes (CO, CO_2, SO, H_2, and H_2S) and plants (hydrocarbons and VOCs) [1,36–39]. Table 1 shows the distinctive features of different types of smog.

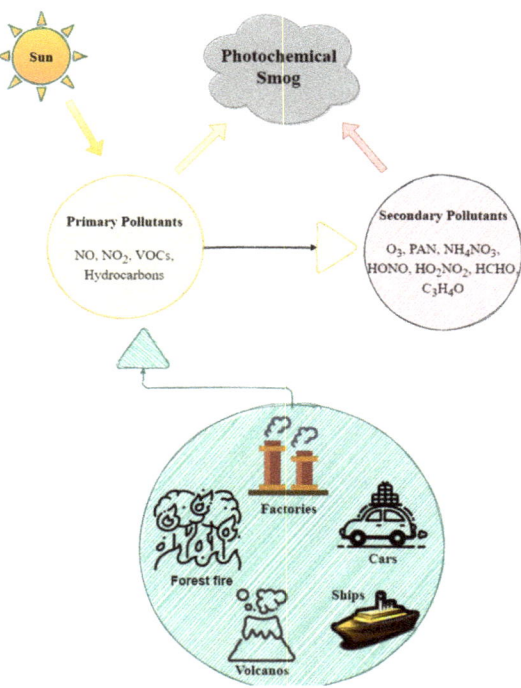

Figure 2. The activities of erupting volcanoes, traffic emissions, forest fires, general combustion, mining, agriculture are directly or indirectly involved in the production of primary pollutants like NO, NO_2, VOCs, and hydrocarbons which are major forerunners of smog. These primary pollutants undergo chemical reactions in presence of sunlight to form secondary pollutants like formaldehyde, peroxyacetyl nitrate (PAN), and O_3 [40,41]. Both primary and secondary pollutants then concoct smog.

Table 1. Distinctive features between London, Photochemical and Natural smog.

Characters	London Smog (Sulfurous Smog)	Polish Smog	Photochemical Smog (Los Angeles Smog or Summer Smog)	Natural Smog	References
Definition	Develops due to high concentration of sulfur oxides in the air	When the temperature drops, inversion takes place and a low-level cloud of pollutants form a dusty cloud	It is produced when sunlight reacts with oxides of nitrogen or at least one VOC [1]	It may result due to volcanoes also known as acid smog (vog) and by plants i.e., natural sources of hydrocarbons and volatile organic compounds	[36,42–44]
Occurrence	It occurs in cold, humid climates	It occurs in the winter seasons	It occurs in a warm, dry, and sunny climate	It occurs mostly in warm, humid, and summer climate	[36,37,45,46]
Effects	It irritates the eyes, causes bronchitis and lung problems	It affects the lungs, causes asthma and cardiovascular diseases	It irritates the eyes, causes obstructive pulmonary disease, cardiovascular disease, and asthma.	Irritation and inflammation of eyes, dry cough, anterior uveitis, breathing difficulties, asthma, subconjunctival hemorrhage.	[45,47–49]

[1] VOC: Volatile organic compound.

4. Some Major Smog Affected Populations

Smog has affected developing as well as under-developing countries likewise. The air quality of any region is estimated by Air Quality Index (AQI). The more the AQI of a region more is pollution in the environment. The AQI values are compared with the units described in Figure 3. There are environment protection agencies that work for the improvement of air quality in the region because it affects nature as well as humans. Therefore, the implication of these standards and regulations during a pandemic is important as they help to monitor the air quality of different regions. These standards make sure that pollutants concentrations do not cross the threshold levels i.e., maximum permitted level (MPL), and if some have already crossed that limit then how could we reduce their concentration to MPLs. Air pollution has become a global problem but we can see that policies regarding control of air pollution vary from region to region. Developed countries like the United States (US) and European Union (EU) have adopted more advanced technologies while developing countries like India and China have just started to build their legislation regarding air pollution.

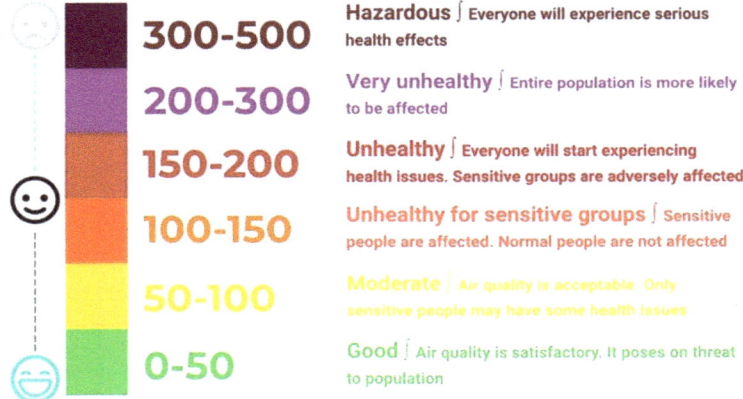

Figure 3. Air Quality Index Chart.

4.1. China

Air pollution has become a most concerning affair in China. Urbanization is considered the most detrimental cause of air pollution in which rural and agricultural land is converted to urban and non-agricultural land. Moreover, natural habitats are metamorphosed into cities. The enormously increasing Chinese economy, industrialization, and urbanization come at the cost of severe air pollution especially smog pollution [41]. After smoking, high blood pressure, and dietary risks, ambient $PM_{2.5}$, and PM_{10} have become the fourth leading cause of death in China [50]. Nonetheless, the population affected by the recent events of air pollutions in China is phenomenal. Each year 350,000 to 400,000 deaths are attributed to air pollution in China [51]. Beijing faced multiple periods of prolonged air pollution in January 2013. The $PM_{2.5}$ was calculated 32 times higher in Beijing (i.e., 800 mg/m^3) than that recommended by World Health Organization (WHO) (i.e., 23 mg/m^3) [52]. Similarly, another episode of smog stuck in Beijing for six days in February 2014. These smog spells affected not only Beijing but also nearby cities forcing the people to stay indoors to prevent adverse health effects [53]. The air quality index (AQI) is the unit used to measure the quality of air in a particular region. The AQI between 0 and 50 is considered good, 50 to 100 is moderate while 101 to onwards is considered unhealthy. Shahecheng (156), Nantong (140), Luancheng (134), Wuda (133), Handan (132), Yangliuqing (127), Dawakou (124), Yigou (122), and Zibo (119) are currently the most polluted cities of China [54]. Being an industrial country China has begun to endorse the policies regarding control of air pollution. Even after the implementation of the Action Plan, 2013 as a strategy to control air pollution, the levels of smog in the atmosphere are still concerning [55]. The evolution of Chinese air pollution control legislation and the standard sets for air pollutants are described in Tables 2 and 3.

Table 2. Evolution of Chinese legislation for Air pollution control [56].

Year	Law or Action	Description
1979	Environmental Protection Law	First legislation related to environmental pollution was established
1987	Air pollution prevention and control Law	For the control of pollution emissions from industries in specific areas
1989	Environmental Protection Law (EPL)	For the very first time, institutional buildings were constructed for the enforcement of law
1998	Establishing acid rain and sulfur dioxide (SO_2) control areas	Measures are developed to reduce the acid rain and SO_2 pollutants in specific areas
2000	Amendment of Air Pollution Prevention and Control Law	Data related to air pollution was linked with AQI [1] which was classified as natural, urban, and industrial. Major pollutants were targeted i.e., SO_2, NO_2, and PM in 42 cities
2002	Environmental Impact Assessment (EIA) law	"Pollute first, clean up later" model was developed to highlight the sources of pollution
2008	Ministry of Environmental Pollution (MEP)	State administration of Environmental Protection was upgraded to a ministry
2010	ODS [2] regulation	Control of ozone by ODS
2013	Air pollution prevention and control action plan	Its purpose was to reduce pollution in specific regions. It aimed to reduce PM by 10% by 2017.
2015	Amendment of EPL	According to these amendments, non-compliance is punished with a high price, EIAs plans should be made mandatory and public awareness programs be done
2016	2nd amendment in Air Pollution Prevention and Control Law	A system for co-operation between regions was introduced. Limits of vehicle emissions were set and involvement of local government was enhanced
2016	Amendment in EIA law	Increases the facilities and planning of EIA
2018	Ministry of Ecology and Environment	The working structure of MEP is enhanced
2018	Environmental Protection Tax law	To replace old pollution fee system
2018	Blue sky war-winning action plan	The second phase of the 2013 plan targets reduction of VOCs, NOx, and ozone in more cities in China

[1] AQI: Air Quality Index, [2] ODS: Ozone-Depleting Substance.

Table 3. National Ambient Air Quality Standards (NAAQSs) of China [57].

Year	No. of Standards	Grade [1]	CO [2]	NO_2 [3]	SO_2 [3]	O_3 [4]	TSP [5]	$PM_{2.5}$ [6]	PM_{10} [3]
1982	GB3095–82	I	100	50	50	120	150	-	50
		II	100	100	150	160	300	-	150
		III	200	150	250	200	500	-	250
1996	GB3095–1996	I	100	40	20	120	80	-	40
		II	100	40	60	160	200	-	100
		III	200	80	100	200	300	-	150
2000	Amended GB3095–1996	I	100	40	20	160	80	-	40
		II	100	80	60	200	200	-	100
		III	200	80	100	200	300	-	150
2016	GB3095–2012	I	100	40	20	160	80	15	40
		II	100	40	60	200	200	35	70

[1] Grade I: Places like forests and national parks, II: Rural, urban, industrial and commercial areas included, III: Heavy industry areas, [2] CO: mg/m^3, 1 h average, [3] NO_2, SO_2, PM_{10}: μg/m^3, 24 h average, [4] O_3 μg/m^3, 1 h average, [5] TSP: Total Suspended Particle, [6] $PM_{2.5}$ μg/m^3, 1-year average.

4.2. United Kingdom

The Great Smog of London 1952, lessoned the people about the long term health consequences of air pollution. In 1956, Clean Air Act was introduced in England to cope with air pollution [58]. Smokeless burning facilities were announced in heavily polluted cities. Reforestation and the use of eco-friendly fuels are encouraged to reduce air pollution [59]. Despite efforts Ashford (109), Crowborough (108), Faversham (107), Ealing (106), London (104), Shenley (104), Cambridge (103), East Ham (103), Cranbrook (102), and Lewes (102) are most polluted cities of England [60]. United Kingdom followed the European Union laws and standards regarding air pollution as shown in Tables 4 and 5.

Table 4. Evolution of European Union legislation on air pollution [61,62].

Year	Law of Action	Description
1979	Convention on Long-range Transboundary Air Pollution	Focused mainly on pollutants that cause eutrophication and acidification i.e., NOx, cadmium (Cd), lead (Pb), mercury (Hg), NH_3, PM, SO_2, and VOCs [1].
1980	Directive 80/779/EEC [2]	This directive dictates the limitation levels of SO_2 and PM
1982	Directive 82/884/EEC	Lead limitations were set
1985	Directive 85/203/EEC	This directive highlighted the NO_2 limitation levels. It did not apply to the inside buildings
1988	Directive 88/609/EEC	The purpose of this Council directive was to limit the emissions of certain pollutants i.e., NOx and SO_2 for large combustion plants. It helped in the reduction of these pollutants.
1992	Directive 92/72/EEC	It introduced provisions related to tropospheric O_3. It holds the Environment Protection Agency (EPA) responsible for measuring O_3 concentrations and defining the threshold levels of O_3 for industries.
1996	Directive 96/61/EC	It's a directive on Ambient Air Quality Assessment and Management which aims at preventing the harmful effects of pollutants on the environment as well as human health. As this directive failed four daughter directives with more specificity were introduced
1999	1st daughter directive 1999/30/EC	It focused on the limit levels of NO, NO_2, SO_2, lead (Pb), and dust. It aimed to protect the ecosystem, plants, and humans.
2000	2nd daughter directive 2000/69/EC	It defined the benzene and CO acceptable levels. Aims at the protection of humans
2002	3rd daughter directive 2002/3/EC	Ozone levels in ambient air. Aims at the long-term protection of plants and humans.
2004	4th daughter directive 2004/107/EC	It defined the acceptable levels of nickel, cadmium, arsenic, and PAHs [3]. Aims to protect humans.
2008	Directive 2008/50/EC	It's a directive on ambient air quality and cleaner air for Europe. It replaced the directives from 1996 to 2002. It ensures the enforcement of laws regarding air pollution. It urges regional authorities to take measures according to their environmental conditions. If any region surpasses the threshold level of pollutants, this directive provides a deadline for reducing the pollutant levels to the threshold.

[1] VOCs: Volatile organic compounds, [2] EEC: European Environment Agency, [3] PAHs: Polycyclic aromatic hydrocarbons.

Table 5. Ambient Air Quality Standards of European Union [63].

Pollutants	Average Time	Concentration	Exceed Permitted Each Year
Carbon monoxide (CO)	8 h	10 mg/m^3	-
Ozone (O$_3$)	8 h	120 μg/m^3	Average of 25 days in 3 years
Sulfur dioxide (SO$_2$)	1 h	350 μg/m^3	24
	24 h	125 μg/m^3	3
Lead (Pb)	1 year	0.5 μg/m^3	-
Nitrogen dioxide (NO$_2$)	1 h	200 μg/m^3	18
	1 year	40 μg/m^3	-
PM$_{2.5}$	1 year	25 μg/m^3	-
PM$_{10}$	24 h	50 μg/m^3	35
	1 year	40 μg/m^3	-
Arsenic (As)	1 year	6 ng/m^3	-
Benzene	1 year	5 μg/m^3	-
Nickel (Ni)	1 year	20 ng/m^3	-

4.3. The USA

Everybody has noticed the effects of the horrible brown haze in urban communities like Shanghai, China, or New Delhi, India. However, it is observed that there are issues with air contamination in the USA as well, particularly on the off chance that you live in California, as per the American Lung Association's 2018. California's Bay area encounters undeniable degrees of both smog and particulate matter contamination. In the colder time of year, wood smoke from chimneys causes significant degrees of smog [64]. In the USA, North fork (186), Oakhurst (186), Kamiah (184), Orofino (170) Hamilton (164), Moscow (162), McCall (160), La Jolla Shores (158), Lewiston (158), and Pullman (158) are worst cities in context to air pollution [65]. Other than these, Krasnoyarsk-Russia (169), Lima-Peru (163), Kabul-Afghanistan (156), Jakarta-Indonesia (152), Santiago-Chile (152), Tehran-Iran (108), and London-United Kingdom (104) are the top polluted communities of the world according to live stats of Air quality and pollution city ranking of 2021 [66]. The US legislation related to air pollution control have evolved much and has set some standard values for pollutants as shown in Tables 6 and 7.

Table 6. Evolution of U.S. legislation on air pollution [67,68].

Year	Law or Action	Description
1955	Air Pollution Control Act	In 1948, a 5 days event of smog in Donora, an industrial town, in Pennsylvania prompted the passing of the first air quality act in the U.S. In 1955, air pollution was declared a national problem under Air Pollution Control Act and research on air pollution was funded.
1963	Clean Air Act (CAA) sets Nationwide Air Quality Standards	Under this act, public education programs were carried out and researches regarding control of air pollution were supported. However, it has no intention of reducing the air pollutants
1965	Motor Vehicle Air Pollution Control Act	With some amendments in CAA, standards regarding automobile emissions were laid down.
1967	Air Quality Act (AQA)	This act distributed the responsibilities to the regions to develop and implement control measures against air pollution. However, this wasn't effective
1970	Clean Air Act Amendments of 1970	A new CAA was passed to control six pollutants i.e., CO$_2$, NO$_2$, CO, O$_3$, PM, and lead. It also provided flexibility to Motor Vehicle Air Pollution Control Act. EPA [1] was established to make sure the implementation of the act.
1977	Clean Air Act Amendments of 1977	It is concerned with provisions for the Prevention of Significant Deterioration (PSD) of air quality in areas fulfilling NAAQS [2] as well as areas not attaining NAAQS.
1990	Clean Air Act Amendments of 1990	These revisions expanded the limits and responsibilities of the federal government. New amendments were made regarding control of acid rains, air toxins, O$_3$ depletion, and ground levels of O$_3$. EPA was authorized more responsibilities to enforce air control acts and reduce air pollutants

[1] EPA: Environment Protection Agency, [2] NAAQS: National Ambient Air Quality Standards.

Table 7. National Ambient Air Quality Standards (NAAQSs) of United States [69].

Pollutants	Average Times	Primary Standards [1]	Secondary Standards [2]	Exceed Permitted
Carbon monoxide (CO)	1 h	8 ppm	-	<1 per year
	8 h	35 ppm	-	
Ozone (O$_3$)	8 h	0.070 ppm	0.070 ppm	4th highest average max 8 h concentration, averaged over 3 years
Sulfur dioxide (SO$_2$)	1 h	75 ppb	-	99th% of max 8 h concentration, averaged over 3 years
	3 h	-	0.5 ppm	<1 per year
Lead (Pb)	3 months	0.15 µg/m^3	0.15 µg/m^3	-
Nitrogen dioxide (NO$_2$)	1 h	100 ppb	-	98th% of max 8 h concentration, averaged over 3 years
	1 year	53 ppb	53 ppb	Annual mean
PM$_{2.5}$	24 h	35 µg/m^3	35 µg/m^3	Annual mean
	1 year	12 µg/m^3	15 µg/m^3	Annual mean
PM$_{10}$	24 h	150 µg/m^3	150 µg/m^3	<1 per year

[1] Primary standard: Covers human health and sensitive groups (asthma patients and children), [2] Secondary standards: Protects human welfare (plants, buildings, and animals).

5. COVID-19 Pandemic

The 2019 novel COVID or the extreme intense respiratory condition COVID-19 (SARS-CoV-2) for what it's worth presently called, has quickly spread from its source in Wuhan City to the rest of the world [70]. According to the World Health Organization (WHO) and Center for Disease Control (CDC) around 222 M instances of COVID-19 (Coronavirus) and 4.6 M fatalities have occurred till the 8th of September 2021. Most affected populations of the world are the USA (41 M cases), India (33 M cases), Brazil (20.9 M cases), Russia (7 M cases), UK (7 M cases), France (6.8 M cases), Turkey (6.5 M cases), Argentina (5.2 M cases), Iran (5.1 M cases), Colombia (4.9 M cases) and so on 223 countries of the world are affected [71].

Coronavirus is an RNA virus (enveloped) having a diameter of 60 nm to 140 nm. Spike-like projections are present on its surface due to which it has a crown-like structure when observed under the electron microscope that's why it's named Coronavirus [72]. Pneumonia-like infection was first observed in Wuhan, Hubei region, China in December 2019 in local workers of the Hunan seafood market. Initially, they faced intense acute respiratory distress syndrome (ARDS) and respiratory failure in critical stages [73]. January 7, 2020, marks the day when SARS-CoV-2 was isolated for the very first time from the throat swabs of the patient. After China, it gradually spread in Thailand, Japan, Korea, and the USA. All first cases reported (26 out of 29) had a travel history to China. The remaining 3 had a meet-up or are relatives of the other 26 patients. This study conducted by WHO members confirmed that the seafood market of China was the epidemiological source of COVID-19 [74]. Moreover, they also concluded that coronavirus spread through human-to-human contact, and no intermediary live host is involved in transmission. Coronavirus infection spreads from symptomatic people through droplets produced from coughing or sneezing as well as asymptomatic people [75]. The disease can also be attained by rubbing your nose, eyes after touching virus-contaminated surfaces. The stool of patients also contains the virus that results in contamination in the water supply [76].

6. Smog and Coronavirus

The correlation between air pollution and COVID-19 has pros and cons. Studies have backed both the aspects that COVID-19 mortality rates are high in highly polluted regions while the lockdown during the pandemic may lower the air pollution rates and thus lower the infection rates. Previous studies have proved that smog is a risk factor for respiratory infections by carrying microorganisms to humans and distressing the body's immunity to make people more vulnerable to pathogens [77,78].

Smog effects on our health depend on several different factors, including the level of air pollutants, types of air pollutants, age and health conditions, exposure time, and where you live. Smog affects different organs of the body as shown in Figure 4 and Table 8. It can irritate our eyes, nose, and throat and can also cause existing heart and lung problems in people to worsen or lead to lung cancer if the exposure time of smog is long [3,79]. It also leads to premature death. Studies on ozone have shown that once it gets into your lungs, it can cause damage even when you are feeling well. It affects mainly those people who are at risk or suffer from heart and lung diseases. Children are most sensitive to smog because their respiratory systems are still underdeveloped and they have an active lifestyle [80]. However, these effects vary from person to person and exposure time. Healthy people who are exposed to smog for short period do not get long-term effects but in comparison, if a person is immunocompromised the effects will be long-term and might get worsen if the time of exposure is long and the dose is higher. Children are at more risk than adults, even if a low dose is present [81].

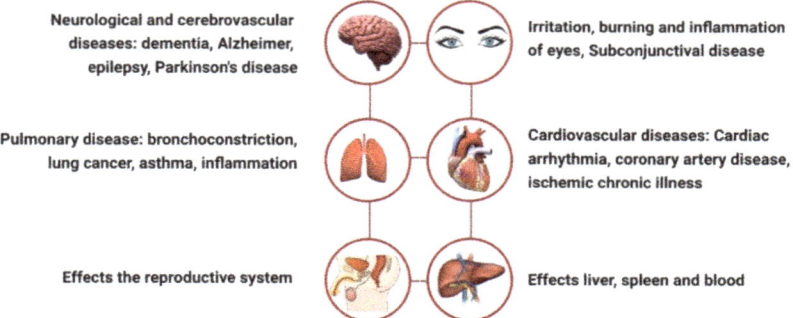

Figure 4. Effect of smog particles on different organs (nervous system, eyes, throat, lungs, heart, liver, spleen, and reproductive system) of the human body and the problems associated with it.

Table 8. Sources and diseases associated with sulfur dioxide, hydrocarbons, peroxyacetyl nitrate, nitrogen oxide, tropospheric ozone, and particulate matter i.e., different components of smog.

Smog Components	Source	Effect	References
Sulfur dioxide	Industries, burning of fossil fuels, electric generation plant, volcanic eruption	Respiratory problems i.e., irritation, inflammation, and infection. Asthma and reduced lung function. Chronic obstructive pulmonary disease. Cardiovascular disease, cardiac arrhythmias, hemorrhagic stroke	[82–84]
Hydrocarbons	Automobile exhaust and industries	Carcinogenic, may cause leukemia, lung cancer	[85]
PAN [1]	Photochemical reaction of hydrocarbons and nitrogen oxide	Irritation in the eye. nose and throat, breathing problems, damage to proteins	[86]
Nitrogen oxide	Combustion of fossil fuels, volcanic action, lightning, forest fires	Effects liver, spleen, and blood, kidney cancer, prostate cancer, brain cancer, reduce the birth length	[87]
Tropospheric ozone	Formed as a by-product of photochemical smog	Eye and respiratory irritation, cardiovascular disease, heart failure, breast cancer, fatal bladder cancer. Effects growth and bodyweight of the baby throughout pregnancy.	[88–90]
PM [2]	Vehicles, industries	Particles penetrate deep into the lungs, affect the reproductive system, cause Parkinson's disease, low birth weight, and halt fetal growth.	[91,92]

[1] PAN: peroxyacetyl nitrate, [2] PM: Particulate matter.

The pathogenesis of SARS-CoV-2 is similar to its closely related SARS-CoV-1 with an exception of the S-protein of SAR-CoV-2 that has a more binding affinity for Angiotensin Converting Enzyme-2 (ACE-2) receptors. Excess of plasma angiotensin-II is accumulated because of down-regulation of ACE2 leading to ARDS and myocarditis making other organs like the esophagus, kidney, lungs, heart, and ileum more vulnerable to SARS-CoV-2 [93]. Children under 5 years have low numbers of ACE2 receptors which probably makes them less susceptible to the disease [94].

The symptoms of the coronavirus vary from asymptomatic to severe respiratory diseases and organ damage. Some common symptoms include fever, fatigue, cough, headache, loss of smell and taste. Some people also suffer from acute lung injury (ALI) and impairment in blood clotting. Despite pulmonary damage being the cause of fatality, elderly patients also develop coronary heart diseases, atherosclerosis, ischemic cardiomyopathy, or hypertension. Apart from pulmonary damage COVID-19 is also involved in extra-pulmonary disorders like lymphopenia (67–91% of COVID-19 cases), proteinuria (87%), hepatocellular injuries (14–53%), gastrointestinal damage (12–61%), thrombotic complications (30%) and acute kidney injury (0.5–29%) [95]. The death rate in elder people is more than that of young people [96]. The death rate of adult patients in hospitals ranges from 4–11%, while the overall death rate is considered to range from 2–3%.

7. Amalgamation of Smog and COVID-19

Since COVID-19 is a respiratory disease, it is investigated that smog results in the transmission of coronavirus, and SARS-CoV-2 can remain feasible in the air for hours [97]. Short-term exposure to elevated concentrations of air pollutants results in an increased risk of coronavirus infection. The significance of lessening air contamination is perceived under its notable effect on environmental change and its impact on wellbeing because of expanded bleakness and mortality related to smog and air pollution [98]. As per late investigations, smog appears to support the spread of coronavirus disease. As the viral particle is airborne, the impact of COVID-19 is exasperated by smog [99]. Even though there are opposing sentiments on the transmission of SARS-CoV-2, it appears that one can obtain the disease through the air [16] because of its strength in mist concentrates [97] and the reality that the pollutant cloud and its payload (microbe bearing droplets) can travel 7–8 m [100]. In a recent experiment, aerosols containing SARS-CoV-2 were created using three jet Collison nebulizers to mimic the aerosolized atmosphere. The viral load remained active for 3 h even though their virulent capacity was reduced [97]. Similarly, a double hit hypothesis has also been proposed initially in which NO_2 and $PM_{2.5}$ are considered responsible for coronavirus spread [19]. Particulate matter ($PM_{2.5}$) stabilizes the exhaled droplets in the air after fusing with them. The droplet would have evaporated rapidly in the atmosphere under normal air conditions but in high PM concentration, PM stabilizes the droplet and reduces its diffusion coefficient making it more transmissible. Moreover, a study conducted on mice supported the hypothesis that increased exposure to PM promoted the ACE2 and transmembrane-protease serine2 (TMPRSS2) production in macrophages and angiotensin-receptor type 2 (AT2) in lung tissues. This increase made the mice more susceptible to SARS-CoV-2 [101]. The studies conducted here supported the hypothesis that regions with a high concentration of air pollution are more affected by the coronavirus. Some of these studies are listed in Table 9.

From the above studies, it can be summarized that pollutants especially NO_2 and PM are strongly responsible for respiratory disorders in humans. Similarly, SARS-CoV-2 is also associated with respiratory disorders. Therefore, the existence of air pollutants and coronavirus at a time can prove to be fatal as described in the earlier studies.

Table 9. Studies correlating high COVID-19 incidences to the high rates of air pollution.

Region	Study	References
England	This study suggested that people who have been exposed to chronic levels of air pollution may have a high instance of contracting severe COVID-19. This may be attributed to the weakening of immune defense protocol by air pollution. It has also been suggested that mortality of COVID-19 may also be associated with cytokine storm syndrome, a response of the immune system that ascends to the chain of destructive events in the body and eventually causes death.	[102]
France	A correlation between air pollution and COVID-19 hospitalization maps has been studied. It was evident that areas with high requirements of hospitalization due to COVID-19 have also profound levels of $PM_{2.5}$.	[103]
Czech Republic	In industrialized regions, high air pollution trends correlate with COVID-19 hospitality.	[103]
Poland	Mazowieckie Voivodship, Upper Silesian Voivodship, and Lower Silesian Voivodship hold a maximum number of COVID-19 cases. All these regions have $PM_{2.5}$ concentrations in the range 19.58–29.84 $\mu g/m^3$ which is higher than those set by WHO i.e., 25$\mu g/m^3$.	[104]
United States	Just 1 $\mu g/m^3$ increase in $PM_{2.5}$ concentration causes a 15% increase in COVID-19 fatality rates.	[105]
United States	The increase of 4.6 ppb in a concentration of NO_2 caused an increase in the mortality rate of COVID-19 up to 16.2%. If this 4.6 ppb concentration could been reduced it would have prevented 14,000 deaths of COVID-19 patients.	[106]
United Kingdom	Out of the first 44,000 deaths of COVID-19, 6,100 (14%) deaths could be attributed to air pollution.	[107]
Germany	Long term exposure to air pollution is involved in 26% of COVID-19 fatalities.	[108]
Lima	A higher concentration of $PM_{2.5}$ is responsible for the increase in COVID-19 cases however it does not affect the rate of COVID-19 fatalities.	[109]
Italy	Most COVID-19 affected regions had a high concentration of $PM_{2.5}$ and PM_{10} during February 2020.	[110]

8. Impact of Lockdown on Smog

Since the 15th of December 2019, transmission from patients to medical care staff has happened, which shows that human-to-human transmission has occurred through close contact [111]. Most nations have forced city lockdown also, quarantine measures to diminish transmission to manage the epidemic. Public danger correspondence exercises have been performed to improve public attention to self-insurance [112]. The Chinese government has step by step executed a severe lockdown on Wuhan and encompassing urban areas as of 23 January 2020. Not before long, the Government of India also reported a total cross-country lockdown, from the 24th of March 2020. All industries, entertainment centers have been temporarily shut down. Domestic as well as all international flights have been suspended, trains and public transport have been temporarily banned [113].

The lockdowns imposed by governments all around the world have caused economical and financial instability. However, due to lockdowns 30% reduction in air pollutants have been evident in COVID-19 epicenters like Brazil, the USA, Spain, Italy, Wuhan according to reports of the Center for Research on Energy and Clean Air (CREA), European Space Agency (ESA), and National Aeronautics and Space Administration (NASA). NASA and ESA have reported a substantial drop of 2.5µ diameter in ($PM_{2.5}$ and PM_{10}) in Beijing, China where most of the pollution comes from heating instruments in the winters and heavy industrialization [24]. During the time of lockdown, air quality and smog conditions would be predicted to have improved in favor of life being. Due to traffic and industrial lockdown, a fall of ~63% in the concentration of NO_2 is evident in Wuhan, China. This fall in NO_2 concentration resulted in fewer deaths of people in Wuhan (496 deaths prevented), Hubei (3368 deaths prevented), and in China (10,822 deaths prevented). Similarly, a shortfall of 20 $\mu g/m^3$ in PM_{10} concentration is also observed in Wuhan. However, no reduction was noticed in SO_2 and CO concentration because of the dependence of the country on coal-based energy plants [114].

Another study conducted over Pakistan stated a decrease of 7.39% in $PM_{2.5}$ and 4.13–5.78% drop in column aerosol optical thickness (AOT) [115]. Hernandez-Paniagua and his colleagues concluded that due to the lockdown of motor vehicles, the concentration of NO_2 and $PM_{2.5}$ decrease significantly in Mexico. However, other pollutants concentration remains almost undisturbed except for an increase in O_3 concentration [116]. In Ontario, Canada NO and NO_2 concentration decreased rapidly while O_3 concentration decreased slowly but $PM_{2.5}$ remained the same [117]. Madrid, Spain faced a downfall in NO_2 concentration by 62% [118]. In Gujarat, India 30–84% reduction in NO_2 occurred while O_3 increased by 16–58% [119]. The atmosphere of Delhi, India got rid of 55% of PM_{10}, 49% of $PM_{2.5}$, 60% of NO_2, and 19% of SO_2 while Mumbai, India got rid of 44% of PM_{10}, 37% of $PM_{2.5}$, 78% of NO_2 and 39% of SO_2 [120]. Some figures before and after lockdown are listed in Table 10.

Table 10. Relative percentage difference of pollutants before and during the lockdown in different regions of the world [115].

Pollutants	Region	Before Lockdown	During Lockdown	Relative Percentage Difference (%)
SO_2 ($\mu g/m^3$)	Hubei (China)	15.81	13.83	−13.36
SO_2 (DU) [1]	Malaysia	1.42	0.99	−35.68
	Sale (Morocco)	6.6	3.3	−0.49
	Chennai (India)	44.1	45.2	−2.46
	Delhi (India)	1.03	0.72	−30.35
CO (ppbv) [2]	Hubei (China)	1.207	1.02	−16.79
	Kolkata (India)	0.6	0.5	−18.18
	Malaysia	0.8	0.49	−48.06
	Chennai (India)	29.38	27.33	−7.23
	Delhi (India)	80.51	37.75	−53.11
$PM_{2.5}$	Hubei (China)	81.83	65.81	−21.70
	Malaysia	32.3	22.34	−36.46
	Sao Paulo (Brazil)	12.9	12.5	−3.6
	Wuhan (China)	65.5	40.11	−48.08

[1] DU: Dosbin Unit, ppbv: [2] Parts per billion by volume

After the lockdown of city traffic, workforce stream control turned into the main perspective. Traffic contamination produces NO, NO_2, CO, CO_2, hydrocarbons, and toxins that are injurious to health [121]. There was a distinguishable relationship between traffic-associated air contamination and early mortality, and the danger of respiratory and cardiovascular diseases enlarged in people living close to elevated traffic polluted places [122]. Decreasing the outflows from engine vehicles, particularly trucks and transports, could deliver extensive medical advantages [123]. After lockdown, many surveys were done in hospitals which showed that after a consecutive lockdown of 14 days there was seen a major decline in children in hospitals complaining of asthma problems [124]. In accretion, the decrease in industrial actions after the lockdown also forces definite environmental and health effects. The lockdown has caused financial downfalls in many countries and cities, but it also has given clean air to residents of some of the world's most contaminated cities. The coronavirus pandemic has led to the decrease in the concentration of pollutants like SO_2, NO_2, CO, $PM_{2.5}$ that contribute to smog all over the world and to some extend have enhanced the air quality in most of the polluted cities of the world [125,126].

9. Limitations of the Study

This is a narrative literature review that provides a simple insight into the relation between air pollution and coronavirus in large representative populations. The key limitation of this review is that the individual-level risk factors like race, age, and smoking status are not included. Moreover, chances of miscalculation are always there because during the study we assumed that all people in the region are exposed to equal concentrations of air pollution. The relation between smog and COVID-19 is based on area-level studies so the data is useful to develop coping strategies against the situation in a specific area.

10. Conclusions

Human activities like the burning of fossil fuels, coal combustion, and the smoke from exhausts of automobiles release toxic gases which react in the atmosphere and give rise to secondary pollutants. All these pollutants collectively contribute to smog. Each year rise in respiratory disease is related to smog episodes. Moreover, cardiovascular diseases, neurological disorders, underdevelopment of fetuses, and cancer are the major diseases that are related to smog pollution. Smog episodes can have deleterious effects amidst the COVID-19 pandemic. When a person is long exposed to air pollution, the coronavirus would have an additive effect on the respiratory and cardiovascular systems of the human. From the studies conducted it seems that particulate matter and nitrogen oxides increase the activity and production of ACE2 which in turn enhances the chances of uptake of SARS-CoV-2 and could damage lungs, heart, and blood vessels. However, the relation between smog and coronavirus isn't this. They share an ambiguous relation where on the one hand air pollution may worsen the COVID-19 mortality rate, the lockdown imposed because of a pandemic may have some positive aspects as well. During the lockdown periods, a significant decrease in some of the pollutants like NO_2, SO_2, and PM have been recorded. For a better future, anthropogenic emissions need to be controlled because vaccines are effective against pandemics and not against air pollution.

Author Contributions: Writing—review and editing, A.J. and F.A.; visualization, A.J. and F.A.; supervision, U.F.G. and R.A.M.; project administration, H.M.; investigation, M.Z.-U.-H. and M.O.A.; formal analysis, M.N.B.-J. and O.L.P. All authors have read and agreed to the published version of the manuscript.

Funding: This research was partially funded by UEFISCDI, grant number PN-III-P4-IDPCE-2020-2126 and FDI-0013.

Institutional Review Board Statement: Not applicable.

Informed Consent Statement: Not applicable.

Data Availability Statement: No new data were created or analyzed in this study. Data sharing does not apply to this article.

Acknowledgments: We thank the Institute of Industrial Biotechnology, Government College University Lahore, Pakistan for providing moral and technical support.

Conflicts of Interest: The authors declare no conflict of interest.

References

1. Ali, Y.; Razi, M.; De Felice, F.; Sabir, M.; Petrillo, A. A VIKOR based approach for assessing the social, environmental and economic effects of "smog" on human health. *Sci. Total Environ.* **2019**, *650*, 2897–2905. [CrossRef]
2. Laskin, D. The Great London Smog. *Weatherwise* **2006**, *59*, 42–45. [CrossRef]
3. Shah, A.S.V.; Langrish, J.P.; Nair, H.; McAllister, D.A.; Hunter, A.L.; Donaldson, K.; Newby, D.E.; Mills, N.L. Global association of air pollution and heart failure: A systematic review and meta-analysis. *Lancet* **2013**, *382*, 1039–1048. [CrossRef]
4. Ashraf, A.; Butt, A.; Khalid, I.; Alam, R.U.; Ahmad, S.R. Smog analysis and its effect on reported ocular surface diseases: A case study of 2016 smog event of Lahore. *Atmos. Environ.* **2019**, *198*, 257–264. [CrossRef]

5. Hidy, G.M. An historical experiment: Los Angeles smog evolution observed by blimp. *J. Air Waste Manag. Assoc.* **2018**, *68*, 643–655. [CrossRef]
6. Gohar, U.F.; Iqbal, I.; Shah, Z.; Mukhtar, H.; Zia-Ul-Haq, M. COVID-19: Recent Developments in Therapeutic Approaches. In *Alternative Medicine Interventions for COVID-19*; Zia-Ul-Haq, M., Bin-Jumah, M.N., Alothamn, S.I., Henidi, H.A., Eds.; Springer: Cham, Switzerland, 2021; pp. 249–274.
7. Soto-Coloballes, N. The Development of Air Pollution in Mexico City. *SAGE Open* **2020**, *10*, 2158244020931072. [CrossRef]
8. Tang, D. A Comparison of Control Methods of Air Pollution in London and Beijing. *Int. J. Environ. Sci. Dev.* **2019**, *10*, 141–150. [CrossRef]
9. Yadav, S.; Rawal, G. The great Delhi smog. *Indian J. Immunol. Respir. Med.* **2016**, *1*, 78–79.
10. Mishra, S. Is smog innocuous? Air pollution and cardiovascular disease. *Indian Heart J.* **2017**, *69*, 425–429. [CrossRef]
11. Stafoggia, M.; Schwartz, J.; Forastiere, F.; Perucci, C.A. Does temperature modify the association between air pollution and mortality? A multicity case-crossover analysis in Italy. *Am. J. Epidemiol.* **2008**, *167*, 1476–1485. [CrossRef]
12. Yang, H.; Li, S.; Sun, L.; Zhang, X.; Cao, Z.; Xu, C.; Cao, X.; Cheng, Y.; Yan, T.; Liu, T.; et al. Smog and risk of overall and type-specific cardiovascular diseases: A pooled analysis of 53 cohort studies with 21.09 million participants. *Environ. Res.* **2019**, *172*, 375–383. [CrossRef]
13. Altindag, D.T.; Baek, D.; Mocan, N. Chinese Yellow Dust and Korean infant health. *Soc. Sci. Med.* **2017**, *186*, 78–86. [CrossRef]
14. Maher, A.; Abdel Rahman, M.F.; Gad, M.Z. The role of nitric oxide from neurological disease to cancer. *Adv. Exp. Med. Biol.* **2017**, *1007*, 71–88. [CrossRef]
15. Ontawong, A.; Saokaew, S.; Jamroendararasame, B.; Duangjai, A. Impact of long-term exposure wildfire smog on respiratory health outcomes. *Expert Rev. Respir. Med.* **2020**, *14*, 527–531. [CrossRef]
16. Cao, Y.; Chen, M.; Dong, D.; Xie, S.; Liu, M. Environmental pollutants damage airway epithelial cell cilia: Implications for the prevention of obstructive lung diseases. *Thorac. Cancer* **2020**, *11*, 505–510. [CrossRef]
17. Zia-Ul-Haq, M. Past, present and future of Carotenoids Research. In *Carotenoids: Structure and Function in the Human Body*; Zia-Ul-Haq, M., Dewanjee, S., Riaz, M., Eds.; Springer: Cham, Switzerland, 2021; pp. 827–854.
18. Conticini, E.; Frediani, B.; Caro, D. Can atmospheric pollution be considered a co-factor in extremely high level of SARS-CoV-2 lethality in Northern Italy? *Environ. Pollut.* **2020**, *261*, 114465. [CrossRef]
19. Paital, B.; Kumar, P. Air pollution by NO_2 and $PM_{2.5}$ explains COVID-19 infection severity by overexpression of angiotensin—converting enzyme 2 in respiratory cells: A review. *Environ. Chem. Lett.* **2021**, *19*, 25–42. [CrossRef]
20. Mele, M.; Magazzino, C.; Schneider, N.; Strezov, V. NO_2 levels as a contributing factor to COVID-19 deaths: The first empirical estimate of threshold values. *Environ. Res.* **2021**, *194*, 110663. [CrossRef]
21. Zia-Ul-Haq, M. Historical and introductory aspects of carotenoids. In *Carotenoids: Structure and Function in the Human Body*; Zia-Ul-Haq, M., Dewanjee, S., Riaz, M., Eds.; Springer: Cham, Switzerland, 2021; pp. 1–42.
22. Leung, W.W.F.; Sun, Q. Electrostatic charged nanofiber filter for filtering airborne novel coronavirus (COVID-19) and nano-aerosols. *Sep. Purif. Technol.* **2020**, *250*, 116886. [CrossRef]
23. Domingo, J.L.; Rovira, J. Effects of air pollutants on the transmission and severity of respiratory viral infections. *Environ. Res.* **2020**, *187*, 109650. [CrossRef]
24. Dutheil, F.; Navel, V.; Clinchamps, M. The Indirect Benefit on Respiratory Health From the World's Effort to Reduce Transmission of SARS-CoV-2. *Chest* **2020**, *158*, 467–468. [CrossRef] [PubMed]
25. Nemery, B.; Hoet, P.H.M.; Nemmar, A. Department of medical history The Meuse Valley fog of 1930: An air pollution disaster. *Lancet* **2001**, *357*, 704–708. [CrossRef]
26. Firket, J. Fog along the Meuse valley. *Cornell Univ. Libr.* **1978**, *68*, 1421–1448. [CrossRef]
27. Tim, B.Y.; St, O.N. 28 November 1939: The Day "Black Tuesday" Rolled into St. Louis. Available online: https://www.stltoday.com/news/local/history/nov-28-1939-the-day-black-tuesday-rolled-into-st-louis/article_00c3b6cd-ba69-5a19-b498-fbc29f9630c4.html (accessed on 20 October 2021).
28. Johnson, H.R.; Johnson, H.R. *$PM_{2.5}$ Pollution and Temperature Inversions: A Case Study in St. Louis, MO*; Iowa State University: Ames, IA, USA, 2018.
29. Tucker-, R.R. Smoke prevention in St. Louis. *Ind. Eng. Chem.* **1941**, *33*, 836–839. [CrossRef]
30. Hoffman, D.G. Three Ballads of the Donora Smog. *N. Y. Folkl. Q.* **1949**, *5*, 51.
31. Helfand, W.H.; Lazarus, J.; Theerman, P. Donora, Pennsylvania: An environmental disaster of the 20th century. *Am. J. Public Health* **2001**, *91*, 553. [CrossRef]
32. Zia-Ul-Haq, M.; Riaz, M.; Ahmedah, H.T. Carotenoids and Periodontal Diseases. In *Carotenoids: Structure and Function in the Human Body*; Zia-Ul-Haq, M., Dewanjee, S., Riaz, M., Eds.; Springer: Cham, Switzerland, 2021; pp. 715–720.
33. Ball, A. Air pollution, foetal mortality, and long-term health: Evidence from the Great London Smog. *Munich Pers. RePEc Arch. Eurpean Univ. Inst.* **2015**.
34. Polivka, B.J. The Great London Smog of 1952. *Am. J. Nurs.* **2018**, *118*, 57–61. [CrossRef]
35. Bell, M.L.; Davis, D.L. Reassessment of the lethal London fog of 1952: Novel indicators of acute and chronic consequences of acute exposure to air pollution. *Environ. Health Perspect.* **2001**, *109*, 389–394. [CrossRef]
36. Czerwińska, J.; Wielgosiński, G. The effect of selected meteorological factors on the process of "Polish smog" formation. *J. Ecol. Eng.* **2020**, *21*, 180–187. [CrossRef]

37. Czerwińska, J.; Wielgosiński, G.; Szymańska, O. Is the Polish Smog a New Type of Smog? *Ecol. Chem. Eng. S* **2019**, *26*, 465–474. [CrossRef]
38. Loyola, D.; Van Geffen, J.; Valks, P.; Erbertseder, T.; Van Roozendael, M.; Thomas, W.; Zimmer, W.; Wißkirchen, K. Satellite-based detection of volcanic sulphur dioxide from recent eruptions in Central and South America. *Adv. Geosci.* **2008**, *14*, 35–40. [CrossRef]
39. Vecchiato, M.; Bonato, T.; Bertin, A.; Argiriadis, E.; Barbante, C.; Piazza, R. Plant Residues as Direct and Indirect Sources of Hydrocarbons in Soils: Current Issues and Legal Implications. *Environ. Sci. Technol. Lett.* **2017**, *4*, 512–517. [CrossRef]
40. Dewulf, J.; Langenhove, H. Van Hydrocarbons in the atmosphere. In *Environmental and Ecological Chemistry; Encyclopedia of Life Support Systems (EOLSS)*; Unesco: Paris, France, 2000; Volume 2.
41. Hallquist, M.; Munthe, J.; Hu, M.; Wang, T.; Chan, C.K.; Gao, J.; Boman, J.; Guo, S.; Hallquist, A.M.; Mellqvist, J.; et al. Photochemical smog in China: Scientific challenges and implications for air-quality policies. *Natl. Sci. Rev.* **2016**, *3*, 401–403. [CrossRef]
42. Zia-Ul-Haq, M.; Riaz, M.; Modhi, A.O. Carotenoids and Bone Health. In *Carotenoids: Structure and Function in the Human Body*; Zia-Ul-Haq, M., Dewanjee, S., Riaz, M., Eds.; Springer: Cham, Switzerland, 2021; pp. 697–713.
43. Tofte, K.; Chu, P.S.; Barnes, G.M. Large-scale weather patterns favorable for volcanic smog occurrences on O'ahu, Hawai'i. *Air Qual. Atmos. Health* **2017**, *10*, 1163–1180. [CrossRef]
44. Wang, H.; Wang, Q.; Gao, Y.; Zhou, M.; Jing, S.; Qiao, L.; Yuan, B.; Huang, D.; Huang, C.; Lou, S.; et al. Estimation of Secondary Organic Aerosol Formation During a Photochemical Smog Episode in Shanghai, China. *J. Geophys. Res. Atmos.* **2020**, *125*, 1–14. [CrossRef]
45. Yin, S.; Zhang, X.; Yu, A.; Sun, N.; Lyu, J.; Zhu, P.; Liu, C. Determining $PM_{2.5}$ dry deposition velocity on plant leaves: An indirect experimental method. *Urban For. Urban Green.* **2019**, *46*, 126467. [CrossRef]
46. Carmona-Cabezas, R.; Gómez-Gómeiaz, J.; Gutiérrez de Ravé, E.; Jiménez-Hornero, F.J. Checking complex networks indicators in search of singular episodes of the photochemical smog. *Chemosphere* **2020**, *241*, 125085. [CrossRef]
47. Read, C.; Parton, K.A. The impact of the 1952 London smog event and its relevance for current wood-smoke abatement strategies in Australia. *J. Air Waste Manag. Assoc.* **2019**, *69*, 1049–1058. [CrossRef] [PubMed]
48. Burchard-Dziubińska, M. Air pollution and health in Poland: Anti-smog movement in the most polluted Polish cities. *Ekon. Sr.* **2019**, *2*, 76–90. [CrossRef]
49. Karmakar, A.; Das, A.K.; Ghosh, S.; Sil, P.C. Carotenoids as Coloring Agents. In *Carotenoids: Structure and Function in the Human Body*; Zia-Ul-Haq, M., Dewanjee, S., Riaz, M., Eds.; Springer: Cham, Switzerland, 2021.
50. Yu, Y.; Shen, M.; Shen, W.; Zhang, X. Effects of land urbanization on smog pollution in China: Estimation of spatial autoregressive panel data models. *Land* **2020**, *9*, 337. [CrossRef]
51. Air Pollution Linked to 1.2 Million Deaths in China—The New York Times. Available online: https://www.nytimes.com/2013/04/02/world/asia/air-pollution-linked-to-1-2-million-deaths-in-china.html (accessed on 13 July 2021).
52. Xu, Q.; Li, X.; Wang, S.; Wang, C.; Huang, F.; Gao, Q.; Wu, L.; Tao, L.; Guo, J.; Wang, W. Fine particulate air pollution and hospital emergency room visits for respiratory disease in urban areas in Beijing, China, in 2013. *PLoS ONE* **2016**, *11*, e0153099. [CrossRef]
53. Zhou, M.; He, G.; Fan, M.; Wang, Z.; Liu, Y.; Ma, J.; Ma, Z.; Liu, J.; Liu, Y.; Wang, L.; et al. Smog episodes, fine particulate pollution and mortality in China. *Environ. Res.* **2015**, *136*, 396–404. [CrossRef] [PubMed]
54. China Air Quality Index (AQI) and Air Pollution information | AirVisual. Available online: https://www.iqair.com/us/china (accessed on 13 July 2021).
55. Maji, K.J.; Li, V.O.K.; Lam, J.C.K. Effects of China's current Air Pollution Prevention and Control Action Plan on air pollution patterns, health risks and mortalities in Beijing 2014–2018. *Chemosphere* **2020**, *260*, 127572. [CrossRef] [PubMed]
56. Trnka, D. Policies, regulatory framework and enforcement for air quality management: The case of Korea. *OECD Environ. Work. Pap.* **2020**. [CrossRef]
57. Jin, Y.H.; Cai, L.; Cheng, Z.S.; Cheng, H.; Deng, T.; Fan, Y.P.; Fang, C.; Huang, D.; Huang, L.Q.; Huang, Q.; et al. A rapid advice guideline for the diagnosis and treatment of 2019 novel coronavirus (2019-nCoV) infected pneumonia (standard version). *Mil. Med. Res.* **2020**, *7*, 4. [CrossRef]
58. Longhurst, J.W.S.; Barnes, J.H.; Chatterton, T.J.; Hayes, E.T.; Williams, W.B. Progress with air quality management in the 60 years since the UK clean air act, 1956. Lessons, failures, challenges and opportunities. *Int. J. Sustain. Dev. Plan.* **2016**, *11*, 491–499. [CrossRef]
59. Burakowski, E.A.; Ollinger, S.V.; Bonan, G.B.; Wake, C.P.; Dibb, J.E.; Hollinger, D.Y. Evaluating the climate effects of reforestation in New England using a Weather Research and Forecasting (WRF) model multiphysics ensemble. *J. Clim.* **2016**, *29*, 5141–5156. [CrossRef]
60. England Air Quality Index (AQI) and United Kingdom Air Pollution | AirVisual. Available online: https://www.iqair.com/uk/england (accessed on 13 July 2021).
61. Crippa, M.; Janssens-Maenhout, G.; Dentener, F.; Guizzardi, D.; Sindelarova, K.; Muntean, M.; Van Dingenen, R.; Granier, C. Forty years of improvements in European air quality: Regional policy-industry interactions with global impacts. *Atmos. Chem. Phys.* **2016**, *16*, 3825–3841. [CrossRef]
62. Bin-Jumah, M.; Alwakeel, S.S.; Moga, M.; Buvnariu, L.; Bigiu, N.; Zia-Ul-Haq, M. Application of Carotenoids in Cosmetics. In *Carotenoids: Structure and Function in the Human Body*; Zia-Ul-Haq, M., Dewanjee, S., Riaz, M., Eds.; Springer: Cham, Switzerland, 2021.

63. EU: Air Quality Standards | Transport Policy. Available online: https://www.transportpolicy.net/standard/eu-air-quality-standards/ (accessed on 7 September 2021).
64. Air Pollution Facts, Causes and the Effects of Pollutants in the Air | NRDC. Available online: https://www.nrdc.org/stories/air-pollution-everything-you-need-know (accessed on 13 July 2021).
65. USA Air Quality Index (AQI) and Air Pollution Information | AirVisual. Available online: https://www.iqair.com/usa (accessed on 13 July 2021).
66. World Air Quality Index (AQI) Ranking | AirVisual. Available online: https://www.iqair.com/world-air-quality-ranking (accessed on 13 July 2021).
67. Kuklinska, K.; Wolska, L.; Namiesnik, J. Air quality policy in the U.S. and the EU—A review. *Atmos. Pollut. Res.* **2015**, *6*, 129–137. [CrossRef]
68. Evolution of the Clean Air Act | US EPA. Available online: https://www.epa.gov/clean-air-act-overview/evolution-clean-air-act (accessed on 7 September 2021).
69. NAAQS Table | US EPA. Available online: https://www.epa.gov/criteria-air-pollutants/naaqs-table (accessed on 7 September 2021).
70. Wang, C.; Horby, P.W.; Hayden, F.G.; Gao, G.F. A novel coronavirus outbreak of global health concern. *Lancet* **2020**, *395*, 470–473. [CrossRef]
71. COVID Live Update: 222,812,592 Cases and 4,601,142 Deaths from the Coronavirus—Worldometer. Available online: https://www.worldometers.info/coronavirus/#countries (accessed on 7 September 2021).
72. Richman, D.; Whitely, R.; Hayden, F.G. *Clinical Virology*, 4th ed.; Wiley: Hoboken, NJ, USA, 2016.
73. Chen, N.; Zhou, M.; Dong, X.; Qu, J.; Gong, F.; Han, Y.; Qiu, Y.; Wang, J.; Liu, Y.; Wei, Y.; et al. Epidemiological and Clinical Characteristics of 99 Cases of 2019 Novel Coronavirus Pneumonia in Wuhan, China: A Descript. *Lancet* **2020**, *395*, 507–513. [CrossRef]
74. Muralidar, S.; Visaga, S.; Sekaran, S. Since January 2020 Elsevier has created a COVID-19 resource centre with free information in English and Mandarin on the novel coronavirus COVID-19. The COVID-19 resource centre is hosted on Elsevier Connect, the company's public news and information. *Biochimie* **2020**, *179*, 85–100. [CrossRef]
75. Rothe, C.; Schunk, M.; Sothmann, P.; Bretzel, G.; Froeschl, G.; Wallrauch, C.; Zimmer, T.; Thiel, V.; Janke, C.; Guggemos, W.; et al. Transmission of 2019-nCoV Infection from an Asymptomatic Contact in Germany. *N. Engl. J. Med.* **2020**, *382*, 970–971. [CrossRef]
76. World Health Organization. *Clinical Management of Severe Acute Respiratory Infection When Novel Coronavirus (2019-nCoV) Infection Is Suspected: Interim Guidance 28 January 2020*; WHO: Geneva, Switzerland, 2020; p. 10.
77. Becker, S.; Soukup, J.M. Exposure to urban air particulates alters the macrophage-mediated inflammatory response to respiratory viral infection. *J. Toxicol. Environ. Health-Part A* **1999**, *57*, 445–457. [CrossRef]
78. Cai, Q.C.; Lu, J.; Xu, Q.F.; Guo, Q.; Xu, D.Z.; Sun, Q.W.; Yang, H.; Zhao, G.M.; Jiang, Q.W. Influence of meteorological factors and air pollution on the outbreak of severe acute respiratory syndrome. *Public Health* **2007**, *121*, 258–265. [CrossRef]
79. Valavanidis, A.; Vlachogianni, T.; Fiotakis, K.; Loridas, S. Pulmonary oxidative stress, inflammation and cancer: Respirable particulate matter, fibrous dusts and ozone as major causes of lung carcinogenesis through reactive oxygen species mechanisms. *Int. J. Environ. Res. Public Health* **2013**, *10*, 3886–3907. [CrossRef] [PubMed]
80. Coneus, K.; Spiess, C.K. Pollution exposure and child health: Evidence for infants and toddlers in Germany. *J. Health Econ.* **2012**, *31*, 180–196. [CrossRef]
81. Gehring, U.; Wijga, A.H.; Hoek, G.; Bellander, T.; Berdel, D.; Brüske, I.; Fuertes, E.; Gruzieva, O.; Heinrich, J.; Hoffmann, B.; et al. Exposure to air pollution and development of asthma and rhinoconjunctivitis throughout childhood and adolescence: A population-based birth cohort study. *Lancet Respir. Med.* **2015**, *3*, 933–942. [CrossRef]
82. Camara, J.G.; Lagunzad, J.K.D. Ocular findings in volcanic fog induced conjunctivitis. *Hawaii Med. J.* **2011**, *70*, 262–265.
83. Longo, B.M. Adverse Health Effects Associated with Increased Activity at Kīlauea Volcano: A Repeated Population-Based Survey. *ISRN Public Health* **2013**, *2013*, 475962. [CrossRef]
84. Williams-Jones, G.; Rymer, H. *Hazards of Volcanic Gases*, 2nd ed.; Elsevier Inc.: Amsterdam, The Netherlands, 2015; ISBN 9780123859389.
85. Folabi, T.; Phan, T. Evaluation of Volatile Organic Compounds and Polyaromatic Hydrocarbons in Barker Reservoir in Houston, Texas after the 2017 Hurricane Harvey. *Am. J. Anal. Chem.* **2020**, *11*, 376–388. [CrossRef]
86. Zhang, B.; Zhao, B.; Zuo, P.; Huang, Z.; Zhang, J. Influencing factors and prediction of ambient Peroxyacetyl nitrate concentration in Beijing, China. *J. Environ. Sci.* **2019**, *77*, 189–197. [CrossRef] [PubMed]
87. Munawer, M.E. Human health and environmental impacts of coal combustion and post-combustion wastes. *J. Sustain. Min.* **2018**, *17*, 87–96. [CrossRef]
88. Lai, L.W. Effect of photochemical smog associated with synoptic weather patterns on cardiovascular and respiratory hospital admissions in metropolitan Taipei. *Int. J. Environ. Health Res.* **2012**, *22*, 287–304. [CrossRef] [PubMed]
89. Samet, J.M. Ozone and respiratory health the story continues. *Am. J. Respir. Crit. Care Med.* **2015**, *192*, 272–273. [CrossRef] [PubMed]
90. Zhang, J.; Chen, Q.; Wang, Q.; Ding, Z.; Sun, H.; Xu, Y. The acute health effects of ozone and $PM_{2.5}$ on daily cardiovascular disease mortality: A multi-center time series study in China. *Ecotoxicol. Environ. Saf.* **2019**, *174*, 218–223. [CrossRef]
91. Mukherjee, A.; Agrawal, M. World air particulate matter: Sources, distribution and health effects. *Environ. Chem. Lett.* **2017**, *15*, 283–309. [CrossRef]

92. Liao, B.Q.; Liu, C.B.; Xie, S.J.; Liu, Y.; Deng, Y.B.; He, S.W.; Fu, X.P.; Fu, B.B.; Wang, Y.L.; Chen, M.H.; et al. Effects of fine particulate matter ($PM_{2.5}$) on ovarian function and embryo quality in mice. *Environ. Int.* **2020**, *135*, 105338. [CrossRef]
93. Zou, X.; Chen, K.; Zou, J.; Han, P.; Hao, J.; Han, Z. Single-cell RNA-seq data analysis on the receptor ACE2 expression reveals the potential risk of different human organs vulnerable to 2019-nCoV infection. *Front. Med.* **2020**, *14*, 185–192. [CrossRef]
94. Bunyavanich, S.; Do, A.; Vicencio, A. Nasal Gene Expression of Angiotensin-Converting Enzyme 2 in Children and Adults. *JAMA—J. Am. Med. Assoc.* **2020**, *323*, 2427–2429. [CrossRef] [PubMed]
95. Zheng, K.I.; Feng, G.; Liu, W.-Y.; Targher, G.; Byrne, C.D.; Zheng, M.-H. Extrapulmonary complications of COVID-19: A multisystem disease? *J. Med. Virol.* **2021**, *93*, 323–335. [CrossRef] [PubMed]
96. Brooke, J.; Jackson, D. Older people and COVID-19: Isolation, risk and ageism. *J. Clin. Nurs.* **2020**, *29*, 2044–2046. [CrossRef] [PubMed]
97. Van Doremalen, N.; Bushmaker, T.; Morris, D.H.; Holbrook, M.G.; Gamble, A.; Williamson, B.N.; Tamin, A.; Harcourt, J.L.; Thornburg, N.J.; Gerber, S.I. Aerosol and surface stability of SARS-CoV-2 as compared with SARS-CoV-1. *N. Engl. J. Med.* **2020**, *382*, 1564–1567. [CrossRef] [PubMed]
98. Manisalidis, I.; Stavropoulou, E.; Stavropoulos, A.; Bezirtzoglou, E. Environmental and Health Impacts of Air Pollution: A Review. *Front. Public Health* **2020**, *8*, 14. [CrossRef] [PubMed]
99. Gupta, A.; Bherwani, H.; Gautam, S.; Anjum, S.; Musugu, K.; Kumar, N.; Anshul, A.; Kumar, R. Air pollution aggravating COVID-19 lethality? Exploration in Asian cities using statistical models. *Environ. Dev. Sustain.* **2020**, *23*, 6408–6417. [CrossRef] [PubMed]
100. Bourouiba, L. Turbulent Gas Clouds and Respiratory Pathogen Emissions: Potential Implications for Reducing Transmission of COVID-19. *JAMA—J. Am. Med. Assoc.* **2020**, *323*, 1837–1838. [CrossRef] [PubMed]
101. Sagawa, T.; Tsujikawa, T.; Honda, A.; Miyasaka, N.; Tanaka, M.; Kida, T.; Hasegawa, K.; Okuda, T.; Yatuka, K.; Takano, H. Exposure to particulate matter upregulates ACE2 and TMPRSS2 expression in the murine lung. *Environ. Res.* **2021**, *195*, 110722. [CrossRef]
102. Travaglio, M.; Yu, Y.; Popovic, R.; Selley, L.; Leal, N.S.; Martins, L.M. Links between air pollution and COVID-19 in England. *Environ. Pollut.* **2021**, *268*, 115859. [CrossRef] [PubMed]
103. Why Air Pollution Is Linked to a Faster Spread of Coronavirus—AirQualityNews. Available online: https://airqualitynews.com/2020/04/09/why-air-pollution-is-linked-to-a-faster-spread-of-coronavirus/ (accessed on 9 September 2021).
104. Urrutia-Pereira, M.; Mello-da-Silva, C.A.; Solé, D. COVID-19 and air pollution: A dangerous association? *Allergol. Immunopathol. (Madr).* **2020**, *48*, 496–499. [CrossRef]
105. Wu, X.; Nethery, R.C.; Sabath, B.M.; Braun, D.; Dominici, F. Exposure to air pollution and COVID-19 mortality in the United States: A nationwide cross-sectional study. *medRxiv Prepr. Serv. Health Sci.* **2005**. [CrossRef]
106. Understanding the Link between COVID-19 Mortality and Air Pollution | American Lung Association. Available online: https://www.lung.org/blog/covid-19-mortality-and-air-pollution (accessed on 9 September 2021).
107. Air Pollution as Co-Factor of Covid-19 Mortality | Max-Planck-Gesellschaft. Available online: https://www.mpg.de/15952279/1028-chem-099020-air-pollution-as-co-factor-of-covid-19-mortality (accessed on 9 September 2021).
108. Pozzer, A.; Dominici, F.; Haines, A.; Witt, C.; Münzel, T.; Lelieveld, J. Regional and global contributions of air pollution to risk of death from COVID-19. *Cardiovasc. Res.* **2020**, *116*, 2247–2253. [CrossRef]
109. Vasquez-Apestegui, B.V.; Parras-Garrido, E.; Tapia, V.; Paz-Aparicio, V.M.; Rojas, J.P.; Sanchez-Ccoyllo, O.R.; Gonzales, G.F. Association between air pollution in Lima and the high incidence of COVID-19: Findings from a post hoc analysis. *BMC Public Health* **2021**, *21*, 1161. [CrossRef] [PubMed]
110. Martelletti, L.; Martelletti, P. Air pollution and the novel Covid-19 disease: A putative disease risk factor. *SN Compr. Clin. Med.* **2020**, *2*, 383–387. [CrossRef]
111. Huang, C.; Wang, Y.; Li, X.; Ren, L.; Zhao, J.; Hu, Y.; Zhang, L.; Fan, G.; Xu, J.; Gu, X.; et al. Clinical features of patients infected with 2019 novel coronavirus in Wuhan, China. *Lancet* **2020**, *395*, 497–506. [CrossRef]
112. Hui, D.S.; Azhar, E.I.; Madani, T.A.; Ntoumi, F.; Kock, R.; Dar, O.; Ippolito, G.; Mchugh, T.D.; Memish, Z.A.; Drosten, C.; et al. The continuing 2019-nCoV epidemic threat of novel coronaviruses to global health—The latest 2019 novel coronavirus outbreak in Wuhan, China. *Int. J. Infect. Dis.* **2020**, *91*, 264–266. [CrossRef]
113. Wu, J.T.; Leung, K.; Leung, G.M. Nowcasting and forecasting the potential domestic and international spread of the 2019-nCoV outbreak originating in Wuhan, China: A modelling study. *Lancet* **2020**, *395*, 689–697. [CrossRef]
114. Cole, M.A.; Elliott, R.J.R.; Liu, B. The Impact of the Wuhan Covid-19 Lockdown on Air Pollution and Health: A Machine Learning and Augmented Synthetic Control Approach. *Environ. Resour. Econ.* **2020**, *76*, 553–580. [CrossRef]
115. Khan, R.; Kumar, K.R.; Zhao, T. The impact of lockdown on air quality in Pakistan during the covid-19 pandemic inferred from the multi-sensor remote sensed data. *Aerosol Air Qual. Res.* **2021**, *21*, 1–18. [CrossRef]
116. Hernández-Paniagua, I.Y.; Valdez, S.I.; Almanza, V.; Rivera-Cárdenas, C.; Grutter, M.; Stremme, W.; García-Reynoso, A.; Ruiz-Suárez, L.G. Impact of the COVID-19 Lockdown on Air Quality and Resulting Public Health Benefits in the Mexico City Metropolitan Area. *Front. Public Health* **2021**, *9*, 1–19. [CrossRef] [PubMed]
117. Adams, M.D. Air pollution in Ontario, Canada during the COVID-19 State of Emergency. *Sci. Total Environ.* **2020**, *742*, 140516. [CrossRef] [PubMed]

118. Baldasano, J.M. COVID-19 lockdown effects on air quality by NO_2 in the cities of Barcelona and Madrid (Spain). *Sci. Total Environ.* **2020**, *741*, 140353. [CrossRef]
119. Selvam, S.; Muthukumar, P.; Venkatramanan, S.; Roy, P.D.; Manikanda Bharath, K.; Jesuraja, K. SARS-CoV-2 pandemic lockdown: Effects on air quality in the industrialized Gujarat state of India. *Sci. Total Environ.* **2020**, *737*, 140391. [CrossRef] [PubMed]
120. Kumari, P.; Toshniwal, D. Impact of lockdown measures during COVID-19 on air quality—A case study of India. *Int. J. Environ. Health Res.* **2020**, 1–8. [CrossRef]
121. Beckerman, B.; Jerrett, M.; Brook, J.R.; Verma, D.K.; Arain, M.A.; Finkelstein, M.M. Correlation of nitrogen dioxide with other traffic pollutants near a major expressway. *Atmos. Environ.* **2008**, *42*, 275–290. [CrossRef]
122. Brugge, D.; Durant, J.L.; Rioux, C. Near-highway pollutants in motor vehicle exhaust: A review of epidemiologic evidence of cardiac and pulmonary health risks. *Environ. Health A Glob. Access Sci. Source* **2007**, *6*, 1–12. [CrossRef] [PubMed]
123. Kheirbek, I.; Haney, J.; Douglas, S.; Ito, K.; Matte, T. The contribution of motor vehicle emissions to ambient fine particulate matter public health impacts in New York City: A health burden assessment. *Environ. Health A Glob. Access Sci. Source* **2016**, *15*, 89. [CrossRef]
124. Lee, J.T.; Son, J.Y.; Cho, Y.S. Benefits of mitigated ambient air quality due to transportation control on childhood asthma hospitalization during the 2002 Summer Asian Games in Busan, Korea. *J. Air Waste Manag. Assoc.* **2007**, *57*, 968–973. [CrossRef]
125. Berman, J.D.; Ebisu, K. Changes in U.S. air pollution during the COVID-19 pandemic. *Sci. Total Environ.* **2020**, *739*, 139864. [CrossRef] [PubMed]
126. Ju, M.J.; Oh, J.; Choi, Y.H. Changes in air pollution levels after COVID-19 outbreak in Korea. *Sci. Total Environ.* **2021**, *750*, 141521. [CrossRef]

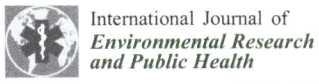

International Journal of *Environmental Research and Public Health*

Article

An Empirical Perception of Economic Resilience Responded to the COVID-19 Epidemic Outbreak in Beijing–Tianjin–Hebei Urban Agglomeration, China: Characterization and Interaction

Yaping Zhang [1], Jianjun Zhang [1,2,*], Ke Wang [1] and Xia Wu [1]

1. School of Land Science and Technology, China University of Geosciences (Beijing), Beijing 100083, China; zhangyp1007@163.com (Y.Z.); wangke11260@163.com (K.W.); alisonwuxia@126.com (X.W.)
2. Land Consolidation and Rehabilitation Center, Ministry of Natural and Resource, Beijing 100083, China
* Correspondence: zhangjianjun_bj@126.com or zhangjianjun@cugb.edu.cn

Citation: Zhang, Y.; Zhang, J.; Wang, K.; Wu, X. An Empirical Perception of Economic Resilience Responded to the COVID-19 Epidemic Outbreak in Beijing–Tianjin–Hebei Urban Agglomeration, China: Characterization and Interaction. *Int. J. Environ. Res. Public Health* **2021**, *18*, 10532. https://doi.org/10.3390/ijerph181910532

Academic Editor: Dirga Kumar Lamichhane

Received: 8 September 2021
Accepted: 3 October 2021
Published: 7 October 2021

Publisher's Note: MDPI stays neutral with regard to jurisdictional claims in published maps and institutional affiliations.

Copyright: © 2021 by the authors. Licensee MDPI, Basel, Switzerland. This article is an open access article distributed under the terms and conditions of the Creative Commons Attribution (CC BY) license (https://creativecommons.org/licenses/by/4.0/).

Abstract: The COVID-19 has caused a serious impact on the global economy, and all countries are in a predicament of fighting the epidemic and recovering their economies. Aiming to discuss the impact of the COVID-19 on the economic resilience of urban agglomerations, the economic data of each quarter from June 2019 to September 2020 of the Beijing–Tianjin–Hebei Urban Agglomeration are selected, and the economic development index (EDI) is calculated based on the entropy method. Combining the fundamental conditions of urban agglomerations and industrial policies during the COVID-19, urban economic resilience is discussed by the changing trend of the economic development index (EDI) and dividing into resistance and restoration. The results show that: (1) The economic development level of the urban agglomeration has been affected by the epidemic and has changed significantly. The change of endogenous power is the main cause of change; (2) During the outbreak of the COVID-19, the economic resilience of the Beijing–Tianjin–Hebei urban agglomeration shows four different development types: high resistance and restoration, high resistance but low restoration, low resistance but high restoration, low resistance and restoration cities; (3) High resistance but low restoration, low resistance but high restoration, and low resistance and restoration cities influence each other, but the relationship between cities is mainly dependent; (4) The economic restoration within the urban agglomeration forms a synergy, which promotes the economic recovery and development of the urban agglomeration during the recovery period of the COVID-19. Urban agglomerations should enhance the combined effect of resistance and increase the impact of high resistance and restoration cities on surrounding cities in the future.

Keywords: COVID-19; economy resilience; economy resistance; economy restoration; China

1. Introduction

As a particularly major public health emergency, the COVID-19 became a global pandemic, which made a severe impact on global national economic and social development [1,2]. In China, due to the outbreak of the COVID-19 on the eve of the Spring Festival, the large flow of people returned home before the holiday, which has increased the difficulty of prevention and control of the epidemic [3]. The home quarantine policy had caused an impact on the tourism, transportation, catering, wholesale, retail, entertainment, and other service industries in various regions. The resumption of work after the holiday was also greatly delayed, which caused the national economic development to be obstructed [4]. The urban agglomeration is a unique organizational construction formed with the new urbanization, which plays an important role in promoting the development of various cities [5]. Meanwhile, the urban agglomeration has a high level of economic development, advanced transportation construction, high population density, and close inter-regional relations [6]. Therefore, economic exchanges and frequent population movements have accelerated the spread of the epidemic. While the global epidemic is still in progress [7], analyzing the differences in resilience shown by different cities in responding to the COVID-19 and studying the economic recovery process of urban agglomerations is important for balancing and improving the quality of regional economic development [8].

The outbreak of the COVID-19 in 2020 is a major public health emergency with the fastest spread, the widest range of infections, and the most difficult prevention and control in the world [9]. It has brought a huge impact on the economic development of the world and it caused a huge test of urban economic resilience. Foster [10] and Hill. E [11] think that economic resilience mainly refers to the ability of the economic system to recover from shocks or destruction. Hassink [12] define economic resilience as an important part of urban resilience, is mainly reflected in the ability to continuously adjust its industrial structure and social relations, which can adapt to changes in the external environment and ensure the smooth operation of the economy. The difference in urban economic resilience determines whether a city can recover quickly or fall into a long-term stagnation in the face of a crisis.

2. Literature Review

In recent years, natural and artificial disasters have occurred frequently, and urban safety needs in various countries have intensified [13]. Many cities at home and abroad have successively launched resilient city construction. Metropolises in various countries have successively proposed new development concepts to enhance urban resilience in urban planning. Resilience includes not only the ability to resist in the face of crises, but also the restoration to respond to crises. Cellini pointed out that resilience should not only discuss restoration behaviors [14]. Resilience structure can be explained by the adaptation–adaptability relationships between competing, Separated and Reciprocal, etc. [15] This also illustrates the necessity of studying resilience from the perspective of resistance. Research on urban economic resilience has attracted attention after the global financial crisis in 2008. The outbreak of the COVID-19 in 2020 has caused a huge impact on the world economy and a test of urban economic resilience [16,17]. Research on urban economic resilience has received more attention [18]. Di Pietro et al. measured the vulnerability, resistance and recoverability of regions to discuss the resilience and identify key regional features [19]. Islam et al. found that severe adverse impact of the pandemic on global production, employment, and prices [20]. Zhang K. et al. found that the outbreak of the COVID-19 has the greatest impact on the service industry [21]. Many researchers have selected indicators to measure economic resilience. Brown et al. found that industry structures and concentration in particular industries influence economic resilience [22]. Pretorius et al. indicated that economic openness, export market dynamics and sectoral composition may influence economic resilience [23]. Simmie et al. found that regional innovation systems policies can contribute to their economic resilience [24]. Tan J. found that economic development, labor conditions, and the industrial structure had a statistically significant negative effect on economic resilience [25]. Liu et al. pointed out that there are significant differences in economic resilience revealed by multi-dimensional indicators [26]. It provides a reference for constructing an index to measure economic resilience.

The current research scale for analyzing urban economic resilience in the context of the COVID-19 focuses on the world [20], countries [17,21,27], and cities, while there is relatively little research from the perspective of urban agglomerations. Research dimension on resilience needs to further rise from the "urban resilience" to "urban agglomeration resilience" [5]. It is of great significance for improving the emergencies governance level of urban agglomerations to identify the main characteristics of economic resilience of different types of cities. Meanwhile, clarifying the economic resilience of different cities can provide strong support for judgment of the economic situation and urban recovery in the normalized epidemic prevention and control stage [26].

Based on previous research, we discuss the difference of economic resilience by classifying cities from two aspects of resistance and restoration by calculating the economic development index (EDI). The reasons for the differences are analyzed from urban fundamentals, policies and the relationship between urban agglomerations. In addition, suggestions are made for the future development of urban agglomeration under the normalization of epidemic prevention and control. The remainder of this paper is organized as follows. The research framework, methods, and data are introduced in Section 3. Section 4 presents and discusses the resilience results and reasons by modeling analysis and spatial analysis. Based on the analysis results, Sections 5 and 6 discusses and concludes this study.

3. Materials and Methods

3.1. Study Area

The Beijing–Tianjin–Hebei urban agglomeration is one of the regions with the most dynamic economy, the highest degree of openness, the strongest innovation capabilities, and the largest population absorption in China [28,29]. It is also the main area of China to participate in regional cooperation in Northeast Asia, which consists of the municipalities of Beijing and Tianjin, along with 11 cities in Hebei Province (Shijiazhuang, Langfang, Qinhuangdao, Hengshui, Chengde, Xingtai, Baoding, Tangshan, Zhangjiakou, Cangzhou, and Handan) (Figure 1). With the continuous advancement of the Beijing–Tianjin–Hebei coordinated development strategy in 2014, the Beijing–Tianjin–Hebei urban agglomeration has achieved industrial agglomeration and in-depth cooperation [30]. Beijing has the ripe high-end manufacturing, while Tianjin and Hebei have strong industrial bases in traditional industries such as heavy and chemical industries, logistics and ports. This urban agglomeration has the national political center, the Chinese–foreign cultural exchange center, and the economic center in the north. To a large extent, it represents the economic development level of China's well-developed urban agglomeration and plays a pivotal role in China's economic development.

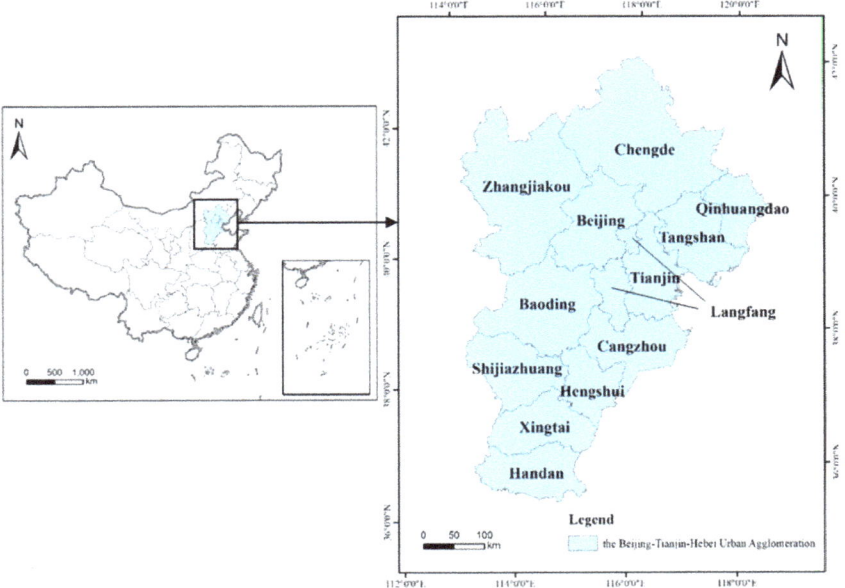

Figure 1. The location and range of the Beijing–Tianjin–Hebei urban agglomeration. Data Source: http://bzdt.ch.mnr.gov.cn/ (accessed on 23 June 2021).

As the main economic development center, the Beijing–Tianjin–Hebei urban agglomeration is one of the earliest urban agglomerations established in China. With the implementation of the regional coordinated development strategy, Beijing, Tianjin, and Hebei have strengthened their construction of transportation interconnection, comprehensive environmental improvement, and industrial coordination [31]. Meanwhile, the population density of the urban agglomeration is high, the economic industry is developed. The outbreak of the COVID-19 has affected many aspects of the agglomeration such as population flow, industrial division of labor, and urban development in the urban agglomeration, which in turn becomes a threat to urban economic resilience.

3.2. Data Sources

The COVID-19 is fast and lasts a long time [32], so this paper selects quarterly economic data before and after the COVID-19(September 2019 to December 2020). The data used for calculating the economic indicators were obtained from the Statistical Yearbook of Beijing, Tianjin and Hebei Province. The local epidemic data come from the real-time updated data of the official websites of the health commissions of the localities, and the policy data come from the policy documents of the official websites of the local governments. For individual missing data, data with the same nature and meaning are used to make up for it.

3.3. Methods

3.3.1. Research Framework

The level of urban economic resilience is reflected in the timely and effective use of existing resources to respond to emergencies, and to further repair the dynamic process of economic development in a certain period in the future [12,14,19,33,34]. Research on urban resilience needs to consider both the city's resistance and the city's restoration. Firstly, the trend of the economic development index (EDI) is the performance of the city's economic level under the influence of the epidemic. Therefore, the change in the EDI in the short term caused by the epidemic can be used as dynamic indicators of the city's economic resilience level. Cities can be divided into different development types based on the results of their resilience. Secondly, economic resilience cannot be measured in a single dimension. A multi-dimensional examination can clarify the nature of economic resilience [26]. Affected by economic resource endowment, infrastructure construction, and the degree of perfection of policies and systems, cities have different performances in adapting to pressures. Due to this, this paper takes the urban fundamentals and industrial policies during the COVID-19 as the primary cause of the differences in urban economic resilience levels under the influence of emergencies. Thirdly, due to the high integration of the cities in the urban agglomeration, the strong economic foundation, and the strong spatial interaction [35], the role of urban agglomerations needs to be considered when discussing the differences in resilience of various cities [36]. So, the spatial correlation characteristics of the economic resilience of various cities is discussed. The research framework of this study is shown in Figure 2.

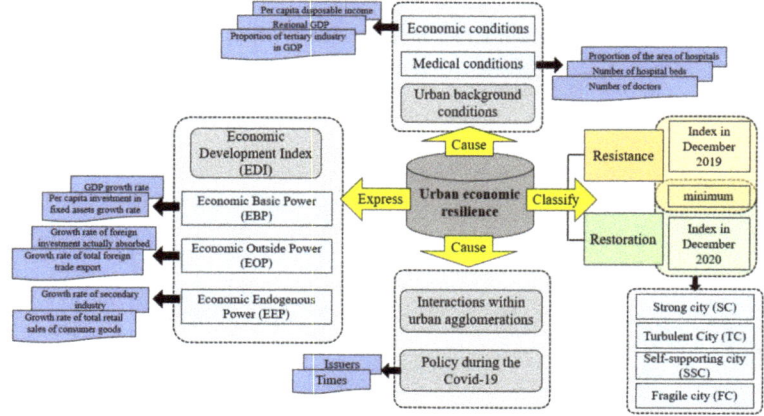

Figure 2. The research framework of this study.

3.3.2. Selection and Calculation of Urban Fundamentals

Urban economic fundamentals reflect the prosperity of the urban economy [37,38], which are of great significance for measuring economic resilience. What is more, there are differences in medical facilities in cities of different scales, resulting in cities showing different economic resilience in response to the COVID-19. The impact of the COVID-19 on the economy reflects the important role of the city's economic fundamentals and medical fundamentals in the city's response to the crisis. Urban economic fundamentals are the support to ensure the survival and sustainable development of the city. Urban medical fundamentals are the most important material bases for the construction of urban. This paper selects economic and medical fundamentals to measure the urban fundamentals, and analyzes the causes of the differences in urban economic resilience.

1. Indicator system establishment

Considering the accuracy, rationality, and availability of the indicators, this paper selects per capita disposable income, regional GDP, and proportion of tertiary industry in GDP to measure the economic fundamentals of the Beijing–Tianjin–Hebei urban agglomeration [26,39–42]. The allocation indicators of medical facilities are selected to measure the background of the medical conditions in the urban agglomeration, including the proportion of the area of hospitals, number of hospital beds and number of doctors. Finally, the weight ratios of specific indicators are integrated to determine the differences in urban economic resilience in different urban fundamentals. The specific indicators and their meanings are shown in Table 1.

Table 1. The indicator system of the urban fundamentals of the Beijing–Tianjin–Hebei urban agglomeration.

Criterion Layer	Indicator Layer	Indicator Interpretation	Data Source
Economic fundamentals	Per capita disposable income Regional GDP Proportion of tertiary industry in GDP	Regional economic strength and market size, the level of consumer spending in the regional economy and the degree of economic development of the region	Statistical yearbooks and statistical bulletins of Beijing, Tianjin, and Hebei
Medical fundamentals	Proportion of the area of hospitals Number of hospital beds Number of doctors	The configuration of medical facilities in cities of different sizes	Statistical yearbooks and statistical bulletins of Beijing, Tianjin, and Hebei

2. Calculation of indicators

In order to ensure the accuracy of the conclusions, this paper standardizes the indicators. Positive indicators:

$$X_{ij} = \frac{x_{ij} - x_{min}}{x_{max} - x_{min}} \quad (1)$$

Negative indicators:

$$X_{ij} = \frac{x_{max} - x_{ij}}{x_{max} - x_{min}} \quad (2)$$

where x_{ij} refers to the initial value of indicator i (i = 1, 2, 3, ..., m) in the j (j = 1, 2, 3, ..., n) year, and X_{ij} is the normalized value, $X_{ij} \in [0, 1]$.

3.3.3. Establishment of Economic Development Index (EDI)

Urban economic resilience can be characterized by index changes in a certain period under the influence of emergencies [43,44]. Therefore, the changing trend of the EDI before and after the COVID-19 can reflect the strength of economic resilience. From the perspective of quantity, space and structure, the economic level of a city is affected by the city's basic industrial structure, geographical location factors, foreign trade as well as the radiation of the surrounding cities (Figure 3). Therefore, based on the development background of the Beijing–Tianjin–Hebei urban agglomeration, this paper selects quarterly data from the basic driving force, external driving force, and endogenous driving force of regional economic development to construct the EDI.

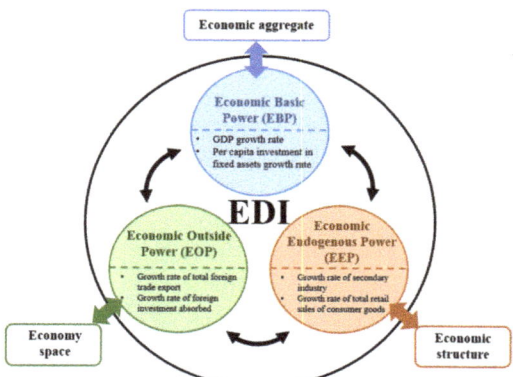

Figure 3. The EDI Frame of Beijing–Tianjin–Hebei Urban Agglomeration.

1. Indicator System Establishment

When calculating the EDI, based on the characteristics of the spatial structure of the Beijing–Tianjin–Hebei urban agglomeration, as well as the connotation of economic basic power (EBP), outside power (EOP), and endogenous power (EEP) [40,45]. GDP growth rate and fixed asset investment growth rate are selected as indicators to measure the EBP; the growth rate of total foreign trade exports and the growth rate of foreign investment absorbed are selected as indicators to measure the EOP; the output value of the secondary industry and the growth rate of total retail sales of social consumer goods are selected to measure the EEP. The specific indicators and their meanings are shown in Table 2.

Table 2. The EDI System of Beijing–Tianjin–Hebei Urban Agglomeration.

Criterion Layer	Indicator Layer	Indicator Interpretation	Data Source
Economic Basic Power (EBP)	GDP growth rate Per capita investment in fixed assets growth rate	The economic development status of a region over a period of time	Statistical yearbooks and monthly reports of Beijing, Tianjin, and Hebei
Economic Outside Power (EOP)	Growth rate of foreign investment absorbed Growth rate of total foreign trade export	The level and trend of regional foreign economy	Statistical yearbooks and monthly reports of Beijing, Tianjin, and Hebei
Economic Endogenous Power (EEP)	Growth rate of secondary industry Growth rate of total retail sales of consumer goods	The economic development mode of a region and the vitality of regional economic development	Statistical yearbooks and monthly reports of Beijing, Tianjin, and Hebei

2. Calculation of Indicator Weight

The entropy evaluation method determines the relative importance of different indicators based on the information entropy implied by the indicator data to calculate indicator weights [46].

Standardization of indicators (Refer to formulas (1) and (2)).

$$f_{ij} = \frac{X_{ij}}{\sum_{j=1}^{n} X_{ij}} \tag{3}$$

$$E_i = -\frac{1}{\ln(n)} \sum_{j=1}^{n} f_{ij} \ln(f_{ij}) \quad (4)$$

$$w_i = \frac{1 - E_i}{m - \sum_{i=1}^{m} E_i} \quad (5)$$

$$\text{EDI} = \sum X_{ij} \times w_i \quad (6)$$

where f_{ij} is the rate of the x_{ij} in the sum of the standardized values of the indicator, E_i is the information entropy of x_{ij}, and w_i is the indicator weight of indicator, $w_i \in [0, 1]$, EDI $\in [0, 1]$.

3.3.4. The Resilience of Urban Economy

In the part of framework designing, we construct a model named urban economic resilience model in the crisis through economic resistance and restoration (Figure 4). The curve simulates the trend of economic development index. The resistance is $f(x)$, which is the minimum EDI change rate (k_1) from before the outbreak of the crisis to the study period. The restoration is $g(x)$, which is the maximum EDI change rate (k_2) from the study period after the crisis broke out.

$$f(x) = \min(k_1) = \frac{EDI_1 - EDI_{min}}{t_1 - t_{min}} \quad (7)$$

$$g(x) = \max(k_2) = \frac{EDI_2 - EDI_{min}}{t_2 - t_{min}} \quad (8)$$

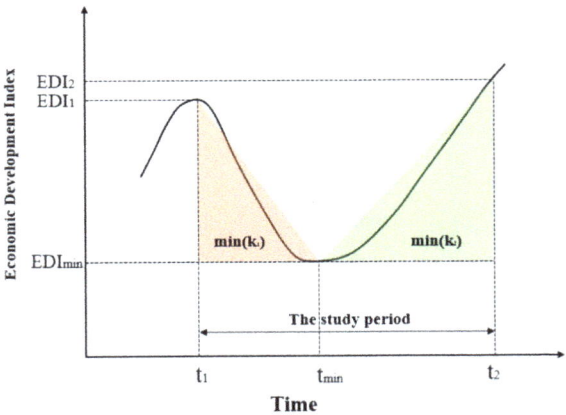

Figure 4. Conceptual Diagram of Economic Resilience Model.

This paper uses the rate of change of the EDI to measure the economic resilience of different cities. In order to be comparable, based on the first, middle, and last three time points of the crisis. The lowest critical point of the EDI, the EDI in December 2019, and the December index in the same period of 2020 are selected. This paper calculates the two-point slope of the difference between the data in December 2019 and the critical index point as the city's resistance to judge the city's ability to resist the impact of the epidemic, and calculates the two-point slope of the difference between the data in December 2020 and the critical index point as the city's restoration to judge the city's ability to recover after the epidemic.

$$r_1 = f(x) = \frac{EDI_1 - EDI_{min}}{t_1 - t_{min}} \quad (9)$$

$$r_2 = g(x) = \frac{EDI_2 - EDI_{min}}{t_2 - t_{min}} \quad (10)$$

where r_1 is the city's resistance. r_2 is the city's restoration. EDI_1 is the EDI in December 2019 and t_1 is December 2019, EDI_2 is the EDI in December 2020 and t_2 is December 2020, EDI_{min} is the minimum of the EDI and t_{min} is the time of the lowest critical point.

4. Results
4.1. Urban Fundamentals

By calculating the economic fundamentals and medical fundamentals of each city in the Beijing–Tianjin–Hebei urban agglomeration, the results are shown in the Figure 5. Beijing and Tianjin show the strongest level of economic and medical fundamentals. Other cities belong to Hebei Province, which economic fundamentals are similar, but the medical fundamentals are quite different. The urban fundamentals of the Beijing–Tianjin–Hebei urban agglomeration show great differences, and there is an imbalance in the allocation of regional resources in the urban agglomeration. Besides, the overall urban medical fundamentals and economic fundamentals show a relatively significant positive correlation. Cities with better economic fundamentals have relatively better medical fundamentals. It shows that as the economic development shifts from high-speed development to high-quality development, the urban medical basic security system is becoming more excellent, turning to the overall high-quality development of the city.

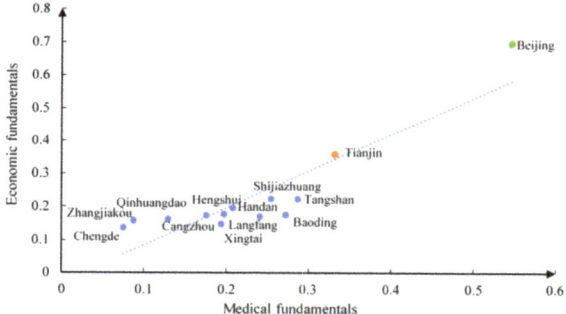

Figure 5. Urban fundamentals of the Beijing–Tianjin–Hebei urban agglomeration.

4.2. Economic Performance under the Influence of the COVID-19
4.2.1. Economic Performance of the Beijing–Tianjin–Hebei Urban Agglomeration

By calculating the changes in the indicators, and combining local epidemic data from the real-time update data of the official websites of the health commissions of the localities and policies from the policy documents of the official websites of the local governments, we draw the trend of the economic development index before and after the COVID-19 (Figure 6). The EDI of the Beijing–Tianjin–Hebei urban agglomeration has been greatly affected by the COVID-19. With the outbreak stage from December 2019 to March 2020, the EDI showed a significant downward trend. Local governments have actively taken corresponding measures to respond to the COVID-19, and timely promulgated epidemic prevention and control policies to prevent the further spread of the epidemic. The number of newly diagnosed patients began to decline after the peak in March 2020, and the COVID-19 was brought under control. Due to the lag effect in the policy response of some cities, the EDI of the Beijing–Tianjin–Hebei urban agglomeration showed a certain downward trend after March 2020. However, the downward trend has obviously slowed down, and after June it began to show an upward trend, and the rising rate has gradually increased.

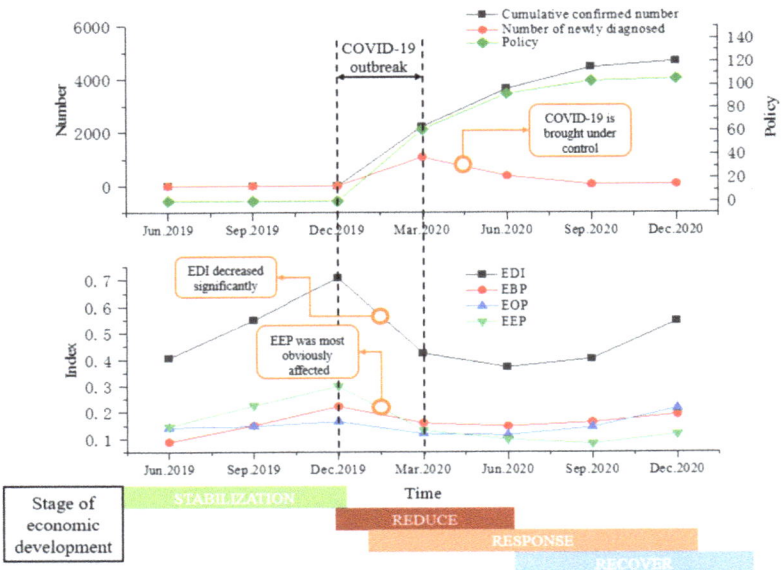

Figure 6. The EDI of the Beijing–Tianjin–Hebei urban agglomeration, the trend of confirmed number and industrial policy before and after the COVID-19.

After the outbreak of the COVID-19, the main influencing factor that led to a significant downward trend in the EDI was the significant decline in the EEP. Because the impact of the COVID-19 caused the suspension of work and production, which had a larger impact on the production and sales of industrial enterprises, and caused a significant decline in the output value of the secondary industry. Coupled with the suspension of traffic during the epidemic, many laborers were unable to return to work in time, which also greatly affected the resumption of work and production. In addition, the spread of the COVID-19 throughout the country during the Spring Festival has led to a reduction in population flow. Service industries and retail industries such as tourism and catering are also affected to a certain extent.

4.2.2. Economic Performance of Each City in the Beijing–Tianjin–Hebei Urban Agglomeration

By calculating the changes in the indicators, we draw the trend of the economic development index before and after the COVID-19 in different cities (Figure 7). The overall EDI of the cities in the Beijing–Tianjin–Hebei urban agglomeration shows relatively similar trend, but the magnitudes of change are significantly different. Before the outbreak of the COVID-19 (December 2019), the EDI of the urban agglomeration showed a relatively stable upward trend. The coordinated development and cooperation between cities in the urban agglomeration has been further deepened, and the overall competitiveness of the urban agglomeration has been further improved. After the outbreak of the COVID-19 in early 2020, the EDIs of various regions showed downward trends. Until the epidemic was controlled in the second quarter, the EDIs of some cities began to rise. There are differences in the basic level of economic development, urban fundamentals, and industrial policies between cities. Therefore, the impact of the COVID-19 has caused different change ranges in the EDIs. The difference in the degree of decline and the speed of recovery in the EDI of each city reflects the difference in economic resilience in the event of a public health crisis.

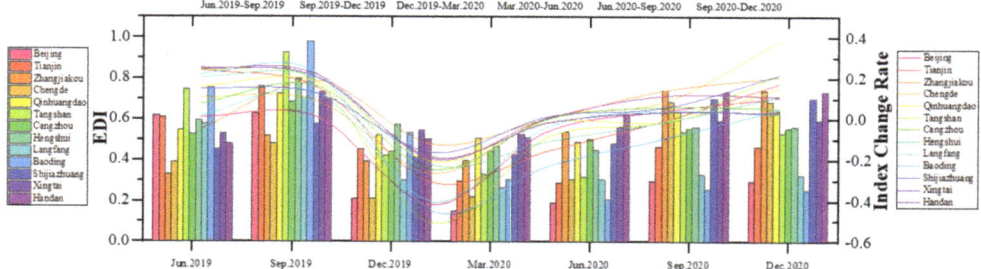

Figure 7. Changes in the EDI of each city in the urban agglomeration before and after the COVID-19.

4.3. Economic Resilience of the Beijing–Tianjin–Hebei Urban Agglomeration

4.3.1. Types of Economic Resilience of the Beijing–Tianjin–Hebei Urban Agglomeration

Based on the definition of economic resilience, this paper summarizes it as resistance and restoration. We divide resilience into four types, including strong cities (SC), turbulent cities (TC), self-supporting cities (SSC) and fragile cities (FC) (Table 3). Using the economic resilience model, this paper calculates the resilience and restoration of the cities in the Beijing–Tianjin–Hebei urban agglomeration (Figure 8).

Table 3. Types of Economic Resilience.

Types of Economic Resilience	Resistance Level	Restoration Level	Resilience Characteristics
Strong Cities (SCs)	high	high	Respond quickly and recover in time
Turbulent Cities (TCs)	high	low	Respond quickly and recover slowly
Self-supporting Cities (SSCs)	low	high	Respond overwhelmingly and recover in time
Fragile Cities (FCs)	low	low	Respond overwhelmingly and recover slowly

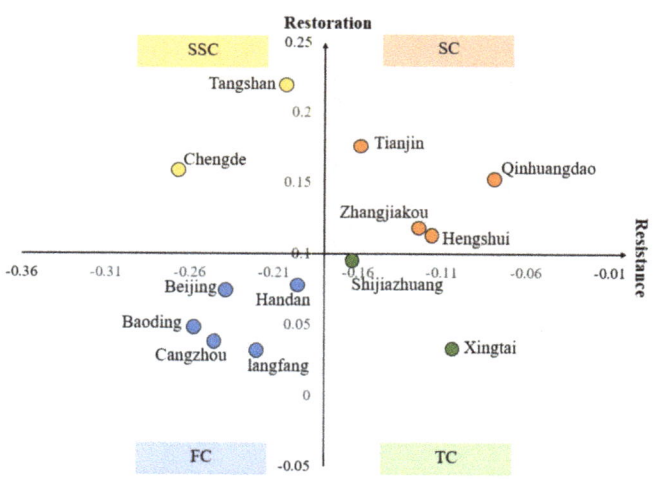

Figure 8. The distribution of economic resilience of the Beijing–Tianjin–Hebei urban agglomeration.

1. The Characteristics of Strong Cities (SCs)

SCs can effectively resist the impact of the epidemic, while being able to recover and adjust in time. It is mainly because of the improvement of the coordinated promotion of epidemic prevention and control as well as economic and social development basis. After the outbreak of the COVID-19, those cities took some policies to respond quickly in time, which can ensure the stable operation of the economy. Ensuring the supply of materials during the epidemic, supporting the resumption of work and production of enterprises, increasing fiscal, taxation and financial support, and supporting the development of key industries helped the economy recover quickly. Zhangjiakou, Tianjin, Qinhuangdao, and Hengshui belong to SCs. Tianjin has a strong economic and industrial structure, and the economic fundamentals are relatively stable. Despite the poor urban fundamentals, Zhangjiakou, Qinhuangdao, and Hengshui can respond quickly in the face of crisis, which also reflects the importance of emergency management for urban development.

2. The Characteristics of Turbulent Cities (TCs)

TCs are less affected by the epidemic, and rely on their fundamentals to cope with the spread of the epidemic in the short term. These cities have certain industrial or economic and political advantages, which can withstand a crisis with sufficiently strong fundamentals. However, the development of urban economy is unstable, the transformation and upgrading of urban pillar industries and traditional industries are lacking. The lack of digital technology-supported new industries and new business formats can timely "supplement" economic development. It is difficult for these cities to recover in time from economic turmoil when facing the long-term impact of the crisis. The COVID-19 has continuous impacts on the EDI, resulting in low restoration. Shijiazhuang and Xingtai are TCs.

3. The Characteristics of Self-Supporting Cities (SSCs)

SSCs lacked emergency management capabilities in responding to the epidemic after the outbreak of the COVID-19, resulting in low resistance. The relatively large number of confirmed cases of the epidemic has caused a greater impact on their economy. As time goes by, the strong fundamentals in cities and the implementation of subsequent epidemic prevention and control mechanisms have enabled the epidemic to be effectively controlled. Policies on the resumption of work and production of enterprises, support for small and micro-enterprises, and strengthening of employment security have been introduced to help the resumption of economy. Including important port city Tangshan, the urban fundamentals are developed. Chengde's urban fundamentals are poor, so it is difficult to fight the epidemic. However, influenced by Tangshan, its economic development gradually recovered.

4. The Characteristics of Fragile Cities (FCs)

FCs have been severely affected by the COVID-19 for a long time, which has a greater impact on the city's economy. During the epidemic, the suspension of work and production as well as the reduction of population movement caused the economic industry to be stagnant. The epidemic has caused a continuous impact on the urban economy, leading to a slower recovery and development of economic industries. Beijing, Baoding, Langfang, Cangzhou and Handan are FCs. Differences in economic resilience cannot be explained simply by geographical location and political advantage. Baoding, Langfang, Cangzhou, and Handan with poor urban fundamentals are greatly affected by the industrial transfer in Beijing. As the world's urbanization process, large cities are becoming an important focus of spreading infectious diseases [13]. Beijing is relatively special, the risk of epidemic spread is high, and the prevention and control of the epidemic is difficult. As a result, its EDI declines quickly and rebounds slowly. This also reflects that, compared with the urban fundamentals, the management ability with an urban emergency response is more important in the face of major health emergencies.

We visualize cities with different types of economic resilience (Figure 9). SSCs, TCs, and FCs show significant spatial agglomeration and the centers are Tangshan, Shijiazhuang, and Beijing, respectively, based on their relatively strong fundamentals. Among them, TCs are mainly distributed in the north of the Beijing–Tianjin–Hebei urban agglomeration. As a port city, Tangshan is close to Beijing and Tianjin, with a superior geographical position and a strong economic foundation, which has a positive effect on the economic development of Chengde. SSCs are mainly distributed in the south of the Beijing–Tianjin–Hebei urban agglomeration. Shijiazhuang, the capital of Hebei Province, is one of the growth poles in the Beijing–Tianjin–Hebei region. It has strong urban fundamentals, and formed "the certain spillover effect." Most of the FCs are located in the central area of the Beijing–Tianjin–Hebei urban agglomeration. With the evacuation of Beijing's non-capital functions, Baoding and Langfang are mainly affected by Beijing's industrial transfer. Therefore, under the influence of the epidemic, the resilience of these cities has shown similar characteristics. At present, the cities relation in the urban agglomeration are mainly dependent on attachment, lack of cooperation, and reciprocity.

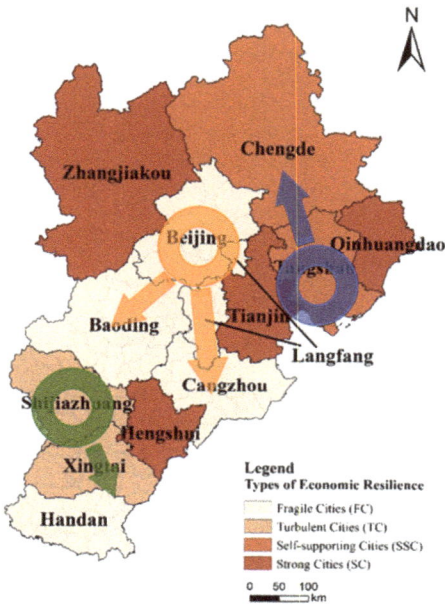

Figure 9. Visualization of economic resilience of Beijing–Tianjin–Hebei urban agglomeration.

4.3.2. Response of Economic Resilience of Beijing–Tianjin–Hebei Urban Agglomeration

As urban agglomerations have close economic exchanges and frequent population movements, the economic impact of the COVID-19 on the Beijing–Tianjin–Hebei urban agglomeration is spatially interactive. This paper discusses the spatial correlation characteristics of economic resilience of Beijing–Tianjin–Hebei urban agglomeration. By calculating the global Moran's I of resilience (Figure 10), the global Moran's I of urban agglomeration economic resistance is -0.189, and the P-value is 0.32. The significance test is not passed, indicating that the urban agglomeration resistance has not yet formed a synergistic effect when faced the COVID-19. A unified "anti-epidemic" response was not reached. The global Moran's I of urban agglomeration economic restoration is 0.435, and the P-value is 0.006, passing the significance test of 0.01. The restoration of the Beijing–Tianjin–Hebei urban agglomeration has positive correlation characteristics. During the period of economic recovery, the Beijing–Tianjin–Hebei urban agglomeration established a joint work mechanism for joint prevention and control of the Beijing–Tianjin–Hebei new crown pneumonia epidemic and achieved positive results.

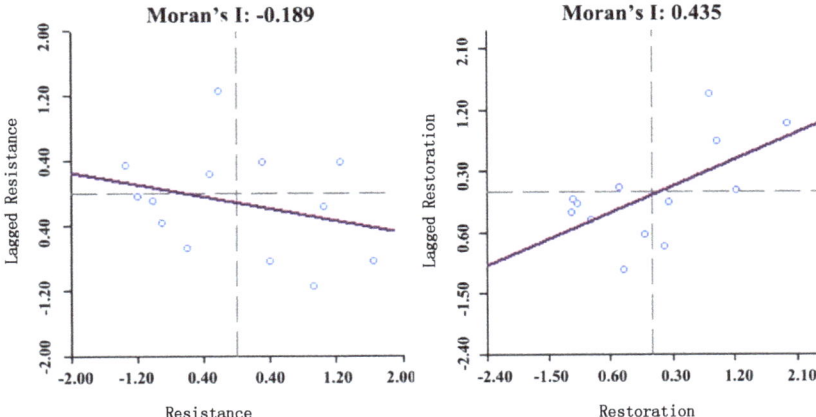

Figure 10. The global Moran's I of resistance and restoration of the Beijing–Tianjin–Hebei urban agglomeration.

5. Discussion

5.1. Main Achievements

From the perspective of economic resilience, this paper provides a case and a new analysis perspective for urban agglomerations to respond and govern the public health emergencies in the future. Affected by economic resource endowment, infrastructure construction, and the degree of perfection of policies and systems, cities have different performances in facing crises. This paper discusses the economic resilience of the Beijing–Tianjin–Hebei urban agglomerations under the impact of the COVID-19 from two perspectives of resistance and restoration, as well as summarizes the urban agglomerations into four types. SCs have high urban resilience both resistance and restoration, which can effectively deal with the impact of the epidemic. TCs have shown strong resistance, but their restoration is relatively weak. The epidemic is not good for their long-term development. SSCs have weak resistance and strong restoration. Due to a lack of emergency management capabilities, the epidemic is likely to cause fluctuations in these cities in the short term. FCs have weak resistance and restoration and the epidemic has hit them harder. This classification method is also consistent with the current common classification of regional economic resilience [47].

5.2. Limitations and Uncertainties

This paper proposed a method to measure the resilience of urban economy under the impact of public health emergencies by using short-term economic development index, which can better reflect the sudden impact of public health emergencies. Because the outbreak has not yet been fully contained globally, the data currently available cannot be used to discuss the lasting impact of the outbreak. Urban economic resilience is a diverse and complex concept, which is affected by multiple factors. After the data are perfected in the future, indicators can be further added to measure the urban EDI, making the measurement of urban economic resilience more accurate. Regardless, our study at least evaluates resilience differences in cities using existing data under the impact of emergencies, and the research conclusion provides a useful diagnosis and helpful information for urban agglomeration construction.

When studying the influencing factors of EDI, this paper draws a statistical conclusion according to the index weight ratio. From a macro perspective, the economic endogenous power is the main reason for the decline of EDI, and urban agglomeration should focus on protecting endogenous power when dealing with emergencies. Only macro statistical laws are shown when showing the internal factors mechanism of the EDI that is a highly susceptible factor, and lack an analysis of the causal relationship between specific indicators and EDI. In the future, this study will be better supported by statistical conclusions by constructing an analysis model of influencing factors. For example, the main influencing factors of urban economic resilience can be analyzed by constructing a regression model.

The current research takes the Beijing–Tianjin–Hebei urban agglomeration as an example to analyze the differences in urban economic resilience within the urban agglomeration under the influence of the COVID-19, and whether the Beijing–Tianjin–Hebei urban agglomeration has played a synergistic role in the economic resilience of each city. The comparison of different urban agglomerations can clarify the differences in the economic resilience of urban agglomerations, thereby promoting the improvement of urban agglomeration governance capabilities. In the future, we can compare the Beijing–Tianjin–Hebei urban agglomerations with other types of urban agglomerations around the world to analyze the differences in economic resilience under the influence of the COVID-19, especially to discuss economic development differences under the normalization of the epidemic. It is conducive to realizing the scientific layout of urban agglomeration functions, space, transportation, and form, and to deal with the relationship between concentration and decentralization [5].

5.3. Implications and Applications

The outbreak of the COVID-19 in early 2020 has had a greater impact on the urban economic development of the Beijing–Tianjin–Hebei urban agglomeration. The COVID-19 epidemic has been brought under control through proactive response measures, and economic activity is slowly recovering. There are certain differences in the change trends of the EDI of each city, which reflect the difference in the level of urban resilience. With the effective control of the COVID-19, the economic level of urban agglomerations will continue to rise. The upward trend mainly includes two situations, which are recovery to the pre-recession rate (b) or to a sustained higher (a)/lower (c) growth rate (Figure 11) (Only simulating the trend of change, the curve will fluctuate with the actual situation). Moreover, the economic resilience of each city is one of the main influencing factors. Meanwhile, it is also affected by the extent and duration of the emergency.

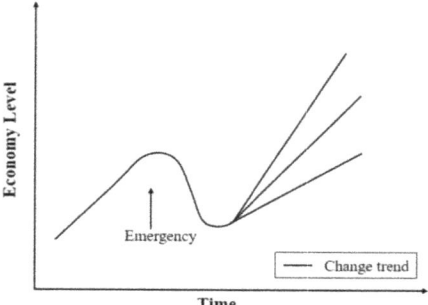

Figure 11. Impacts of an emergency shock on a city's economy: (a) resumption of a unchangeable rate (pre-recession); (b) resumption of a sustained higher growth rate; (c) resumption of a sustained lower growth rate.

The lack of synergy in the resilience of the Beijing–Tianjin–Hebei urban agglomeration after the outbreak of the COVID-19 reflects the inadequate emergency management capacity of the urban agglomeration as an overall economic system. Meanwhile, within the urban agglomeration, there is a lack of cooperation and reciprocity. The epidemic was finally controlled thanks to the relevant prevention and control policies issued by the local government. Urban agglomerations have strong population and economic agglomeration. Therefore, local government should actively play the joint role of urban agglomerations when responding to the crisis. In the future, urban agglomeration construction should not only focus on restoration improvement, but also further strengthen resistance construction.

On the one hand, urban agglomeration should actively promote medical and health cooperation, share medical and health resources, build medical and health informatization, and improve medical service application system. On the other hand, a global crisis such as the COVID-19 pandemic requires a global response, not only on health but also on trade, finance, and macroeconomic policies [48]. To cope with the economic construction under the normal situation of epidemic prevention and control, urban agglomerations need to build a moderately gradient industrial division structure, and further rely on industrial clusters to form synergistically supported industrial clusters, which can help the agglomeration form more cooperative relations.

By classifying cities according to the characteristics of economic resilience, it helps local governments to better formulate relevant economic policies in the future. Different cities in the urban agglomeration have their development characteristics, especially facing crisis. Although SCs have a strong industrial foundation and emergency response capabilities, which can resist the impact of the epidemic, they have not played a spreading role and have no positive impact on the surrounding cities. In the future, those cities should further strengthen their ties with neighboring cities to enhance their joint efforts to cope with the crisis. SSCs have economic and industrial foundations, while the epidemic embodies the lack of urban emergency management capacity. Therefore, an effective public health early warning system should be built in the future, the early warning responsibility mechanism of all levels of departments should be strengthened and the regional economic resistance to pressure. Most of TCs are less affected by the epidemic and can resist the epidemic in the short term. After the epidemic is controlled, TCs are difficult to resume development promptly and lack certain innovation capabilities. It is necessary to build pillar industries in the city, vigorously promote the development of new technologies, promote sustained and stable economic recovery, as well as enhance the development of foreign trade. FCs are supposed to be the focus of the future construction of urban agglomerations. It is necessary to promote the development of new technologies, and promote sustained economic recovery in most of FCs. Besides, those cities should enhance the city's emergency management capabilities and improve the early warning system.

6. Conclusions

Taking the Beijing–Tianjin–Hebei urban agglomeration as an example, this paper combined traditional epidemiological survey data, short-term economic development level data, and urban development background data to calculate economic development index (EDI). Based on the differences of resource endowments, development models, policies, and background conditions of each city, the reasons for differences in urban economic resilience were discussed.

The urban fundamentals of the Beijing–Tianjin–Hebei urban agglomeration have significant internal differences, and there is still a certain gap in the background conditions of Hebei Province with Beijing and Tianjin. In the future, the central city must play a leading role in the coordinated development of the region to achieve the coordination of urban fundamentals of the urban agglomeration background. Based on the changing trend of the economic development index (EDI), we discussed economic resilience in terms of resistance and restoration, and divided cities into four types, including Strong Cities (SCs), Turbulent Cities (TCs), Self-supporting Cities (SSCs), Fragile Cities (FCs). It provides a research idea for studying the economic resilience of different cities in urban agglomerations, and is conducive to making development suggestions tailored to local conditions. Additionally, we found that the central cities of FCs, SSCs and TCs affect surrounding cities and urban agglomeration played a synergistic role in economic recovery after the epidemic was brought under control. In the future, the urban agglomeration needs to play a synergistic role after the outbreak of the crisis to improve urban resilience.

Author Contributions: Conceptualization, Y.Z.; methodology, Y.Z. and X.W.; software, Y.Z. and K.W.; validation, Y.Z., K.W., and X.W.; formal analysis, Y.Z.; investigation, K.W.; resources, X.W.; data curation, Y.Z.; writing—original draft preparation, Y.Z.; writing—review and editing, Y.Z.; visualization, Y.Z.; supervision, Y.Z. and J.Z.; project administration, J.Z.; funding acquisition, J.Z. All authors have read and agreed to the published version of the manuscript.

Funding: This article is supported by the Fundamental Research Funds for the Central Universities.

Institutional Review Board Statement: Not applicable.

Informed Consent Statement: Not applicable.

Data Availability Statement: The datasets used in this research are available upon request.

Acknowledgments: We thank to all the participants involved in the projects for their contribution in our research data.

Conflicts of Interest: The authors declare no conflict of interest. The funders had no role in the design of the study; in the collection, analyses, or interpretation of data; in the writing of the manuscript, or in the decision to publish the results.

References

1. Lin, Q.; Zhao, S.; Gao, D.; Lou, Y.; Yang, S.; Musa, S.S.; Wang, M.H.; Cai, Y.; Wang, W.; Yang, L.; et al. A conceptual model for the coronavirus disease 2019 (COVID-19) outbreak in Wuhan, China with individual reaction and governmental action. *Int. J. Infect. Dis.* **2020**, *93*, 211–216. [CrossRef] [PubMed]
2. Ibn-Mohammed, T.; Mustapha, K.B.; Godsell, J.; Adamu, Z.; Babatunde, K.A.; Akintade, D.D.; Acquaye, A.; Fujii, H.; Ndiaye, M.M.; Yamoah, F.A.; et al. A critical analysis of the impacts of COVID-19 on the global economy and ecosystems and opportunities for circular economy strategies. *Resour. Conserv. Recycl.* **2021**, *164*, 105169. [CrossRef]
3. Wang, Q.; Zhang, F. What does the China's economic recovery after COVID-19 pandemic mean for the economic growth and energy consumption of other countries? *J. Clean. Prod.* **2021**, *295*, 126265. [CrossRef] [PubMed]
4. Sun, Y.; Zeng, X.; Zhao, H.; Simkins, B.; Cui, X. The impact of COVID-19 on SMEs in China: Textual analysis and empirical evidence. *Financ. Res. Lett.* **2021**, 102211. [CrossRef]
5. Wang, J.; Du, D.; Wei, Z.; Yang, H. The development of COVID-19 in China: Spatial diffusion and geographical pattern. *Geogr. Res.* **2020**, *39*, 1450–1462.
6. Yang, Z. Comparison and empirical analysis of the urban economic development level in the Yangtze River urban agglomeration based on an analogical ecosystem perspective. *Ecol. Inform.* **2021**, *64*, 101321. [CrossRef]
7. Phiri, D.; Salekin, S.; Nyirenda, V.R.; Simwanda, M.; Ranagalage, M.; Murayama, Y. Spread of COVID-19 in Zambia: An assessment of environmental and socioeconomic factors using a classification tree approach. *Sci. Afr.* **2021**, *12*, e00827. [CrossRef]
8. Zhou, Q.; Zhu, M.; Qiao, Y.; Zhang, X.; Chen, J. Achieving resilience through smart cities? Evidence from China. *Habitat Int.* **2021**, *111*, 102348. [CrossRef]
9. Si, D.-K.; Li, X.-L.; Xu, X.; Fang, Y. The risk spillover effect of the COVID-19 pandemic on energy sector: Evidence from China. *Energy Econ.* **2021**, *102*, 105498. [CrossRef]
10. Foster, K.A. *A Case Study Approach to Understanding Regional Resilience*; University of California: Oakland, CA, USA, 2007.
11. Hill, E.; Clair, T.S.; Wial, H.; Wolman, H.; Friedhoff, A. Economic shocks and regional economic resilience. In *Urban and Regional Policy and Its Effects: Building Resilient Regions*; Brookings Institution Press: Washington, DC, USA, 2012.
12. Hassink, R. Regional resilience: A promising concept to explain differences in regional economic adaptability? *Camb. J. Reg. Econ. Soc.* **2010**, *3*, 45–58. [CrossRef]
13. Alirol, E.; Getaz, L.; Stoll, B.; Chappuis, F.; Loutan, L. Urbanisation and infectious diseases in a globalised world. *Lancet Infect. Dis.* **2011**, *11*, 131–141. [CrossRef]
14. Cellini, R.; Torrisi, G. Regional Resilience in Italy: A Very Long-Run Analysis. *Reg. Stud.* **2014**, *48*, 1779–1796. [CrossRef]
15. Hu, X.; Hassink, R. Exploring adaptation and adaptability in uneven economic resilience: A tale of two Chinese mining regions. *Camb. J. Reg. Econ. Soc.* **2017**, *10*, 527–541. [CrossRef]
16. Batool, M.; Ghulam, H.; Hayat, M.A.; Naeem, M.Z.; Ejaz, A.; Imran, Z.A.; Spulbar, C.; Birau, R.; Gorun, T.H. How COVID-19 has shaken the sharing economy? An analysis using Google trends data. *Econ. Res.-Ekon. Istraživanja* **2021**, *34*, 2374–2386. [CrossRef]
17. Wang, Y.; Gao, J. Shocks of 2019-nCoV, Economic Resilience and China's High Quality Development. *Bus. Manag. J.* **2020**, *42*, 5–17.
18. Martin, R.; Sunley, P. On the notion of regional economic resilience: Conceptualization and explanation. *J. Econ. Geogr.* **2015**, *15*, 1–42. [CrossRef]
19. Di Pietro, F.; Lecca, P.; Salotti, S. Regional economic resilience in the European Union: A numerical general equilibrium analysis. *Spat. Econ. Anal.* **2021**, *16*, 287–312. [CrossRef]
20. Islam, A.M. Impact of Covid-19 pandemic on global output, employment and prices: An assessment. *Transnatl. Corp. Rev.* **2021**, *13*, 189–201.

21. Zhang, K.; Qian, Q. The impact of COVID-19 on China's economy and discussions of policies—Evidence from listed companies. *Trop. Geogr.* **2020**, *40*, 396–407.
22. Brown, L.; Greenbaum, R.T. The role of industrial diversity in economic resilience: An empirical examination across 35 years. *Urban Stud.* **2017**, *54*, 1347–1366. [CrossRef]
23. Pretorius, O.; Drewes, E.; van Aswegen, M.; Malan, G. A Policy Approach towards Achieving Regional Economic Resilience in Developing Countries: Evidence from the SADC. *Sustainability* **2021**, *13*, 2674. [CrossRef]
24. Simmie, J. Regional Economic Resilience: A Schumpeterian Perspective. *Raumforsch. Und Raumordn.* **2014**, *72*, 103–116. [CrossRef]
25. Tan, J.; Zhao, H.; LIu, W.; Zhang, P.; Chou, F. Regional Economic Resilience and Influential Mechanism During Economic Crises in China. *Sci. Geogr. Sin.* **2020**, *40*, 173–181.
26. Liu, Y.; Ji, J.; Zhang, Y.; Yang, Y. Economic resilience and spatial divergence in the Guangdong-Hong Kong-Macao Greater Bay Area in China. *Geogr. Res.* **2020**, *39*, 2029–2043.
27. Qin, Y.; Li, G. Study on the Impact on China's Economy from the Novel Coronavirus Pneumonia Based on the Perspective of Questionnaire Analysis. *Reg. Econ. Rev.* **2020**, 146–156. [CrossRef]
28. Yang, Z.; Yang, H.; Wang, H. Evaluating urban sustainability under different development pathways: A case study of the Beijing-Tianjin-Hebei region. *Sustain. Cities Soc.* **2020**, *61*, 102226. [CrossRef]
29. Adzania, F.H.; Fauzia, S.; Aryati, G.P.; Mahkota, R. Sociodemographic and environmental health risk factor of COVID-19 in Jakarta, Indonesia: An ecological study. *One Health* **2021**, *13*, 100303. [CrossRef]
30. Fang, C. Strategic choice of integrated development of Beijing-Tianjin-Hebei urban agglomeration. *Reform* **2017**, *5*, 54–63.
31. Chen, Y. Conditions, characteristics and dynamic mechanism of formation of urban agglomeration. *Urban Probl.* **2009**, *1*, 18–22, 34. [CrossRef]
32. Kanagarathinam, K.; Algehyne, E.A.; Sekar, K. Analysis of 'earlyR' epidemic model and time series model for prediction of COVID-19 registered cases. In *Materials Today: Proceedings*; Elsevier: Amsterdam, The Nederlands, 2020. [CrossRef]
33. Martin, R. Regional economic resilience, hysteresis and recessionary shocks. *J. Econ. Geogr.* **2012**, *12*, 1–32. [CrossRef]
34. Slocum, S.; Kline, C. Regional resilience: Opportunities, challenges and policy messages from Western North Carolina. *Anatolia* **2014**, *25*, 403–416. [CrossRef]
35. Dube, J.; Polese, M. Resilience Revisited: Assessing the Impact of the 2007-09 Recession on 83 Canadian Regions with Accompanying Thoughts on an Elusive Concept. *Reg. Stud.* **2016**, *50*, 615–628. [CrossRef]
36. Cao, Q.; Shi, M.J. Research on spatial resilience characteristics and response mechanism of Chengdu-Chongqing urban agglomeration based on power-law. In Proceedings of the International Workshop on Green Energy, Environment and Sustainable Development (G2ESD), Weihai, China, 28–30 August 2020.
37. Bai, L.; Xiu, C.; Feng, X.; Mei, D.; Wei, Z. A comprehensive assessment of urban resilience and its spatial differentiation in China. *World Reg. Stud.* **2019**, *28*, 77–87.
38. Xu, Z.; Tian, J.; Zhang, J. Urban resilience evaluation system and optimization strategy from the perspective of disaster prevention. *China Saf. Sci. J.* **2019**, *29*, 1–7.
39. Cao, L.; Zhou, Z.; Wang, K. Coupling and coordinated evolution of public health infrastructure and high-quality economic development: A case study of the Yangtze River Economic Belt. *Stat. Decis.* **2021**, *17*, 140–144. [CrossRef]
40. Ma, D.; Shen, Z. Research on Coupling Coordination of Urban Resilience and Economic Development Level—Taking Beijing-Tianjin-Hebei Urban Agglomeration as an Example. *Resour. Dev. Mark.* **2021**, *37*, 820–827.
41. Qian, Y.; Yang, J. Analysis on Equity of Health Resources Allocation in Gansu Province Based on Gini coefficient and Agglomeration degree. *Med. Soc.* **2021**, *34*, 11–16.
42. Yang, S.; Yao, J. Equalization Measurement and Optimization of Public Service Resources in Beijing-Tianjin-Hebei Urban Agglomeration. *Public Adm. Policy Rev.* **2021**, *10*, 123–133.
43. Tong, Y.; Ma, Y.; Liu, H. The short-term impact of COVID-19 epidemic on the migration of Chinese urban population and the evaluation of Chinese urban resilience. *Acta Geogr. Sin.* **2020**, *75*, 2505–2520.
44. Wei, S.; Jinghu, P. Network structure resilience of cities at the prefecture level and above in China. *Acta Geogr. Sin.* **2021**, *76*, 1394–1407.
45. Xiao, D.; Yu, F. A Measurement and Comparative Analysis of High Quality Economic Development of Chinese Urban Agglomerations. *J. Macro-Qual. Res.* **2021**, *9*, 86–98.
46. Chen, M.; Lu, D.; Zhang, H. Comprehensive Evaluation and Driving Factors of China' Urbanization. *Acta Geogr. Sin.* **2009**, *64*, 387–398.
47. Briguglio, L.; Cordina, G.; Farrugia, N.; Vella, S. Economic Vulnerability and Resilience: Concepts and Measurements. *Oxf. Dev. Stud.* **2009**, *37*, 229–247. [CrossRef]
48. Padhan, R.; Prabheesh, K.P. The economics of COVID-19 pandemic: A survey. *Econ. Anal. Policy* **2020**, *70*, 220–237. [CrossRef]

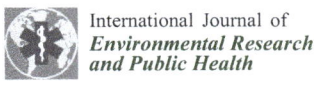 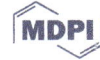

Article

Impact of COVID-19 on Czech Dentistry: A Nationwide Cross-Sectional Preliminary Study among Dentists in the Czech Republic

Jan Schmidt [1,†], Eliska Waldova [2,†], Stepanka Balkova [3], Jakub Suchanek [1,*] and Roman Smucler [3]

1. Department of Dentistry, Charles University, Faculty of Medicine in Hradec Kralove and University Hospital Hradec Kralove, 500 05 Hradec Kralove, Czech Republic; Jan.Schmidt@lfhk.cuni.cz
2. Wald Pharmaceuticals, s.r.o., Detska 37, 100 00 Prague, Czech Republic; eliska.waldova@enzymel.cz
3. Czech Dental Chamber, Slavojova 270/22, 128 00 Prague, Czech Republic; stepabal@gmail.com (S.B.); smucler@dent.cz (R.S.)
* Correspondence: SuchanekJ@lfhk.cuni.cz; Tel.: +420-495-832-634
† Authors contributed equally to this work.

Abstract: This work evaluates the impact of the COVID-19 pandemic on Czech dentistry from March 2020 to March 2021. The assessment was based on questionnaires filled out by 3674 Czech dentists representing 42.6% of practicing dentists in the country. During March–May, 2020 (the first COVID-19 wave), 90.7% of dental practices remained open; however, only 22.8% of the practices continued to operate with no changes, 46.5% had fewer patients, 21.4% treated only acute cases, and 3.8% were closed. During September 2020–May 2021 (the second wave of COVID-19), 96.1% of dental practices remained open, 60.8% operated with no changes, 34.5% had fewer patients, 0.8% treated only acute cases, and 0.5% were closed. The reasons leading to the closure of Czech dental practices during the whole pandemic were a shortage of personal protective equipment (50.5%), a COVID-19 outbreak in the workplace (24.5%), fear of a possible self-infection (24.0%), and quarantine (20.5%). The time range of Czech dental practices closure during the whole pandemic was: 1–2 weeks (49.9%), 2–4 weeks (21.2%), and >1 month (0.8%). The greatest professional difficulties of Czech dentists during the pandemic were crisis operating management (55%), health safety and hygiene concerns (21%), shortage of personal protective equipment (21%), and difficulty working with the protective equipment (15%). In addition, 47.3% of dentists also observed a declining interest in preventive dental care, and 16.9% of them observed worse oral care of patients. These results show that despite the lack of protective equipment, dental care was maintained throughout the pandemic. Additionally, the pandemic negatively affected the patients' approach to dental care, indicating a deterioration in oral health as a possible delayed outcome of the COVID-19 pandemic.

Keywords: COVID-19; dentistry; pandemic; dentist; protective equipment

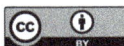

1. Introduction

Coronavirus disease 2019 (COVID-19) is a contagious disease caused by severe acute respiratory syndrome coronavirus 2 (SARS-CoV-2). Symptoms of COVID-19 are variable, ranging from mild to deadly, including fever, cough, headache, fatigue, loss of smell and taste, breathing difficulties, respiratory failure, or acute inflammatory response (cytokine storm) [1–6]. The human-to-human transmission is caused by respiratory droplets, either by being inhaled or deposited on mucosal surfaces and via direct contact of mucous membranes, such as oral, nasal, or eye [7]. It was first reported in Wuhan City, Hubei Province, China, in December 2019 [8]. Since then, COVID-19 has become a worldwide major health concern, and on 11 March 2020, it was declared a pandemic disease [9].

In the Czech Republic, the first laboratory-confirmed case of COVID-19 was announced on 1 March 2020. A state of emergency was declared as of 12 March 2020. The emergency was later extended until 18 May 2020. From 16 March 2020, free movement was limited with the exception of travel to and from work, and essential trips, including grocery shopping, trips to the pharmacy, or aiding elderly members of the family. The key measures issued by the Czech government are described in Table 1 [10–12]. Due to these early precautions, the pandemic was mild in the Czech Republic during the spring of 2020, with a cumulative number of 79 COVID-19 positive cases per 100,000 people at the end of the first state of emergency [13]. During late May and early June 2020, the obligation of social distancing and wearing masks was abolished. This period, from March to May 2020, is also called the "first wave" of COVID-19. For the rest of the summer, the number of new cases was minimal. However, in September, new COVID-19 cases began to rise again. A state of emergency was declared again on 5 October 2020 and was to remain in force until 11 April 2021. The pandemic was most severe from September to March and began to subside in April. At the end of the second emergency, the cumulative number of cases per 100,000 people was 14,308 [13]. This period from September to March 2020 is also called the 'second wave' of COVID-19.

Table 1. Overview of selected key anti-pandemic measures issued by the Czech government.

	Issued on	Effective from	Description of Key Measures
2020	March 12	March 12	Declaration of the state of emergency in the Czech Republic
	March 13	March 14	Prohibition of selected leisure activities; prohibition of retail sales and services
	March 15	March 16	Prohibition of free movement of persons (with exceptions, including healthcare consumption)
	March 18	March 19	Mandatory covering of mouth and nose indoors and outdoors
	April 30	May 18	End of the emergency
	September 30	October 5	Declaration of the state of emergency in the Czech Republic
	September 30	October 5	Prohibition of selected leisure activities
	October 12	October 13	Obligation to use face masks indoors
	October 19	October 21	Obligation to use face masks indoors and outdoors
	October 21	October 22	Prohibition of free movement of persons (with exceptions, including healthcare consumption)
	October 21	October 22	Prohibition of retail sales and services
2021	February 26	April 11	End of the emergency

Healthcare workers were considered particularly vulnerable to the pandemic all around the world, especially those whose work is in close contact with mucus and saliva droplets. Due to their work settings, dentists are one of the most endangered professional groups. At the beginning of the pandemic, the Czech Republic and most European countries lacked protective equipment, even for health professionals. Regardless of the pandemic, according to good medical practice and Czech law, it is the duty of each health care provider to limit the transmission of infectious diseases as much as possible. The same has been true during the pandemic with no exception, leaving health care providers in unprecedented medical and, eventually, legal insecurity. In the case of dentists, the culpable transmission of the disease was at stake. Such conditions were not unique to the Czech Republic and were also faced by health care workers in other European countries [14,15].

These multiple factors, combined with the rapid increase in the number of COVID-19 patients, led to a suspension of non-acute general healthcare in the Czech Republic. However, thanks to the effort of the Czech Dental Chamber and especially its members, dental care was provided throughout the whole pandemic, albeit with some restrictions. As the vast majority of the dental practices in the Czech Republic are private institutions, the anti-epidemic measures specific to dental practice were issued individually by each dental health care provider. Only a limited number of restrictions common for all public places were based on general government regulations, e.g., a limited number of people per area and disinfection being provided after entering interiors. Thus, the measures specific to dental practice were not issued centrally but were given at the individual discretion of the dentists. Such an individual approach was unusual in Europe and specific to the Czech Republic. However, to date, there are no statistics on the impact of the COVID-19 pandemic on dentistry in the Czech Republic. To reflect on it, the Czech Dental Chamber decided to perform a nationwide survey among its members, the results of which are presented in this article.

As membership in this professional chamber is mandatory for practicing dentistry in the Czech Republic, we were able to reach dentists from all around the country. A specific survey design based on a fast completion of the questionnaire resulted in an extraordinary response rate, representing, both relatively and absolutely, one of the most extensive sets of dentists as participants in a COVID-19 survey.

The aim of this work is to evaluate the impact of the COVID-19 pandemic on dental care in the Czech Republic from March 2020 to March 2021.

2. Materials and Methods

2.1. Design

This ad hoc, cross-sectional, self-administered, online survey was developed by the Czech Dental Chamber and performed among volunteers who were recruited from chamber members. All participants were informed about the objective of the study and did not have a patient status. The questionnaire was anonymous; completed questionnaires did not contain any personal information that could identify the participants and did not allow any traceability of the person answering. There were no direct benefits provided for participation. This study was conducted in accordance with the Declaration of Helsinki.

The survey consisted of 7 questions in the Czech native language, of which 6 were closed-ended, and 1 was open-ended. The questions were identified in cooperation with experts from the target population to ensure their clarity and appropriateness. The questionnaire was designed to be completed within 5 min.

The first question (Q1) regarded the impact of the pandemic on dental practices from March to May 2020. The dentists were asked about the opening hours of their practices, the number of patients treated, and the type of care provided. It was a closed-ended question with five single-choice answer options.

The second question (Q2) regarded the impact of the pandemic on dental practices from 1 September 2020, to 9 May 2021. The design was the same as in the first question. The first and the second questions followed the same design to reflect changes between the first and the second waves of COVID-19 in the Czech Republic. It was a closed-ended question with five single-choice answer options.

The third question (Q3) focused on the reasons for the closure of the dental practices during the whole pandemic. Respondents whose practices were not closed were asked to skip this question. It was a closed-ended question, five multiple-choice answer options.

In the fourth question (Q4), the participants were asked to evaluate the time range during which their dental practices were closed. Respondents whose practices were not closed were asked to skip this question. Six closed-ended answers option were provided. It was a closed-ended question with five single-choice answer options.

In the fifth question (Q5), the participants were asked to assess the patients' interest in preventive care using the data retrieved from their dental practice management software. It was a closed-ended question with six single-choice answer options.

In the sixth question (Q6), the participants were asked to evaluate the impact of the pandemic on the oral health of their patients. It was a closed-ended question with four single-choice answer options.

The seventh question (Q7) regarded the participants' greatest professional difficulty for the last year. It was an open-ended question with no limitations.

2.2. Sample

Officially registered e-mail addresses of 9922 Czech Dental Chamber members were addressed with a call for participation in this study focused on the impact of COVID-19 on practicing dentistry in the Czech Republic. Dentists were asked to participate in an online questionnaire from 24 February to 9 March 2021. As membership in this professional institution is mandatory for all practicing dentists in the country, the survey population included all practicing dentists in the Czech Republic. In this study, practicing dentists are defined as all dentists officially classified as Active members of the Czech Dental Chamber. According to the Czech Dental Chamber 2020 Annual Report, the chamber had 8624 Active members as of 31 December 2020 [16]. The rest of the 9922 e-mail addresses include members who are not practicing the dentist profession, including retired persons. Although these persons were not able to contribute to the survey, they are generally included in all full chamber correspondence.

2.3. Sample Size Relevancy

Considering the total number of practicing dentists in the Czech Republic, the minimum number of participants required for a relevant study was set to 368. The minimal sample size needed was calculated by Formula (1) using the online Netquest calculator. The calculation was performed with a study universe of all practicing dentists in the Czech Republic ($N = 8624$), a standard heterogeneity of 50%, a margin of error of 5%, and a confidence level of 95%. As the final sample size was 3674, the data within this study provide significantly relevant results.

$$n = \frac{N \cdot Z^2 \cdot p \cdot (1-p)}{(N-1) \cdot e^2 + Z^2 \cdot p \cdot (1-p)} \quad (1)$$

Formula (1). Relevant sample size calculation. Sample size calculated (n), size of the universe (N), deviation from the mean value (Z), the maximum margin of error tolerated (e), and the expected proportion (p).

2.4. Data Collection

The participants were contacted via e-mail invitation sent by the Czech Dental Chamber to officially registered the e-mail addresses of chamber members ($n = 9922$). The invitation included a link to an electronic questionnaire using a SurveyMonkey Questionnaire (SurveyMonkey, San Mateo, CA, USA). The questionnaire interface was compatible with a cell phone, desktop computer, or laptop to be accessible by as many respondents as possible. All replies were submitted fully completed. No exclusion criteria were applied. The participants' responses were stored in the SurveyMonkey Questionnaire cloud database during the survey process and downloaded at its end.

2.5. Statistical Analysis

Results of closed-ended questions (Q1–6) were downloaded from the SurveyMonkey Questionnaire cloud database. The data representing numbers of responses were analyzed, and the results are presented as the percentage frequency of individual answers within all answers provided. Skipping of a question was not counted as an answer and was not included in the percentage pool.

Each response of Q7 with an open-ended setup was evaluated by the authors individually and classified into one of the 38 general categories. Answers including more than one piece of information were subclassified into several categories. Replies that did not occur repeatedly were included in the "Others" category. Answers that could not be evaluated because they had no content or the content was incomprehensible were included in the category "No reply/do not know/sorting not applicable". Finally, the related categories were merged. The results of Q7 were processed as a table of the four most frequent categories summarizing the greatest professional difficulties among Czech dentists for the last year.

The data were analyzed using custom Microsoft Office Excel formulas (version 2106 for Windows, Microsoft Corporation, Redmond, WA, USA) and GraphPad Prism (version 8.0.0 for Windows, GraphPad Software, San Diego, CA, USA).

3. Results

3.1. Response Rate

Data from 3674 respondents were received. Compared to 9922 e-mails addresses included, the response rate was 37.0%. However, as this survey was addressed to practicing members (n = 8624), 3674 responses represent a 42.6% response rate within this population. Illustrated in Figure 1.

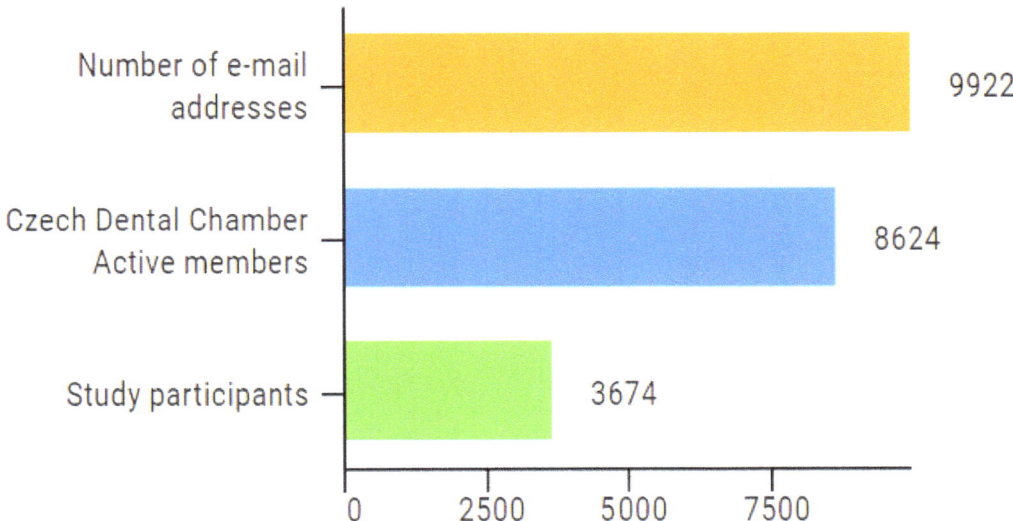

Figure 1. Response rate: 3674 participants represent 37.0% of all e-mail addresses included and 42.6% of practicing dentists in the Czech Republic.

3.2. Impact of the Pandemic on Dental Practices from March to May 2020

Out of 3674 respondents, a significant majority (3334; 90.7%) stated that their practices were open in the spring of 2020. However, almost a quarter of them (788; 21.4%) were open only for urgent and acute cases. At the same time, nearly half of the respondents (1709; 46.5%) reported a decrease in the number of patients. Only a minority of respondents (141; 3.8%) stated that their practices were closed during the pandemic. Other impacts were stated in 201 (5.5%) replies (Figure 2).

These results show that almost all Czech dentists maintained at least basic care for patients, and nearly half of them reported a decrease in patients during the first wave of COVID-19 from March to May of 2020.

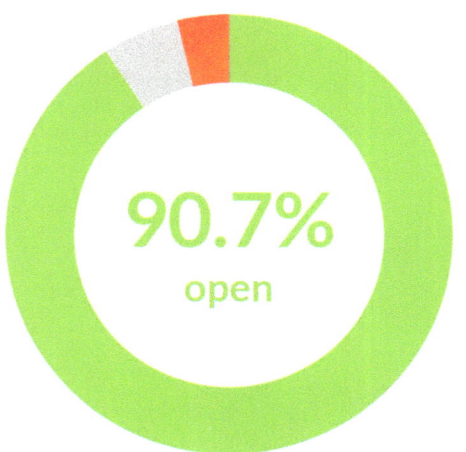

Figure 2. Impact of the pandemic on Czech dental practices from March to May of 2020. More than 90% of them remained open.

3.3. Impact of the Pandemic on Dental Practices from 1 September 2020, to 9 May 2021

Out of 3674 respondents, nearly all (3532; 96.1%) stated that their practices were open from 1 September 2020 to 9 May 2021. A few (31; 0.8%) restricted the care only for acute cases. Approximately one-third (1267; 34.5%) reported a decrease in number of patients. Almost no respondents (19; 0.5%) stated that their practices were closed (Figure 3).

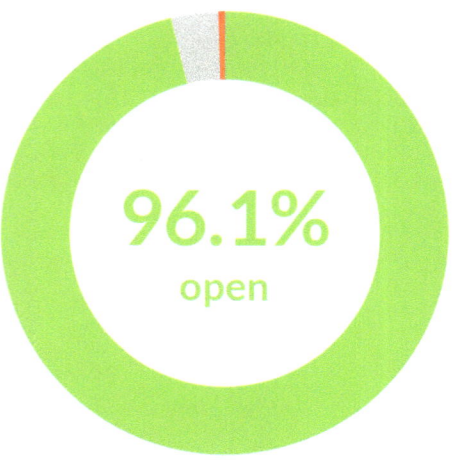

Figure 3. Impact of the pandemic on Czech dental practices from 1 September 2020 to 9 May 2021. More than 96% of them remained open.

These results show that practically all Czech dentists maintained care for patients during the first wave of COVID-19 from 1 September 2020 to 9 May 2021. A third of them reported a decrease in patient numbers.

3.4. Reasons Leading to Dental Practices' Closure during the Whole Pandemic

This question was addressed only to the respondents whose practices were closed at any time during the pandemic. Respondents whose practices were not closed were asked to skip this question. Out of 3674 respondents, 1922 respondents replied to this question, and 1754 respondents skipped it. Multiple answers were allowed.

The 1922 respondents who responded to this question reported 2729 reasons leading to the closure of the dental practice. The results are presented as the number of answers, the percentage of respondents choosing this answer, and the frequency of an answer among all answers, respectively: Shortage of personal protective equipment: 970/50.5%/35.5%; COVID-19 outbreak in the workplace: 471/24.5%/17.3%; Fear of a possible self-infection: 461/24.0%/16.9%; Quarantine: 394/20.5%/14.4%; Other reasons: 433/22.5%/15.9% (Figure 4).

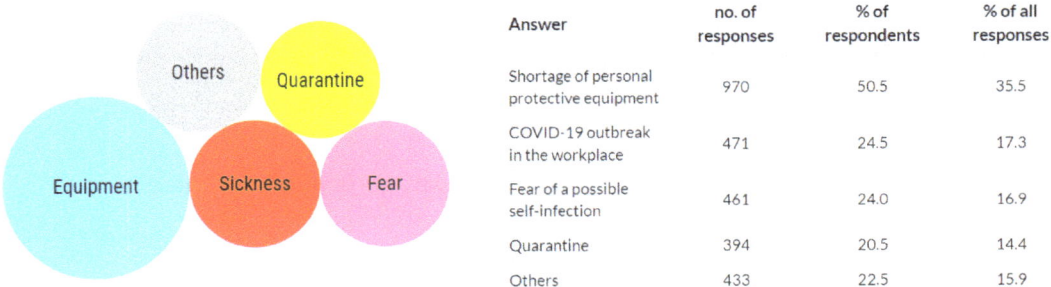

Figure 4. Reasons leading to the closure of Czech dental practices during the whole pandemic.

The data show that if the dental practices were closed, it was mainly due to the lack of personal protective equipment. Out of all reasons, shortage of protective equipment contributed to the closure of the dental practice in half of the cases, followed by the COVID-19 outbreak in the workplace and fear of a possible self-infection in a quarter of the cases, and quarantine in one-fifth of cases.

3.5. Time Range of Dental Practices Closure

This question was addressed only to the respondents whose practices were closed at any time during the pandemic. Respondents whose practices were not closed were asked to skip this question. Out of 3674 respondents, 1551 respondents replied to this question, and 2123 respondents skipped it.

Out of all participants, 1551 (42.2%) responded that their practices were closed during the pandemic. Half of these respondents (774; 49.9%) stated that the closure of their practices was in the range of 1–2 weeks. A total of 328 (21.2%) respondents reported the range of 2–4 weeks, and 152 (9.8%) reported the range longer than 1 month. The other reasons option was chosen by 297 (19.2%) respondents (Figure 5).

The results show that, during the pandemic, dental practices in the Czech Republic were mainly closed only for a short time, and closures longer than 1 month were rare.

Time range of Czech dental practices closure during the whole pandemic

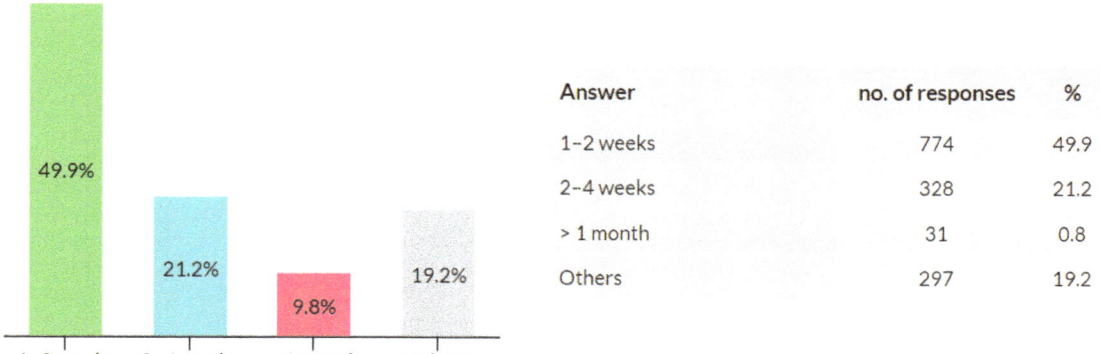

Figure 5. Time range of Czech dental practices closure during the whole pandemic.

3.6. Patients' Interest in Preventive Care during the Pandemic

Out of 3674 respondents, 1498 (40,8%) stated that the patients' interest in preventive care during the pandemic did not decrease at all or decreased by less than 10%, 1155 (31.4%) observed a 10–25% decrease, 474 (12.9%) observed a 26–50% decrease, 72 (2.0%) observed a 51–75% decrease, and 20 (0.5%) observed a >76% decrease, and 457 (12.4%) chose "No reply/do not know" option (Figure 6).

Decline in interest in preventive dental care among Czech patients during the pandemic

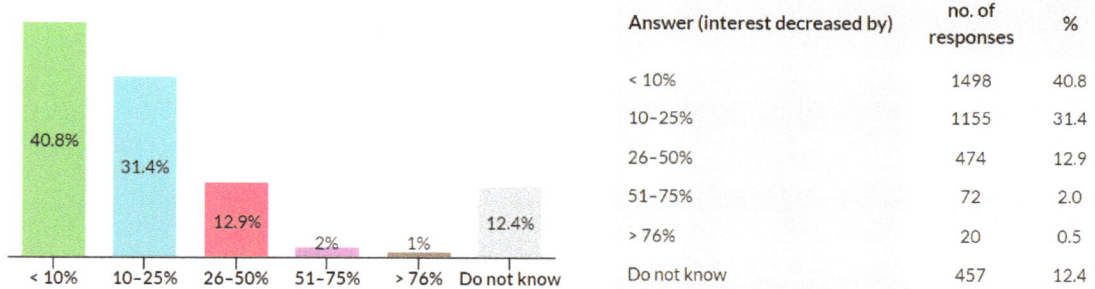

Figure 6. Decline in interest in preventive dental care among Czech patients during the pandemic.

Most dentists observed no decrease or just a minor decrease in patients' interest in preventive care during the pandemic.

3.7. Impact of the Pandemic on the Oral Care of Czech Patients

Out of 3674 respondents, 2852 (77.6%) did not observe any impact of the pandemic on the oral health of their patients, 621 respondents (16.9%) reported that their patients cared less about their oral health, and 61 respondents (1.7%) reported that their patients cared more about their oral health. The "others" option was chosen by 142 (3.9%) of respondents (Figure 7).

The approach to oral care was affected by the pandemic in less than one-fifth of the patients. For most of these, the effect was negative.

Impact of the pandemic on the oral care of Czech patients

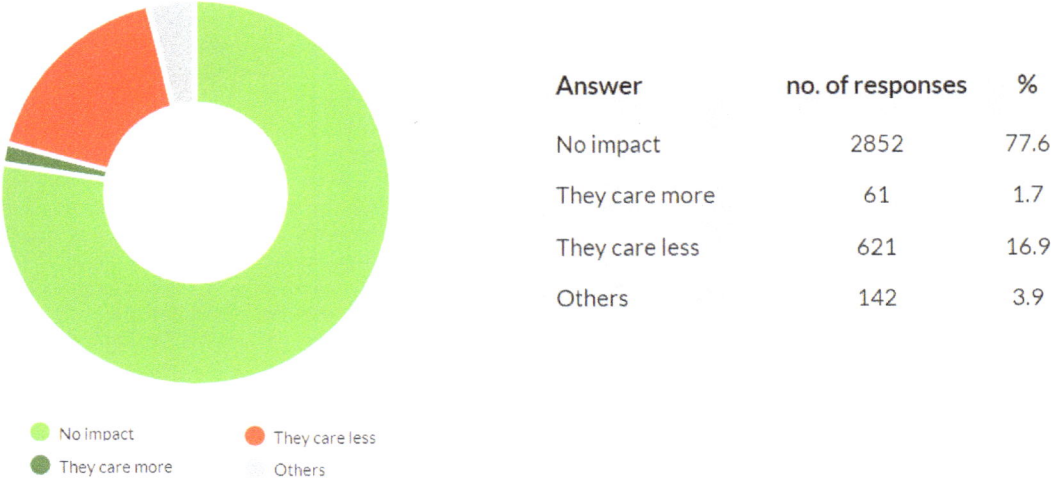

Figure 7. Impact of the pandemic on the oral care of Czech patients.

3.8. Dentists' Greatest Professional Difficulties during the Pandemic

Out of 3674 responses, the most frequent professional difficulties were: difficulties with administration, reorganization, re-ordering due to illness and quarantine of patients, and, in general, crisis operating management (55%); concerns about the safety of staff and patients, difficulties in complying with the strict hygiene measures in the workplace (49%); shortage of personal protective equipment (21%); difficult to work in protective equipment (15%) (Figure 8).

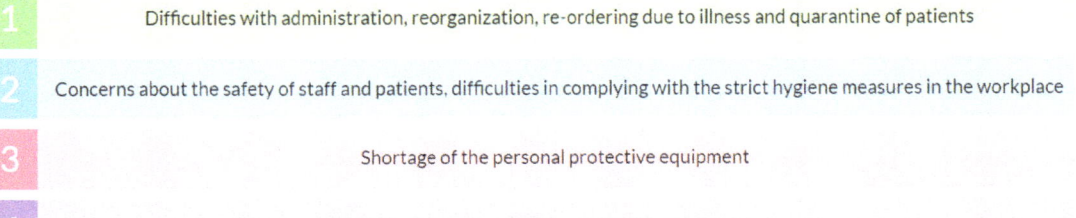

Figure 8. Czech dentists' greatest professional difficulties during the pandemic.

4. Study Limitations

There are three major limitations in this study that could be addressed in future research. First, the presented study includes subjective reports of respondents. Second, the number of questions is limited. Third, some outcomes of this work are not comparable with the pre-pandemic period, as there are no studies or reports containing comparable data from the previous years. These limitations were not accidentally identified during or after the survey but were known to the authors before the research began.

This study provides an insight into the daily difficulties of dental professionals during the pandemic and helps identify the weaknesses of the healthcare system that are usually not retrievable via any other sources. On the other hand, some study outcomes, e.g., the complex quantification of the patients' interest in preventive care (Q5) or impact of the pandemic on oral health (Q6), may be skewed as the quantification is based on the estimation of dental professionals. Although, naturally, the results of questionnaires are based on subjective judgments, we consider it important to comment on this issue and provide future direction for more accurate data acquisition. Q5 was included in the questionnaire mainly to retrieve qualitative results, i.e., whether the respondents observed a decrease in the interest in preventive dental care during the pandemic. The quantification may be considered abundant, the results may be questioned and should be verified by more objective data when available. More accurately quantified outcomes may be retrieved from government health institutions' annual healthcare data reports once released.

Additionally, it is important to discuss the questionnaire extension itself. It may be argued that the questionnaire lacks some information that is commonly included in works of similar focus, such as participants' personal data, dental practice location, or more questions, including those on COVID-19-related data. We agree that more questions would contribute to the informativeness of this study, but we intentionally decided to keep the questionnaire as simple as possible. This study was conducted at the time that the pandemic was escalating, and there were concerns that the respondents' participation would be affected by their different workloads. It was assumed that those who worked during the pandemic had a reduced opportunity and determination to participate in a survey that consisted of many questions due to their extreme workload. Conversely, those who reduced or stopped their work during the pandemic were supposed to have a greater opportunity and determination to participate. Such an outcome would lead to an unequal representation of discrete groups of respondents and biased results. To address this issue, it was necessary to ensure that the survey is as inclusive as possible, i.e., with a time-saving and straightforward design that could be finished within 5 min. Alternatively, it was possible to wait with the survey for the time after the pandemic subsided. At this time, it could be assumed that dentists would have more time to respond. However, such an approach could notably affect the results, as respondents would be interviewed for events several months apart. In conclusion, the questionnaire was purposely developed to provide statistically robust and representative data at the cost of the data extension. This aim was achieved as 3674 participants represent 37.0% of all e-mails sent and 42.6% of practicing dentists in the Czech Republic.

As this study is the first of its kind in the Czech Republic, some data cannot be compared with data from the pre-pandemic period. For instance, the open/closed dental practices during the pandemic cannot be compared to the previous years. However, data of this study can be compared to the results of the studies carried out in the coming years.

5. Discussion

This study was carried out during the second wave of COVID-19 in the Czech Republic. The second wave was the most severe pandemic period regarding the number of new cases and deaths [17]. As there were no official data on the impact of the pandemic on Czech dentistry, the Czech Dental Chamber needed to obtain this information to adequately reflect on the needs of its members. Thus, the chamber decided to address dentists from all over the country with an online survey. As described in the previous chapter, the survey had to be specifically designed to address the broadest possible range of respondents. This unique approach focusing on a limited number of carefully selected questions led to a high participation rate, which accounted for 42.6% of practicing dentists in the Czech Republic. This outcome makes this study one of the largest in terms of the number of participating dentists and especially in terms of the percentage of participating dentists within one country. Furthermore, this is the first study on the COVID-19 impact on dentistry in the Czech Republic. However, although the minimum number of participants required for this study was significantly exceeded, it should be taken into account that the data presented in this study do not represent 100% of Czech dentists, but only those who participated in this study.

Q1 focused on the impact of COVID-19 on dental practices during the first wave of the pandemic (March–May 2020). The results revealed that although dental professionals were considered one of the most vulnerable frontline workers, more than 90% of dental practices were open [18]. Half of them registered fewer patients, about a fifth reduced the care provided only for acute cases, and about a fifth did not report any changes compared to before the COVID-19 outbreak. The number of closed dental practices was minimal. From these results, it is possible to conclude that during the first wave of the pandemic in the spring of 2020 in the Czech Republic:

- 22.8% of dental practices were fully operational with no limitations compared to before the pandemic. The main operating limitation of dental practices (46.5%) was the lower number of patients.
- Acute dental care was provided almost without any restriction.
- Only 3.8% of dental practices were closed.

Q2 focused on the impact of COVID-19 on dental practices during the second pandemic wave (September 2020–May 2021). The percentage of open dental practices did not change significantly (from 90.7% during the first wave to 96.1% during the second wave). However, the results show an increase in dentists who worked without any changes compared to the period before the COVID-19 outbreak (from 22.8% during the first wave to 60.8% during the second wave). Fewer patients were reported by 34.5% of respondents, and only less than 1% of dentists treated only acute cases or closed their practice. It could be hypothesized that this change is probably due to the better availability of protective equipment, which has been identified as a major closure reason (see Q3), as well as a reduction in patients' fear of infection. In summary, during the first wave of the pandemic in the spring of 2020 in the Czech Republic:

- Over 60% of dental practices were fully operational compared to before the pandemic; fewer patients were reported by 34.5%.
- Acute dental care was provided almost without any restriction.
- Only 0.5% of dental practices were closed.

Although these data suggest that access to dental care has not been notably limited, the real impact of a pandemic on oral health may be significant. As shown in the work of Nioi et al., some patients may have delayed treatment due to fear of infection, which could lead to worsening delays [19]. To assess these consequences, it is appropriate to choose a research tool other than a questionnaire, such as analyzing population oral health before, during, and after the pandemic.

In Q3, the dentists who closed their practices anytime during the pandemic were asked about the reasons for closure. The main reason was a shortage of personal protective equipment followed by a COVID-19 outbreak in the workplace, fear of infection, or quarantine. These reasons can be considered interlinked as the shortage of protective equipment may lead to infection, fear of infection, and quarantine. Indeed, most of the multiple answers included a shortage of protective equipment. This finding is in accordance with other studies reporting on the lack of protective equipment as one of the main issues of healthcare providers worldwide during the pandemic [20–24].

Of responders, 42.2% admitted that their practices were closed for some time during the pandemic. Out of these, 49.9% were closed for less than 2 weeks, 21.2% for less than 4 weeks, and 9.8% for more than 1 month (for any reason). These results show that, despite the pandemic, less than 10% of dental practices were closed for more than 1 month between March 2020 and March 2021. As the Czech Republic sets a minimum holiday of 4 weeks by law, Q4 results can be interpreted as showing that the pandemic did not notably extend the total time that dentists were out of work compared to the pre-pandemic years.

In Q5, respondents were asked about the decline in interest in preventive dental care they observed among Czech patients during the pandemic. The results show that

47.3% of dentists observed a decline greater than 10% compared to before the pandemic. As described in the Section 4, Q5 outcomes should be understood as a qualitative indicator of the interest in preventive dental care during the pandemic, and the quantification should be further verified. For accurate quantification, this issue can be addressed by studies covering healthcare data reports for years 2020 and 2021 once available and comparing them with previous years. Another interesting research direction could be the impact of lower interest in preventive dental care on the subsequent deterioration of oral health in the coming years. Additionally, in Q6, dentists were also asked whether they observed any impact of the pandemic on their patients' oral care. More than three-quarters did not observe any impact, and poorer oral care of their patients was reported by 16.9% of dentists, and only 1.9% reported better oral care. Although almost 80% of dentists did not observe a deterioration in their patients' oral care, almost a fifth did the opposite. Such an outcome can significantly contribute to the decline in overall oral health in the Czech Republic. Results of questions Q5 and Q6 indicate a worsening approach of Czech patients to oral health during the pandemic and may affect their oral health in the coming years. These outcomes may indicate the deterioration of oral health as an indirect outcome of the COVID-19 pandemic and serve as an incentive for government health institutions and the Czech Dental Chamber to introduce policies reversing this impact and promoting the oral health of the Czech population.

As revealed in Q7, the greatest professional difficulties of Czech dentists' during May 2020–May 2021 were associated with the COVID-19 pandemic. Crisis operating management was the most significant inconvenience followed by the health concerns, lack of protective equipment, and problems resulting from working in the protective equipment. It is no surprise that all the abovementioned is linked to the pandemic as the dentists had to face this unprecedented situation from the frontline. These findings may indicate that the incidence of COVID-19 among dentists may be higher than in the general population. The notable impact of COVID-19 on the health of the healthcare workers was also reported by other authors; however, thus far, there are no such studies focused on Czech dentists [25]. This topic remains an opportunity for further investigation.

Additional studies with a similar focus reveal that the COVID-19 pandemic has severely affected dentistry globally. A work of Izzeti et al. reporting on dental activity during the pandemic in Italy shows that during the spring of 2020, 99.7% of surveyed dentists reduced their professional activity to urgent treatments or totally stopped working [26]. Another survey focusing on the COVID-19 impact on dental practices in Central Italy during the spring of 2020 reported on very similar trends [27]. In this study, 38.4% of respondents reported that they performed both dental emergencies and urgent care, 26.6% performed only urgent dental care, and 26.4% provided no dental care. In summary, 91.4% of respondents reduced their professional activities to urgent or emergent treatments or totally stopped working. This is in contrast to the reports of Czech dentists. In our survey, 22.8% of respondents admitted that their practices operated with no limitations, only 21.4% reported their practices remained open providing treatment only to acute cases, and 3.8% closed their practices during the spring of 2020. This disparity may be due to a different impact of the pandemic on Italy and the Czech Republic during these months. Italy was one of the most severely affected countries in the whole world; on the other hand, the Czech Republic was affected very mildly [28,29]. An additional study, performed by Miśta et al., focused on professional aspects of dentists in Poland during April 2020 [30]. A total of 71.2% of dentists responded that they decided to suspend their clinical practice. As in our study, the main reasons leading Polish dentists to practice closure were insufficient equipment (63.4%) and fear for their own and their family members' health and life (51.2%, 57.6%, respectively). In June 2020, Ahmadi et al. performed a study among Iranian dentists assessing the pandemic impact on their practices [31]. Seventy percent of the participants admitted they did not perform non-emergency procedures during the pandemic, and 87% had problems finding and providing personal protective equipment. A study by Faccini et al. performed in May 2020 reports that in Brazil, 64.6% of the dentists performed only urgency/emergency dental care, 26.1% maintained routine appointments, and 9.3% closed their dental offices. These results are similar to those of our study. Although there are some methodological differences, our data show that, in comparison to surveys conducted in other countries, Czech dentistry remained more operative during the pandemic and Czech dentists faced similar fears and problems as their colleagues from other countries.

6. Conclusions

This survey conducted among 3674 dentists in the Czech Republic reveals that more than 90% of them worked during the COVID-19 pandemic from March 2020 to March 2021. Out of those who closed their practices, only 9.8% was for more than 1 month. The main reasons leading to the closure were a shortage of protective equipment, COVID-19 infection, fear of infection, or quarantine. The leading professional difficulties of Czech dentists were crisis operating management, a lack of protective equipment, and health safety concerns. Additionally, the respondents observed a declining interest in preventive dental care in 47.3% of patients and worse oral care in 16.9% of patients indicating a deterioration in oral health as a possible delayed outcome of the pandemic.

Author Contributions: Conceptualization J.S. (Jan Schmidt), E.W., and R.S.; methodology E.W. and S.B.; software: E.W.; validation J.S. (Jan Schmidt) and J.S. (Jakub Suchanek); formal analysis, E.W., S.B., and J.S. (Jan Schmidt); investigation E.W., S.B., and R.S.; resources, E.W., S.B., and J.S. (Jan Schmidt); data curation, E.W., S.B., J.S. (Jan Schmidt); writing—original draft preparation, J.S. (Jan Schmidt), and J.S. (Jakub Suchanek); writing—review and editing J.S. (Jan Schmidt), J.S. (Jakub Suchanek), and R.S.; visualization, E.W. and J.S. (Jan Schmidt); supervision J.S. (Jakub Suchanek), R.S.; project administration E.W., S.B., and R.S.; funding acquisition, J.S. (Jakub Suchanek), E.W., and R.S. All authors have read and agreed to the published version of the manuscript.

Funding: This work was supported by the Charles University's program PROGRES Q40/13.

Institutional Review Board Statement: Not applicable.

Informed Consent Statement: Not applicable.

Data Availability Statement: The dataset is available on-demand from the corresponding author.

Acknowledgments: The authors thank Diksha Ghimire for English language editing.

Conflicts of Interest: The authors declare no conflict of interest.

References

1. Islam, M.A.; Alam, S.S.; Kundu, S.; Hossan, T.; Kamal, M.A.; Cavestro, C. Prevalence of Headache in Patients With Coronavirus Disease 2019 (COVID-19): A Systematic Review and Meta-Analysis of 14,275 Patients. *Front. Neurol.* **2020**, *11*, 1492. [CrossRef]
2. Islam, M.A.; Kundu, S.; Alam, S.S.; Hossan, T.; Kamal, M.A.; Hassan, R. Prevalence and characteristics of fever in adult and paediatric patients with coronavirus disease 2019 (COVID-19): A systematic review and meta-analysis of 17515 patients. *PLoS ONE* **2021**, *16*, e0249788. [CrossRef]
3. Saniasiaya, J.; Islam, M.A.; Abdullah, B. Prevalence of Olfactory Dysfunction in Coronavirus Disease 2019 (COVID-19): A Meta-analysis of 27,492 Patients. *Laryngoscope* **2021**, *131*, 865–878. [CrossRef]
4. Saniasiaya, J.; Islam, M.A.; Abdullah, B. Prevalence and Characteristics of Taste Disorders in Cases of COVID-19: A Meta-analysis of 29,349 Patients. *Otolaryngol.—Head Neck Surg.* **2021**, *165*, 33–42. [CrossRef] [PubMed]
5. Hu, B.; Huang, S.; Yin, L. The cytokine storm and COVID-19. *J. Med. Virol.* **2021**, *93*, 250–256. [CrossRef] [PubMed]
6. Li, X.; Ma, X. Acute respiratory failure in COVID-19: Is it "typical" ARDS? *Crit. Care* **2020**, *24*, 198. [CrossRef]
7. Lotfi, M.; Hamblin, M.R.; Rezaei, N. COVID-19: Transmission, prevention, and potential therapeutic opportunities. *Clin. Chim. Acta* **2020**, *508*, 254–266. [CrossRef] [PubMed]
8. Huang, C.; Wang, Y.; Li, X.; Ren, L.; Zhao, J.; Hu, Y.; Zhang, L.; Fan, G.; Xu, J.; Gu, X.; et al. Clinical features of patients infected with 2019 novel coronavirus in Wuhan, China. *Lancet* **2020**, *395*, 497–506. [CrossRef]
9. World Health Organization. WHO Director-General's Opening Remarks at the Media Briefing on COVID-19—11 March 2020. 2020. Available online: https://www.who.int/director-general/speeches/detail/who-director-general-s-opening-remarks-at-the-media-briefing-on-covid-19---11-march-2020 (accessed on 12 July 2021).
10. Government Resolution on Combating the Coronavirus Epidemic—2020/Vládní Usnesení Související s Bojem proti Epidemii Koronaviru—Rok 2020. 2020. Available online: https://www.vlada.cz/cz/epidemie-koronaviru/dulezite-informace/vladni-usneseni-souvisejici-s-bojem-proti-epidemii-koronaviru---rok-2020-186999/#zari (accessed on 16 August 2021).

11. Government Resolution on Combating the Coronavirus Epidemic—2021/Vládní Usnesení Související s Bojem Proti Epidemii Koronaviru—Rok 2021. 2021. Available online: https://www.vlada.cz/cz/epidemie-koronaviru/dulezite-informace/vladni-usneseni-souvisejici-s-bojem-proti-epidemii-180608/ (accessed on 16 August 2021).
12. Czech Government. Measures Adopted by the Czech Government against the Coronavirus. 2021. Available online: https://www.vlada.cz/en/media-centrum/aktualne/measures-adopted-by-the-czech-government-against-coronavirus-180545/ (accessed on 16 August 2021).
13. Global Change Data Lab. Czechia, Coronavirus Cases per Capita. 2021. Available online: https://ourworldindata.org/coronavirus/country/czech-republic (accessed on 12 July 2021).
14. Parisi, S.G.; Viel, G.; Cecchi, R.; Montisci, M. COVID-19: The wrong target for healthcare liability claims. *Leg. Med.* **2020**, *46*, 101718. [CrossRef]
15. d'Aloja, E.; Finco, G.; Demontis, R.; Napoli, P.; Fossarello, M.; Nioi, M. COVID-19 and medical liability: Italy denies the shield to its heroes. *EClinicalMedicine* **2020**, *25*, 100470. [CrossRef]
16. Czech Dental Chamber. Ročenka ČSK 2020 (Czech Dental Chamber 2020 Annual Report). 2021. Available online: https://www.dent.cz/o-nas/rocenky/ (accessed on 10 July 2021).
17. American Library Association. Czechia, Coronavirus Cases. 2021. Available online: https://www.worldometers.info/coronavirus/country/czech-republic/ (accessed on 5 July 2021).
18. Fallahi, H.R.; Keyhan, S.O.; Zandian, D.; Kim, S.-G.; Cheshmi, B. Being a front-line dentist during the Covid-19 pandemic: A literature review. *Maxillofac. Plast. Reconstr. Surg.* **2020**, *42*, 12. [CrossRef] [PubMed]
19. Nioi, M.; Napoli, P.; Finco, G.; Demontis, R.; Fossarello, M.; d'Aloja, E. Fear of the COVID-19 and medical liability. Insights from a series of 130 consecutives medico-legal claims evaluated in a single institution during SARS-CoV-2-related pandemic. *Signa Vitae* **2021**, *17*, 79–85. [CrossRef]
20. Martin-Delgado, J.; Viteri, E.; Mula, A.; Serpa, P.; Pacheco, G.; Prada, D.; Campos de Andrade Lourenção, D.; Campos Pavan Baptista, P.; Ramirez, G.; Mira, J.J. Availability of personal protective equipment and diagnostic and treatment facilities for healthcare workers involved in COVID-19 care: A cross-sectional study in Brazil, Colombia, and Ecuador. *PLoS ONE* **2020**, *15*, e0242185. [CrossRef]
21. Newman, M. Covid-19: Doctors' leaders warn that staff could quit and may die over lack of protective equipment. *BMJ Br. Med. J. (Online)* **2020**, *368*, m1257. [CrossRef] [PubMed]
22. Mantelakis, A.; Spiers, H.V.M.; Lee, C.W.; Chambers, A.; Joshi, A. Availability of Personal Protective Equipment in NHS Hospitals During COVID-19: A National Survey. *Ann. Work Expo. Health* **2021**, *65*, 136–140. [CrossRef] [PubMed]
23. Ahmed, J.; Malik, F.; Bin Arif, T.; Majid, Z.; Chaudhary, M.A.; Ahmad, J.; Malik, M.; Khan, T.M.; Khalid, M. Availability of Personal Protective Equipment (PPE) Among US and Pakistani Doctors in COVID-19 Pandemic. *Cureus* **2020**, *12*, e8550. [CrossRef]
24. Rebmann, T.; Vassallo, A.; Holdsworth, J.E. Availability of personal protective equipment and infection prevention supplies during the first month of the COVID-19 pandemic: A national study by the APIC COVID-19 task force. *Am. J. Infect. Control* **2021**, *49*, 434–437. [CrossRef]
25. Nioi, M.; Napoli, P.E.; Lobina, J.; Fossarello, M.; d'Aloja, E. COVID-19 and Italian Healthcare Workers From the Initial Sacrifice to the mRNA Vaccine: Pandemic Chrono-History, Epidemiological Data, Ethical Dilemmas, and Future Challenges. *Front. Public Health* **2021**, *8*, 1037. [CrossRef]
26. Izzetti, R.; Gennai, S.; Nisi, M.; Barone, A.; Giuca, M.R.; Gabriele, M.; Graziani, F. A perspective on dental activity during COVID-19: The Italian survey. *Oral Dis.* **2021**, *27*, 694–702. [CrossRef]
27. Sinjari, B.; Rexhepi, I.; Santilli, M.; D'Addazio, G.; Chiacchiaretta, P.; Di Carlo, P.; Caputi, S. The Impact of COVID-19 Related Lockdown on Dental Practice in Central Italy—Outcomes of A Survey. *Int. J. Environ. Res. Public Health* **2020**, *17*, 5780. [CrossRef]
28. Smyčka, J.; Levínský, R.; Hromádková, E.; Šoltés, M.; Šlerka, J.; Tuček, V.; Trnka, J.; Šmíd, M.; Zajíček, M.; Diviák, T.; et al. Delays, masks, the elderly, and schools: First COVID-19 wave in the Czech Republic. *medRxiv* **2021**. [CrossRef]
29. Nacoti, M.; Ciocca, A.; Giupponi, A.; Brambillasca, P.; Lussana, F.; Pisano, M.; Goisis, G.; Bonacina, D.; Fazzi, F.; Naspro, R. At the epicenter of the Covid-19 pandemic and humanitarian crises in Italy: Changing perspectives on preparation and mitigation. *NEJM Catal. Innov. Care Deliv.* **2020**, *1*.
30. Tysiąc-Miśta, M.; Dziedzic, A. The Attitudes and Professional Approaches of Dental Practitioners during the COVID-19 Outbreak in Poland: A Cross-Sectional Survey. *Int. J. Environ. Res. Public Health* **2020**, *17*, 4703. [CrossRef] [PubMed]
31. Ahmadi, H.; Ebrahimi, A.; Ghorbani, F. The Impact of COVID-19 Pandemic on Dental Practice in Iran: A questionnaire-based report. *BMC Oral Health* **2020**, *20*, 354. [CrossRef] [PubMed]

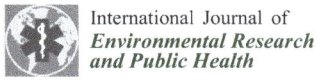

International Journal of
Environmental Research and Public Health

Article

The Impact of the Lockdown Caused by the COVID-19 Pandemic on the Fine Particulate Matter (PM$_{2.5}$) Air Pollution: The Greek Paradigm

Ourania S. Kotsiou [1,2,*], Georgios K. D. Saharidis [3], Georgios Kalantzis [3], Evangelos C. Fradelos [2] and Konstantinos I. Gourgoulianis [1]

1. Respiratory Medicine Department, Faculty of Medicine, University of Thessaly, BIOPOLIS, 41110 Larissa, Greece; kgourg@uth.gr
2. Department of Nursing, Faculty of Nursing, University of Thessaly, GAIOPOLIS, 41110 Larissa, Greece; efradelos@uth.gr
3. Department of Mechanical Engineering, University of Thessaly, Leoforos Athinon, Pedion Areos, 38334 Volos, Greece; saharidis@gmail.com (G.K.D.S.); george.kalantzis4@gmail.com (G.K.)
* Correspondence: raniakotsiou@gmail.com; Tel.: +30-2413-502-812

Abstract: Introduction: Responding to the coronavirus pandemic, Greece implemented the largest quarantine in its history. No data exist regarding its impact on PM$_{2.5}$ pollution. We aimed to assess PM$_{2.5}$ levels before, during, and after lockdown (7 March 2020–16 May 2020) in Volos, one of Greece's most polluted industrialized cities, and compare PM$_{2.5}$ levels with those obtained during the same period last year. Meteorological conditions were examined as confounders. Methods: The study period was discriminated into three phases (pre-lockdown: 7 March–9 March, lockdown: 10 March–4 May, and post-lockdown period: 5 May–16 May). A wireless sensors network was used to collect PM$_{2.5}$, temperature, relative humidity, rainfall, and wind speed data every 2 s. Results: The lockdown resulted in a significant drop of PM$_{2.5}$ by 37.4% in 2020, compared to 2019 levels. The mean daily concentrations of PM$_{2.5}$ exceeded the WHO's guideline value for 24-h mean levels of PM$_{2.5}$ 35% of the study period. During the strictest lockdown (23 March to 4 May), the mean daily PM$_{2.5}$ levels exceeded the standard 41% of the time. The transition from the pre-lockdown period into lockdown or post-lockdown periods was associated with lower PM$_{2.5}$ concentrations. Conclusions: A reduction in the mean daily PM$_{2.5}$ concentration was found compared to 2019. Lockdown was not enough to avoid severe exceedances of air pollution in Volos.

Keywords: air pollution; coronavirus disease 2019; Greece; GreenYourAir; fine particulate matter

Citation: Kotsiou, O.S.; Saharidis, G.K.D.; Kalantzis, G.; Fradelos, E.C.; Gourgoulianis, K.I. The Impact of the Lockdown Caused by the COVID-19 Pandemic on the Fine Particulate Matter (PM$_{2.5}$) Air Pollution: The Greek Paradigm. *Int. J. Environ. Res. Public Health* **2021**, *18*, 6748. https://doi.org/10.3390/ijerph18136748

Academic Editor: Dirga Kumar Lamichhane

Received: 7 May 2021
Accepted: 15 June 2021
Published: 23 June 2021

Publisher's Note: MDPI stays neutral with regard to jurisdictional claims in published maps and institutional affiliations.

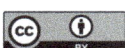

Copyright: © 2021 by the authors. Licensee MDPI, Basel, Switzerland. This article is an open access article distributed under the terms and conditions of the Creative Commons Attribution (CC BY) license (https://creativecommons.org/licenses/by/4.0/).

1. Introduction

The Mediterranean city of Volos is located in Central Greece and situated midway on the Greek mainland. It is the sixth-largest city with the third-largest industrial area. The Volos port is the third-largest port in Greece. Volos is an excellent paradigm of a medium-size city where population shifts and high industrialization in the last decades have resulted in the degradation of the air quality [1]. It is considered among the most polluted cities in Greece, primarily due to domestic heating, traffic, container terminal operations, mineral facilities, and installations for cement and lime production [2].

Air pollutants include gaseous pollutants and particle matters (PM). The pathogenicity of PM is determined by their size, origin, composition, solubility, and ability to produce reactive oxygen species. It has been reported that smog is generally caused by high concentrations of aerosols or fine particles sized less than or equal to 2.5 micrometers, referred to as inhalable fine particulate matter (PM$_{2.5}$) [3–6]. The toxic effects of PMs are mainly attributed to PM$_{2.5}$ [3]. PM$_{2.5}$ pollution is mainly related to anthropogenic emissions from industries, traffic transportation, power plants, and biomass burning [4]. Vehicular traffic constitutes the most important source of particulate pollution in the area under study [1]. More specifically, tourist traffic passing through the city towards the local attractions and the seaport for passengers and commercial use are two factors that aggravate traffic. Among many other sectors, transport is the most hard-hit sector due to lockdown. Road and air transport came to a halt as people were not allowed or hesitate to travel.

The increased industrialization in the city of Volos is strongly related to $PM_{2.5}$ pollution. Cement, steel, and mineral mining industries are making a source of atmospheric pollution in Volos [1,2]. Additionally, there are two relatively small industrial areas to the west and a big cement industry to the east of the study area. Other sources of PM pollutants are the burning of fossil fuels in vehicles and power plants [1,2].

Factors affecting $PM_{2.5}$ mass concentration apart from domestic pollutant emission and external sources [7,8] include the meteorological parameters (relative humidity, wind speed, temperature). These parameters affect pollution concentration, as well as the removal, transportation, and dispersion of airborne particles [9–13]. The climate of Volos is of Mediterranean type with mild, wet winters and hot, dry summers. The average daily temperature for the spring is 15 °C (March, April, May) [1]. The average daily relative humidity varies between 58% in July and 74% in November [14–16]. During 7 March–23 May is a period free from significant activity of residential heating equipment in the city. Also, this period is characterized by the absence of abrupt weather changes and the absence of precipitation which would clean the air, so the local wind system and micro-climate are clearly observable [3].

Saharan dust advection days have been shown to contribute to particulate matter exceeding the daily WHO-recommended limits in the city [17–22]. The cyclones are generated by the thermal contrast between cold Atlantic air and warm continental air that cross North Africa during spring and summer [17–20]. Furthermore, the presence of circumferential, mountainous terrain creates local air turbulences, making air exchange problematic and air polluted with $PM_{2.5}$ may circulate over the region—a condition known as the long-range transport of air pollution. Sea salt emissions (whose growth rate depends on relative humidity) are also a source of PMs and contribute up to 80% of particle levels in the air in the coastal area of Volos [5]. Sea salt contributed by 12.4%, as expected for the maritime location of Volos [6].

The $PM_{2.5}$ air pollution has been associated with an increased risk of acute or chronic respiratory disease and susceptibility to exacerbations given that prolonged exposure to air pollution leads to a chronic inflammatory stimulus, even in young and healthy subjects [23–31]. Particle air pollution has been associated with more medical visits and excess hospitalizations [29–31]. Furthermore, people living in areas with high levels of particular air pollutants are vulnerable to developing respiratory infections [31]. Namely, recent evidence supports that the high pollution level of Northern Italy should be considered an additional co-factor of the high level of COVID-19 death rates recorded in that area [32,33]. Emerging data supporting air pollution exposure is linked to COVID-19 severity, higher morbidity, and mortality [32–34]. Utilizing health information in air pollution health research will result in the achievement of environmental health protection goals.

Globally, interventions to contain the coronavirus disease 2019 (COVID-19) outbreak led to improvements in air quality [35]. The coronavirus pandemic and lockdown slowed business activities, restricted traffic and transportation, and revealed a huge drop in air pollution in affected countries [32]. Responding to the ongoing novel coronavirus outbreak, Greece implemented the largest quarantine in the country's history during the first pandemic wave. A three-phase approach was adopted. On the 10th of March, the operation of educational institutions of all levels was suspended nationwide, and then, on the 13th of March, all commercial stores and entertainment centers were closed down. The Greek authorities announced stringent traffic, transport, and industry restrictions, starting from 6 AM on the 23rd of March. Starting from the 4th of May, after a 42-day lockdown, Greece gradually lifted restrictions on movement and restarted business activity.

The measures put in place in Greece were among the strictest in Europe [32,35]. As Greece went into lockdown, the industrial activities shut down in Volos.

No data exist regarding the impact of the lockdown caused by the COVID-19 pandemic on $PM_{2.5}$ air quality in Greece. The aims of this study were to assess the $PM_{2.5}$ concentrations obtained by a wireless sensors network located at twelve different measurement points in Volos, Greece, before (7 March–9 March), during (10 March–4 May), and after the implementation of lockdown (5 May–16 May), examine to what extent government restrictions affected $PM_{2.5}$ concentrations, and compare $PM_{2.5}$ levels with those obtained from the identical locations during the same period in 2019. Meteorological conditions were also examined as confounders.

2. Materials and Methods

2.1. Network Implementation and Data Collection

The daily 24-h $PM_{2.5}$ air pollution data were collected from twelve fully automated air quality monitoring stations located in the center and the greater area of Volos for the period from 7 March 2020 until 16 May 2020. The selected study period is characterized by the absence of abrupt weather changes and the absence of precipitation which would clean the air, so, the local wind system and micro-climate are clearly observable. Furthermore, this is a period free from significant activity of residential heating equipment in the city [3]. The values of the twelve monitoring devices have been used to calculate the daily mean $PM_{2.5}$ concentration in Volos. The fully automated air quality monitoring network was established by the GreenYourAir research team. The 24-h temperature, relative humidity, rainfall, and wind speed values were also recorded every 2 s along with each $PM_{2.5}$ measurement by the network, for the same period. The higher safe limits for particulates in the air defined as a daily average of 25 $\mu g/m^3$ for $PM_{2.5}$, according to the World Health Organization (WHO) air quality guidelines [36]. More specifically, the GreenYourAir monitoring network consisted of twelve measuring devices (GreenYourAir device 1178/$PM_{2.5}$) (Figure 1) designed and developed by the GreenYourAir research team. The network was developed based on the outcomes of previous EU projects and tests implemented by the team. GreenYourAir projects focus on monitoring the air quality at the city of Volos and especially $PM_{2.5}$, on identifying correlations between medical incidents and levels of $PM_{2.5}$, on quantifying the origins of air pollution in the monitored area, and on suggesting to public authorities and private entities solutions to improve air quality by decreasing the level of $PM_{2.5}$ [37]. The network works 24 h a day and seven days a week since 1 March 2019. Hence, the 2019 data were collected from the same network (GreenYouAir) and devices (GreenYourAir/1178 device) were placed at the same locations. To make day-to-day comparisons between 2019 and 2020 air quality data, we used the means calculated by averaging daily PM levels from all the twelve locations over the sampling duration.

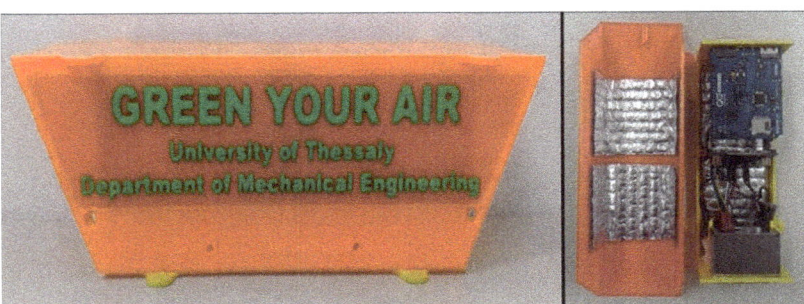

Figure 1. GreenYourAir device 1178/$PM_{2.5}$.

For the data collection, the light-scattering method was utilized. The amount of light scattered by the particles was detected by a photodiode, which translated the signal into electrical pulses. Then, the microprocessor analyzed these signals and calculated the mass concentration based on the amplitude of pulses. The light-scattering method has been widely used in research projects and the development of smart cities. The main parts of the device are: a sensor that provided data for the concertation of $PM_{2.5}$, temperature, and relative humidity, a zero-one integer (I/O) expansion shield, and an Arduino YUN rev. 2. The programming language of the device was C++. The devices were collecting data per second and they were working 24-h per day. In addition, a 3D printed box was designed to install the devices and create the network [20].

The GreenYourAir research team developed a mathematical formula and an optimization model to determine the optimal locations of the twelve sensors and create the sensor network. A mathematical formula was used to divide the city into sub-areas with specific characteristics and determine the number of sensors in each area. An environmental nuisance of 50 squares was calculated based on the source of emissions. In the end, 12 locations with different environmental nuisance were selected in order to represent well the region under study. The data that were introduced as inputs in the mathematical formula were: the five main functional zones of the city, the traffic zones of the city, the existence of bus, train, and boat stations, the presence of schools, parks, the heat sources, and the geomorphological characteristics of the city. In every smaller area created by the formula, a score was assigned regarding the proper number of sensors that should be placed based on its main characteristics.

More specifically, the city of Volos was divided into five functional zones (commercial and recreational zone, high-density residential zone, medium density residential zone, low-density residential zone, and industrial zone) (Figure 2A). The traffic flow of the city was divided into three types according to the density of traffic (high, medium, and low traffic jams), as shown in Figure 2B.

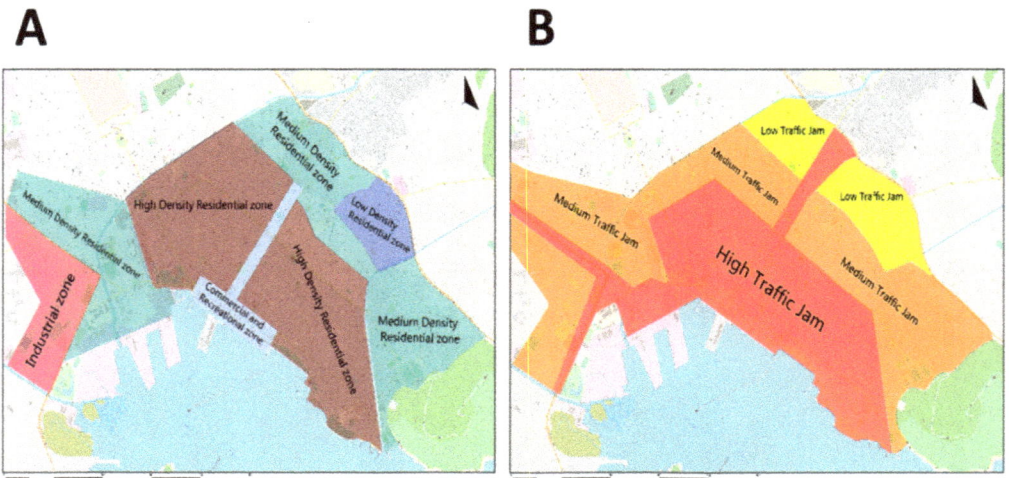

Figure 2. Zones of the city of Volos (**A**) and division into zones according to the density of traffic (**B**).

The city was divided into smaller areas and determined the number of sensors of each area as shown in Figure 3. The 1st industrial zone of Volos is located outside the city to the western suburbs, about 6 km from the center. The Lafarge Cement Volos Plant and the ELINOIL Petroleum company are located outside the city to the eastern suburbs, about 3.5 km from the center of the city. The city's primary sources of heating are oil, natural gas, and fireplaces. The geographical location and the geomorphological features specific to the city were also analyzed.

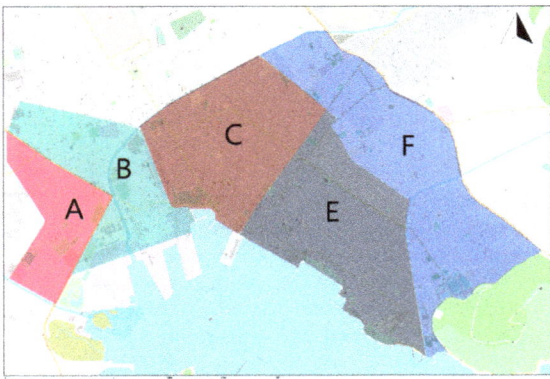

Figure 3. The sub-areas of the city of Volos selected for the placement of the sensors.

The required number of sensors at each sub-area was selected by analyzing the existence of parks, main roads, sports facilities, schools, and universities, the sources of heating, the traffic jam, and the zone within the city. Sensor positioning was the following: one sensor was placed at area A, two sensors at area B, three sensors were placed separately at areas C, E, and F.

The sensor placement locations were strategically placed after an optimization model was developed. The research team formalized the problem by means of a mathematical optimization model guided by the following main parameters: the number of sensors that were placed at each sub-area, the distance between the sensors of the same sub-area, the distance between the sensors of different sub-areas, the specific characteristics of each area and the coverage characteristics among different sub-areas (Figure 4A). The detailed optimization model guided the optimal sensor placement (Figure 4B).

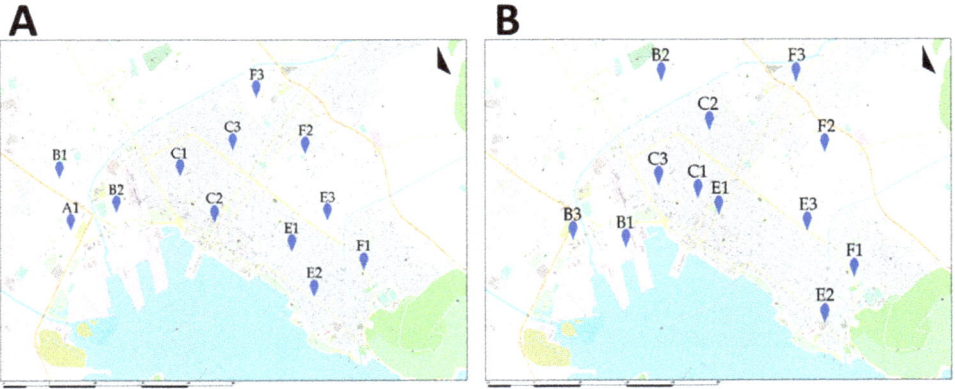

Figure 4. The optimal sensor placement according to the mathematical model (twelve sensors) (**A**) and the actual placement of sensors (twelve sensors) (**B**).

GreenYourAir devices 1178/$PM_{2.5}$ had advantages and disadvantages when compared to the dust samplers. The main advantages of the sensors were the simplicity of real-time measurements, the low cost, and the assessment of board geospatial coverage for the area. The main disadvantage of the sensors, in some cases, could be the accuracy of the measurements. To solve that issue, the GreenYourAir research team developed a calibration methodology.

During the development period, the sensing measurements were tested under laboratory conditions. Their performance was compared to reference instruments. The real-time measurements were compared with the reference instruments to increase accuracy. To this end, real-time air monitoring data is now viewable on the website: http://greenyourair.org/ (accessed on 1 June 2021).

2.2. Statistical Analyses

Spearman's correlation was used for correlation analysis between mean daily concentrations of $PM_{2.5}$ and meteorological variables. Multiple linear analysis and Spearman analysis were used to analyze the correlation between mean daily $PM_{2.5}$ concentrations, meteorological variables, and the three phases of the study. To identify differences between two independent groups, an unpaired t-test was used. Parametric data comparing three or more groups were analyzed with one-way ANOVA and Tukey's multiple comparisons test, while non-parametric data were analyzed with the Kruskal–Wallis test and Dunn's multiple comparison test. A result was considered statistically significant when the p-value was <0.05. Data were analyzed and visualized using SPSS Statistics v.23 (Armonk, NY, USA: IBM Corp.) and Tableau (Tableau Software LLC, Seattle, WA, USA), respectively.

3. Results

3.1. Comparison between the Ambient $PM_{2.5}$ Levels in 2020 and 2019 (7 March 2020 to 16 May 2020)

Daily $PM_{2.5}$ concentrations used in Figure 5 and throughout this study were obtained by averaging 24-h $PM_{2.5}$ measurements monitored at 12 locations in 2019 and 2020. In Volos over the entire sampling period, the mean concentration of $PM_{2.5}$ declined significantly compared with the same 11-week period in 2019 (34.8 ± 11.9 vs. 21.8 ± 9.2, $p < 0.001$), as presented in Figure 5. There was a 37.4% reduction in mean daily $PM_{2.5}$ levels during the COVID-19 period in Volos.

The percentage of days with a mean daily concentration of $PM_{2.5}$ above the safe limit was 80% in 2019, i.e., almost the entire study period except for the last week of April and the first days of May. The $PM_{2.5}$ levels were 30% to 100% higher than the 24-h threshold of 25 $\mu g/m^3$ set by the WHO air quality guidelines. In 2020, the mean daily concentrations of $PM_{2.5}$ exceeded the safe limit of 35% of the study period.

In both years, a significant downward trend of $PM_{2.5}$ concentrations after the 26th of April was observed. In both years, $PM_{2.5}$ level reductions were significant during consecutive phases. In 2019, $PM_{2.5}$ levels significantly decreased from phase 1 to phase 3 (43.65 ± 7.72 vs. 19.24 ± 6.68, $p = 0.001$) and from phase 2 to phase 3 (36.6 ± 9.72 vs. 19.24 ± 6.68, $p < 0.001$). Similarly, in 2020, $PM_{2.5}$ levels significantly decreased from phase 1 to phase 3 (29.67 ± 10.71 vs. 12.57 ± 3.87, $p < 0.001$), from phase 2 to phase 3 (21.98 ± 7.07 vs. 12.57 ± 3.87, $p = 0.001$) as well as from phase 1 to phase 2 (29.67 ± 10.71 vs. 21.98 ± 7.07, $p = 0.015$).

During the strictest period amid phase 2 (23 March to 4 May 2020), when stringent traffic, transport, and industry restrictions were implemented, the mean daily concentrations of $PM_{2.5}$ exceeded the safe limits in 41% of the days.

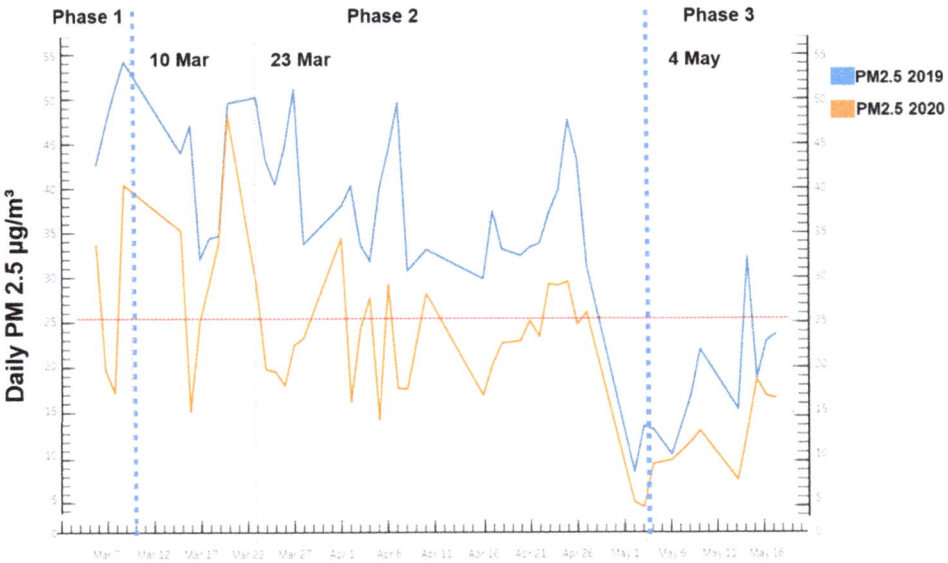

Figure 5. The trend of PM$_{2.5}$ concentration in the city of Volos, Central Greece, from 7 March to 16 May 2020, compared to PM$_{2.5}$ concentrations during the same period in 2019. The horizontal red dashed line identifies the PM$_{2.5}$ concentration at 25 μg/m^3 set as a safe limit by the World Health Organization air quality guidelines. The dotted dash vertical lines indicate the start of each phase of the three-step approach to combat the COVID-19 wave. Phase 1 (pre-lockdown period): 7 March–9 March, Phase 2 (lockdown period): 10 March–4 May, and Phase 3 (post-lockdown period): 5 May–16 May. The vertical black dashed line represents the initiation of the strictest period amid phase 2 (23 March 2020).

3.2. Correlations between Meteorological Variables and PM$_{2.5}$ Air Pollution

We found that PM$_{2.5}$ concentration was negatively correlated with temperature and positively correlated with humidity. No correlation was found between PM$_{2.5}$ concentration and rainfall or wind speed (Figure 6).

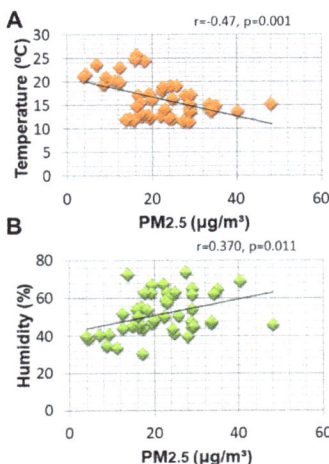

Figure 6. Correlations between meteorological variables and PM$_{2.5}$ air pollution.

3.3. The Impact of Meteorological Variables and Three-Phase Lockdown Approach on $PM_{2.5}$ Air Pollution

A multiple linear regression analysis was conducted with numerical and categorical variables turned into dummy variables. The mean daily temperature, humidity, rainfall, and wind speed, and phase 2 and phase 3 of the study period were used as the independent variables in the prediction of $PM_{2.5}$ air pollution (Table 1). Phase 2 and phase 3 were compared with phase 1, which was used as a reference group. The predictor variables of phase 2 and phase 3 explained 43.5% of the total variance in this regression model. The transition from phase 1 into phase 2 reduced $PM_{2.5}$ levels by 7.694 µg/m^3 and from phase 1 into phase 3 by 14.453 µg/m^3. There was no multicollinearity between the explanatory variables.

Table 1. Multiple linear regression analysis for $PM_{2.5}$ air pollution over the three-phase approach to lifting COVID-19 restrictions in 2020.

Model	Unstandardized Coefficients		Standardized Coefficients	t	Sig.	Collinearity Statistics	
	B	Std. Error	Beta			Tolerance	VIF
(Constant)	21.343	11.088		1.925	0.061		
Mean daily temperature (°C)	−0.058	0.451	−0.025	−0.128	0.899	0.364	2.749
Mean daily humidity (%)	0.158	0.151	0.187	1.052	0.299	0.438	2.281
Mean daily rainfall (inches)	0.251	0.314	0.132	0.799	0.429	0.506	1.975
Phase 2	−7.694	2.966	−0.415	−2.594	0.013	0.539	1.857
Phase 3	−14.453	4.780	−0.625	−3.024	0.004	0.323	3.100

Dependent variable: mean daily $PM_{2.5}$ concentration, R = 65.9%, R^2 = 43.5%, R^2 (adjusted) = 36.6%.

4. Discussion

In this study, for the first time, we assessed the $PM_{2.5}$ concentration before, during, and after lockdown in one of the most polluted cities in Greece, Volos, compared to the same period in 2019. The relationship between $PM_{2.5}$ mass concentration and meteorological conditions was also determined. Our results showed that $PM_{2.5}$ pollution dropped significantly, by 37.4%, during the COVID-19 three-phase period, compared to 2019. The mean daily concentrations of $PM_{2.5}$ exceeded the safe standards of 35% of the study period in 2020, compared to the $PM_{2.5}$ concentration exceeding the limit values over almost the entire study period (80%) in 2019. However, we found that strict lockdown (23 March to 4 May) was not enough to avoid severe exceedances of air pollution in Volos as the mean daily concentrations of $PM_{2.5}$ exceeded the safe limits 41% of the time. In both years, reduction in the $PM_{2.5}$ levels was significant from phase 1 to phase 2, and from phase 1 to phase 3. In both years, a significant downward trend of $PM_{2.5}$ concentrations after the 26th of April was observed. The transition from the pre-lockdown period (phase 1) to the lockdown period (phase 2) and from the pre-lockdown to the post-lockdown period (phase 3) in 2020, contributed to lower $PM_{2.5}$ concentrations, independently of the existing meteorological conditions.

We found that $PM_{2.5}$ concentrations exceeded the limit values over almost the entire study period (80%) in 2019. Our data accorded with earlier observations supporting that average daily $PM_{2.5}$ concentrations exceeded established standard values in the city [1,38]. Previous reports supported a correlation between the number of days exceeding the daily threshold concentration and the annual hospital admission rates for respiratory diseases [1].

However, a significant reduction of 37.4% in mean daily $PM_{2.5}$ concentration during the 2020 three-phase COVID-19 period in Volos, compared to 2019 was recorded. According to data from the Department of Mechanical Engineering of the University of Thessaly, 55 GPS devices installed in city buses demonstrated that, on average, traffic was decreased by 50% on the main roads of Volos during the lockdown in the study period [39]. Similarly, in the two largest cities in Greece, Athens and Thessaloniki, there was 21% and 27% less traffic in 2020 than in 2019, mainly attributed to restriction measures, respectively [40].

While lockdowns have caused the decline of air pollution, this did not seem to be enough to avoid $PM_{2.5}$ air pollution events in Volos due to an extensive network of stationary (industry, central heating) and mobile air pollutant sources. Although stringent traffic, transport, and industry restrictions were implemented during the lockdown period, the mean daily concentrations of $PM_{2.5}$ exceeded the safe limits 41% of the recording days during the strictest period of the lockdown (23 March to 4 May). The long-range dust incidences and sea salt emissions during spring could be partly attributed to this observation [5,6].

Moreover, in both years, a significant parallel downward trend of $PM_{2.5}$ concentration was observed over the spring period in Volos. In both years, $PM_{2.5}$ level reductions were significant from phase 1 to phase 2 and from phase 2 to phase 3. This finding is consistent with previous studies that showed a good overall agreement in $PM_{2.5}$ concentration trend lines during spring and summer [41]. Previous reports well-defined mean seasonal variation of air pollutants concentrations after examining large periods in Volos [42,43]. The spring-summer minimum is due to the reduced domestic heating emissions and private car traffic during vacations and the intense flow of the "Etesian" winds [42,43].

In our study, $PM_{2.5}$ concentration was negatively correlated with temperature and positively correlated with humidity, consistent with previous reports of our team [7,8,33]. Supportive evidence shows that $PM_{2.5}$ emissions increased exponentially as temperature decreased, suggesting a negative correlation between temperature and $PM_{2.5}$. A possible explanation for this finding is that when the temperature is higher, the air convection at the lower surface is stronger, which benefits the upward transport of $PM_{2.5}$ [33]. An increase in relative humidity could aggravate $PM_{2.5}$ pollution through physical and chemical processes, affecting the gas-to-particle conversion rate and wet or dry deposition [33]. No correlation was found between $PM_{2.5}$ concentration and wind speed in the present study.

The COVID-19 pandemic constitutes a multifactorial problem requiring multifactorial responses. Our study provides first-time data regarding one of the most polluted industrialized cities in Greece. However, it has some limitations that need to be acknowledged. Firstly, our analysis did not include all Greek cities. Secondly, this study did not examine the effect of other air pollutants such as carbon monoxide, nitrogen dioxide, and sulfur dioxide, which may increase the risk of respiratory tract infections. Moreover, the comparisons of air quality between different city points would be an important line of study designed to be subject for future study. Our study was designed to focus specifically on to what extent government restrictions affected $PM_{2.5}$ concentrations in one of the most polluted cities in Greece, Volos.

5. Conclusions

Mediterranean urban agglomerates are characterized by relatively high atmospheric pollution due to anthropogenic (urban, industrial) and natural sources (desert dust, biomass burning) and the prevailing atmospheric conditions that favor photochemical production of secondary pollutants. A spring sampling campaign verified a high concentration of $PM_{2.5}$ in the ambient air of the city of Volos in 2019, with a reduction of 37.4% in mean daily $PM_{2.5}$ concentration; without avoiding severe exceedances during the 2020 COVID-19 period. Long-term monitoring of atmospheric pollution should be carried out in Volos and Mediterranean cities of similar characteristics. Continued epidemiological and experimental studies are needed to evaluate the role of atmospheric pollution in specific populations and provide more critical information for better preparedness policies in cases of pandemics.

Author Contributions: Conceptualization, K.I.G. and G.K.D.S.; methodology, G.K.D.S. and G.K.; software, G.K.D.S. and G.K.; validation, G.K.D.S. and G.K.; formal analysis, O.S.K.; investigation, O.S.K., G.K.D.S. and G.K.; resources, G.K.D.S. and G.K.; software, G.K.D.S. and G.K.; writing—original draft preparation, O.S.K.; writing—review and editing, O.S.K., E.C.F., G.K.D.S. and G.K.; visualization, O.S.K.; supervision, K.I.G.; project administration, K.I.G. All authors have read and agreed to the published version of the manuscript.

Funding: This research received no external funding.

Institutional Review Board Statement: The study was conducted according to the guidelines of the Declaration of Helsinki and approved by the Ethics Committee of the University of Thessaly (No2800-1 November 2021). The study was conducted according to the guidelines of the Declaration of Helsinki and approved.

Informed Consent Statement: Not applicable.

Data Availability Statement: The datasets used and/or analyzed during the current study are available from the corresponding author on reasonable request.

Acknowledgments: We thank Vaios S. Kotsios who have helped in data visualization and Thomas Zidros who have helped in carrying out the research.

Conflicts of Interest: The authors declare no conflict of interest.

References

1. Moustris, K.P.; Proias, G.T.; Larissi, I.K.; Nastos, P.T.; Koukouletsos, K.V.; Paliatsos, A.G. Health impacts due to particulate air pollution in Volos City, Greece. *J. Environ. Sci. Health A Tox. Hazard. Subst. Environ. Eng.* **2016**, *51*, 15–20. [CrossRef] [PubMed]
2. The Guardian. Where's the Worst Air Pollution in Europe and How Much Does It Cost Us? 2016. Available online: https://www.theguardian.com/news/datablog/2011/nov/24/cost-of-environmental-pollution (accessed on 10 June 2021).
3. Xing, Y.F.; Xu, Y.-H.; Shi, M.H.; Lian, Y.X. The impact of $PM_{2.5}$ on the human respiratory system. *J. Thorac. Dis.* **2016**, *8*, E69–E74.
4. Katsouyanni, K. Ambient air pollution and health. *Br. Med. Bull.* **2003**, *68*, 143–156. [CrossRef]
5. Lewis, E.R.; Schwartz, S.E. *Sea Salt Aerosol Production: Mechanisms, Methods, Measurements, and Models: A Critical Review*; American Geophysical Union: Washington, DC, USA, 2004.
6. Emmanouil, C.; Drositi, E.; Vasilatou, V.; Diapouli, E.; Krikonis, K.; Eleftheriadis, K.; Kungolos, A. Study on particulate matter air pollution, source origin, and human health risk based of PM_{10} metal content in Volos City, Greece. *Toxicol. Environ. Chem.* **2017**, *99*, 691–709. [CrossRef]
7. Rahman, A.; Luo, C.; Khan, M.J.R.; Ke, J.; Thilakanayaka, V.; Kumar, S. Influence of atmospheric $PM_{2.5}$, PM_{10}, O_3, CO, NO_2, SO_2, and meteorological factors on the concentration of airborne pollen in Guangzhou, China. *Atmos. Environ.* **2019**, *212*, 290–304. [CrossRef]
8. Wang, J.; LI, J.; Peng, Y.; Zhang, M.; Che, H.; Zhang, X. The impacts of the meteorology features on $PM_{2.5}$ levels during a severe haze episode in central-east China. *Atmos. Environ.* **2019**, *197*, 177–189. [CrossRef]
9. Nam, E.; Kishan, S.; Baldauf, R.W.; Fulper, C.R.; Sabisch, M.; Warila, J. Temperature effects on particulate matter emissions from light-duty, gasoline-powered motor vehicles. *Environ. Sci. Technol.* **2010**, *44*, 4672–4677. [CrossRef]
10. Kong, L.; Tan, Q.; Feng, M.; Qu, Y.; An, J.; Liu, X.; Cheng, N.; Deng, Y.; Zhai, R.; Wang, Z. Investigating the characteristics and source analyses of $PM_{2.5}$ seasonal variations in Chengdu, Southwest China. *Chemosphere* **2020**, *243*, 125267. [CrossRef]
11. Wu, J.; Xu, C.; Wang, Q.Z.; Cheng, W. Potential Sources and Formations of the $PM_{2.5}$ Pollution in Urban Hangzhou. *Atmosphere* **2016**, *7*, 100. [CrossRef]
12. Xu, J.; Yan, F.; Xie, Y.; Wang, F.; Wu, J.; Fu, Q. Impact of meteorological conditions on a nine-day particulate matter pollution event observed in December 2013, Shanghai, China. *Particuology* **2015**, *20*, 69–79. [CrossRef]
13. Ouyang, W.; Guo, B.; Cai, G.; Li, Q.; Han, S.; Liu, B.; Liu, X. The washing effect of precipitation on particulate matter and the pollution dynamics of rainwater in downtown Beijing. *Sci. Total Environ.* **2015**, *505*, 306–314. [CrossRef]
14. Papaioannou, A.B.; Viras, L.G.; Nastos, P.T.; Paliatsos, A.G. An analysis of selected air pollutants in the city of Volos, Greece. *Environ. Monit. Assess.* **2010**, *161*, 485–494. [CrossRef] [PubMed]
15. Papanastasiou, D.; Melas, D. Statistical characteristics of ozone and PM_{10} levels in a medium sized Mediterranean city. *Int. J. Environ. Pollut.* **2009**, *36*, 127138. [CrossRef]
16. Papanastasiou, D.K.; Melas, D. Climatology and impact on air quality of sea breeze in an urban coastal environment. *Int. J. Climatol.* **2009**, *29*, 305315. [CrossRef]
17. Antoine, D.; Nobileau, D. Recent increase of Saharan dust transport over the Mediterranean Sea, as revealed from ocean color satellite (SeaWiFS) observations. *JGR* **2006**, *111*, 19. [CrossRef]
18. Barkan, J.; Alpert, P.; Kutiel, H.; Kishcha, P. Synoptics of dust transportation days from Africa toward Italy and central Europe. *JGR* **2005**, *110*, 1–14. [CrossRef]
19. Meloni, D.; di Sarra, A.; Biavati, G.; DeLuisi, J.J.; Monteleone, F.; Pace, G.; Piacentino, S.; Sferlazzo, D.M. Seasonal behavior of Saharan dust events at the Mediterranean island of Lampedusa in the period 1999–2005. *Atmos. Environ.* **2007**, *41*, 3041–3056. [CrossRef]
20. Rodriguez, S.; Querol, X.; Alastuey, A.; Kallos, G.; Kakaliagou, O. Saharan dust contributions to PM10 and TSP levels in Southern and Eastern Spain. *Atmos. Environ.* **2001**, *35*, 2433–2447. [CrossRef]
21. Alessandrini, E.R.; Stafoggia, M.; Faustini, A.; Gobbi, G.P.; Forastiere, F. Saharan Dust and the Association between Particulate Matter and Daily Hospitalisations in Rome, Italy. *Occup. Environ. Med.* **2013**, *70*, 432–434. [CrossRef]

22. Matassoni, L.; Pratesi, G.; Centioli, D.; Cadoni, F.; Malesani, P.; Caricchia, A.M.; di Bucchianico, A.D. Saharan dust episodes in Italy: Influence on PM_{10} daily limit value (DLV) exceedances and the related synoptic. *J. Environ. Monit.* **2009**, *11*, 1586–1594. [CrossRef]
23. Losacco, C.; Perillo, A. Particulate matter air pollution and respiratory impact on humans and animals. *Environ. Sci. Pollut. Res. Int.* **2018**, *25*, 33901–33910. [CrossRef]
24. Pope, C.A., 3rd; Bhatnagar, A.; McCracken, J.P.; Abplanalp, W.; Conklin, D.J.; O'Toole, T. Exposure to fine particulate air pollution is associated with endothelial injury and systemic inflammation. *Circ. Res.* **2016**, *119*, 1204–1214. [CrossRef] [PubMed]
25. Qin, C.; Zhou, L.; Hu, Z.; Zhang, S.; Yang, S.; Tao, Y.; Xie, C.; Ma, K.; Shang, K.; Wang, W.; et al. Dysregulation of immune response in patients with COVID-19 in Wuhan, China. *Clin. Infect Dis.* **2020**, *71*, 762–768. [CrossRef] [PubMed]
26. Radan, M.; Dianat, M.; Badavi, M.; Mard, S.A.; Bayati, V.; Goudarzi, G. Gallic acid protects particulate matter (PM_{10}) triggers cardiac oxidative stress and inflammation causing heart adverse events in rats. *Environ. Sci. Pollut. Res.* **2019**, *26*, 18200–18207. [CrossRef]
27. Tsai, D.H.; Riediker, M.; Berchet, A.; Paccaud, F.; Waeber, G.; Vollenweider, P.; Bochud, M. Effects of short- and long-term exposures to particulate matter on inflammatory marker levels in the general population. *Environ. Sci. Pollut. Res. Int.* **2019**, *26*, 19697–19704. [CrossRef] [PubMed]
28. Yang, J.; Chen, Y.; Yu, Z.; Ding, H.; Ma, Z. The influence of $PM_{2.5}$ on lung injury and cytokines in mice. *Exp. Ther. Med.* **2019**, *18*, 2503–2511. [CrossRef]
29. Berend, N. Contribution of air pollution to COPD and small airway dysfunction. *Respirology* **2016**, *21*, 237–244. [CrossRef]
30. Croft, D.P.; Zhang, W.; Lin, S.; Thurston, S.W.; Hopke, P.K.; Masiol, M.; Squizzato, S.; van Wijngaarden, E.; Utell, M.J.; Rich, D.Q. The Association between Respiratory Infection and Air Pollution in the Setting of Air Quality Policy and Economic Change. *Ann. Am. Thorac. Soc.* **2019**, *16*, 321–330. [CrossRef]
31. Horne, B.D.; Joy, E.A.; Hofmann, M.G.; Gesteland, P.H.; Cannon, J.B.; Lefler, J.S.; Blagev, D.P.; Korgenski, E.K.; Torosyan, N.; Hansen, G.I.; et al. Short-term elevation of fine particulate matter air pollution and acute lower respiratory infection. *Am. J. Respir. Crit. Care Med.* **2018**, *198*, 759–766. [CrossRef]
32. Conticini, E.; Frediani, B.; Caro, D. Can atmospheric pollution be considered a co-factor in extremely high level of SARS-CoV-2 lethality in Northern Italy? *Environ. Pollut.* **2020**, *261*, 114465. [CrossRef]
33. Kotsiou, O.S.; Kotsios, V.; Lampropoulos, I.; Zidros, T.; Zarogiannis, S.G.; Gourgoulianis, K.I. $PM_{2.5}$ pollution strongly predicted COVID-19 incidence in four high-polluted urbanized Italian cities during the pre-lockdown and lockdown periods. *Int. J. Environ. Res. Public Health* **2021**, *18*, 5088. [CrossRef]
34. Brandt, E.B.; Beck, A.F.; Mersha, T.B. Air pollution, racial disparities, and COVID-19 mortality. *J. Allergy Clin. Immunol.* **2020**, *146*, 61–63. [CrossRef]
35. Chen, K.; Wang, M.; Huang, C.; Kinney, P.L.; Anastas, P.T. Air pollution reduction and mortality benefit during the COVID-19 outbreak in China. *Lancet Planet. Health* **2020**, *4*, e210–e212. [CrossRef]
36. World Health Organization. Ambient (Outdoor) Air Pollution. 2018. Available online: https://www.who.int/news-room/fact-sheets/detail/ambient-(outdoor)-air-quality-and-health (accessed on 7 May 2021).
37. Saharidis, G.; Kalantzis, G. Monitoring Network for PM2.5. In Proceedings of the 6th International Conference on "Energy, Sustainability and Climate Change", ESCC 2019, Chania, Greece, 3–7 June 2019; University of Thessaly: Volos, Greece, 2019; p. 11.
38. Antoniadis, V.; Golia, E.E.; Liu, Y.T.; Wang, S.L.; Shaheen, S.M.; Rinkleb, J. Soil and maize contamination by trace elements and associated health risk assessment in the industrial area of Volos, Greece. *Environ. Int.* **2019**, *124*, 79–88. [CrossRef] [PubMed]
39. Taxydromos Newspaper Reporter. 21 May 2021. Available online: https://www.taxydromos.gr/Topika/403457-meiwsh-80-ths-epivatikhs-kinhshs-sto-astiko-ktel-voloy.html?fbclid=IwAR1dUJIRAqVtSogIA0p8gS3caT4FENUZgy3V3wEY-oyHuvMR8N9MRs51ozw (accessed on 2 June 2021). (In Greek).
40. TomTom Traffic Index. Greece Traffic. Available online: https://www.tomtom.com/en_gb/traffic-index/greece-country-traffic/ (accessed on 2 June 2021).
41. Papaioannou, A.B.; Viras, L.G.; Nastos, P.T.; Paliatsos, A.G. Temporal evolution of sulfur dioxide and nitrogen oxides in the city of Volos, Greece. *Environ. Monit. Assess.* **2010**, *161*, 485–494. [CrossRef] [PubMed]
42. Karandinos-Riga, A.N.; Saitanis, C.; Arapis, G. Study of the weekday–weekend variation of air pollutants in a typical Mediterranean coastal town. *Int. J. Environ. Pollut.* **2006**, *27*, 300–312. [CrossRef]
43. Papamanolis, N. On the seasonal dependence of the air pollution in the city of Volos, Greece. *Fresenius Environ. Bull.* **2001**, *10*, 749–754.

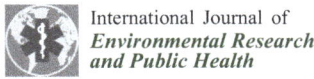

Article

The Economic Burden of Influenza-Like Illness among Children, Chronic Disease Patients, and the Elderly in China: A National Cross-Sectional Survey

Xiaozhen Lai [1,2], Hongguo Rong [2,3], Xiaochen Ma [2], Zhiyuan Hou [4], Shunping Li [5,6], Rize Jing [1,2], Haijun Zhang [1,2], Yun Lyu [1,2], Jiahao Wang [1,2], Huangyufei Feng [1,2], Zhibin Peng [7], Luzhao Feng [8,*] and Hai Fang [2,9,10,*]

1. School of Public Health, Peking University, Beijing 100083, China; laixiaozhen@pku.edu.cn (X.L.); rzjing2015@hsc.pku.edu.cn (R.J.); zhanghj966@bjmu.edu.cn (H.Z.); lydialu1217@hotmail.com (Y.L.); 1510306210@pku.edu.cn (J.W.); yffenghuang@pku.edu.cn (H.F.)
2. China Center for Health Development Studies, Peking University, Beijing 100083, China; hgrong@hsc.pku.edu.cn (H.R.); xma@hsc.pku.edu.cn (X.M.)
3. Institute for Excellence in Evidence-Based Chinese Medicine, Beijing University of Chinese Medicine, Beijing 100029, China
4. School of Public Health, Fudan University, Shanghai 200032, China; zyhou@fudan.edu.cn
5. School of Health Care Management, Cheeloo College of Medicine, Shandong University, Jinan 250012, China; lishunping@sdu.edu.cn
6. NHC Key Laboratory of Health Economics and Policy Research (Shandong University), Jinan 250012, China
7. Division of Infectious Diseases, Chinese Center for Disease Control and Prevention, Beijing 102206, China; pengzb@chinacdc.cn
8. School of Population Medicine and Public Health, Chinese Academy of Medical Sciences & Peking Union Medical College, Beijing 100730, China
9. Peking University Health Science Center—Chinese Center for Disease Control and Prevention Joint Center for Vaccine Economics, Peking University, Beijing 100083, China
10. Key Laboratory of Reproductive Health, National Health Commission of the People's Republic of China, Beijing 100083, China
* Correspondence: fengluzhao@cams.cn (L.F.); hfang@hsc.pku.edu.cn (H.F.); Tel.: +86-10-6525-6093 (L.F.); +86-10-8280-5702 (H.F.)

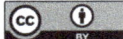

Abstract: Background: The disease burden of seasonal influenza is substantial in China, while there is still a lack of nationwide economic burden estimates. This study aims to examine influenza-like illness (ILI) prevalence, healthcare-seeking behaviors, economic impact of ILI, and its influencing factors among three priority groups during the 2018–19 influenza season. **Methods:** From August to October 2019, 6668 children's caregivers, 1735 chronic disease patients, and 3849 elderly people were recruited from 10 provinces in China to participate in an on-site survey. The economic burden of ILI consisted of direct (medical or non-medical) and indirect burdens, and a two-part model was adopted to predict the influencing factors of total economic burden. **Results:** There were 45.73% children, 16.77% chronic disease patients, and 12.70% elderly people reporting ILI, and most participants chose outpatient service or over-the-counter (OTC) medication after ILI. The average economic burden was CNY 1647 (USD 237.2) for children, CNY 951 (USD 136.9) for chronic disease patients, and CNY 1796 (USD 258.6) for the elderly. Two-part regression showed that age, gender, whether the only child in the family, region, and household income were important predictors of ILI economic burden among children, while age, region, place of residence, basic health insurance, and household income were significant predictors of ILI economic burden among chronic disease patients and the elderly. **Conclusions:** A large economic burden of ILI was highlighted, especially among the elderly with less income and larger medical burdens, as well as children, with higher prevalence and higher self-payment ratio. It is important to adopt targeted interventions for high-risk groups, and this study can help national-level decision-making on the introduction of influenza vaccination as a public health project.

Keywords: economic burden; influenza-like illness; healthcare-seeking behaviors; China

1. Introduction

Annual influenza epidemics result in substantial morbidity and mortality across the globe, with a large share of the total disease burden occurring in low- and middle-income countries (LMICs) [1]. As estimated by the World Health Organization (WHO) in 2018, the annual epidemics of seasonal influenza caused 3–5 million severe cases and 290,000–650,000 deaths [2]. The disease burden of seasonal influenza is also substantial in mainland China, with about 88,000 excess deaths occurring annually [3]. Illness severity and mortality are the greatest in high-risk groups, and so are the associated healthcare costs and productivity losses.

Immunization has been proven to be one of the most cost-effective health investments to prevent and control influenza, with strong positive externalities [4–6], so public intervention is expected to drive vaccine coverage to a socially optimal level [7]. The WHO and Chinese Center for Disease Control and Prevention recommended that children, chronic diseases patients, and the elderly be among the priority groups for influenza vaccination [8,9]. However, influenza vaccination has not been included in China's National Immunization Program (NIP), and the expenses are paid out of pocket on most occasions, even for priority groups. The coverage rate of influenza vaccination in China has been extremely low in the past 15 years, with only 2% of the entire population being immunized, and small-scale policy interventions have failed to increase national uptake of influenza vaccinations [10].

As the WHO reported, as of the end of 2019, 119 out of 194 member states had included influenza vaccination in their NIPs [11], and the economic burden could decrease to a large extent after the introduction of vaccines in NIP. In the United States, a study published early in 2007 estimated the medical and indirect costs attributable to annual influenza epidemics, and found that the total economic burden amounted to USD 87.1 billion annually [12]. More recently, in 2018, researchers provided an updated estimate for the United States after vaccination efforts, and found a substantially lower (approximately half) total cost than previously estimated [13]. By comparison, China has not introduced influenza vaccination into its NIP, so it is even more important to estimate the economic burden of influenza in China to promote decision-making.

Access, affordability, and equity are three basic goals of a well-operated health system [14], so evidence of the economic burden of influenza can help raise awareness in the public and clinical communities of the burden and consequences of this important disease. Additionally, estimating the economic burden of influenza is crucial to support national-level decision-making, while sufficient data to precisely estimate the economic burden of influenza are scarce and incomplete in LMICs [15]. In China, most previous studies were conducted in developed southern areas at the hospital or provincial level, and the economic burden was not evaluated in an all-sided way. Besides, little research was done among different priority groups to make horizontal comparisons, and there also was a lack of national-level community-based estimates of influenza-like illness (ILI) prevalence and healthcare-seeking behaviors.

To address these gaps, the present study collected individual data in 10 provinces in China to examine ILI prevalence in communities, influenza-related healthcare-seeking behaviors, the economic impact of ILI, and its influencing factors among children, chronic disease patients and the elderly during the 2018–2019 influenza season. Among the objectives, the primary goal was to calculate the economic impact of ILI for three priority groups in a national-level community-based survey. We hypothesized that the ILI prevalence, healthcare-seeking behaviors, ILI economic burden, and its composition would vary across different priority groups, and that many sociodemographic factors would have an influence on the economic burden of ILI, such as age, gender, and income. We also paid attention to regional and rural–urban differences in ILI economic burdens, and we hypothesized that patients living in less-developed areas (rural and western) would have a lower economic burden, given the lower lost productivity and direct expenditures [16].

The present study is organized as follows. The first part provides the background information and objectives of the study; the second part presents a literature review on the economic burden of influenza in China; the third part elaborates on the materials and methods adopted in the present study; the fourth part displays the statistical description and study results; the fifth part discusses the results, gives some policy implications, and puts forward the limitations of this study; and the sixth part briefly summarizes the present study.

2. Literature Review

Influenza can impose a substantial socioeconomic burden on families and society. Table 1 summarizes the studies conducted in China that explored the economic burden of influenza, but most of them were done at the hospital or provincial level, and direct non-medical costs or indirect costs were often missed [16–20]. In 2007, a household survey conducted in Guangdong Province found that the cost for an ILI episode was about one-fifth of monthly per capita income, but the study did not ask for the direct non-medical costs of respondents [16]. Similarly, a prospective study conducted in Zhuhai City during 2008–2009 found that direct medical costs of influenza created a substantial economic burden in the outpatient setting, but it did not examine the direct non-medical costs and family labor losses [17]. In Shanghai, a study estimated only the direct medical costs of influenza among the elderly aged over 60 years, and found that the average outpatient and inpatient direct costs were USD 47 and USD 1601, respectively [18]. In Suzhou, two studies were performed to explore the economic burden of influenza in outpatient and inpatient settings, respectively, and both of them focused on children aged less than 5 years [19,20]. The former reported the healthcare-seeking behaviors of outpatients, and collected non-medical or indirect costs via telephone surveys. It found that influenza would impose a heavy economic burden on children's families [19]. The latter collected medical costs and hospital length of stay for pneumonia and influenza inpatients, but did not access non-medical or indirect costs [20].

Besides those at the hospital or provincial level, there were two cross-province studies on the economic burden of influenza [21,22]. One examined the direct medical cost of influenza-related hospitalizations in three provinces, in which non-medical or indirect costs were not examined [21]. The other was a telephone survey in 10 provinces to collect costs in an all-sided way, but it was conducted among the general population [22]. Overall, there were some studies concerning the economic burden of ILI or influenza in China, and they could help in developing influenza control policies. However, most of them were conducted in developed southern China, and did not report the healthcare-seeking behaviors, non-medical costs, indirect costs, or over-the-counter (OTC) medication costs of targeted high-risk groups. In this case, we conducted this survey, trying to fill these gaps.

Table 1. Summary of studies on the economic burden of influenza conducted in China.

Research Articles	Study Sites	Age Groups	Settings	Data Sources	Study Period	Composition of Economic Burden [a]	Whether Healthcare-Seeking Behaviors Reported	Whether OTC Medication Costs Reported [b]
Guo et al. (2011) [16]	Zhuhai and Zhaoqing cities in Guangdong province	All age groups	Population-based	Household survey	2006–2007	DM + I	No	No
Guo et al. (2012) [17]	Zhuhai city in Guangdong province	All age groups	Hospital-based (Outpatient)	Hospital diagnosis and telephone survey	2008–2009	DM + DnM	No	Yes
Chen et al. (2015) [18]	Shanghai city	The elderly aged ≥60 years	Hospital-based	Hospital diagnosis and follow-up survey	2009	DM	Yes	No
Wang et al. (2013) [19]	Suzhou city in Zhejiang province	Children aged <5 years	Hospital-based (Outpatient)	Hospital system and telephone survey	2011–2012	DM + DnM + I	Yes	No
Zhang et al. (2017) [20]	Suzhou city in Zhejiang province	Children aged <5 years	Hospital-based (Inpatient)	Hospital system	2005–2011	DM	No	No
Zhou et al. (2013) [21]	Three hospitals in Sichuan, Hunan and Shandong provinces	All age groups	Hospital-based (Inpatient)	Hospital system	2009–2011	DM	No	No
Yang et al. (2015) [22]	10 hospitals in 10 provinces and municipalities	All age groups	Hospital-based	Hospital diagnosis and telephone survey	2013–2014	DM + DnM + I	Yes	Yes

[a] DM, direct medical burden; DnM, direct non-medical burden; I, indirect burden. [b] OTC, over-the-counter.

3. Materials and Methods

3.1. Study Population and Sampling

In August to October 2019, a total of 12,252 participants in 148 community health centers from 10 provinces in China were approached to join the national survey on the economic burden of seasonal influenza, including 6668 children aged 6–59 months, 1735 chronic disease patients aged 18–59 years, and 3849 elderly people aged above 60 years (Financing Strategies of Influenza Vaccination in China, NCT04038333) [23]. For children aged 6–59 months, we asked their parents or grandparents who accompanied them to health centers to finish the compulsory immunization procedure [9]. For chronic disease patients and the elderly, we asked them in health centers or gathered them in neighborhood committees. This study was ethically reviewed and approved by the Peking University Institutional Review Board (IRB00001052-19076), and written informed consent was obtained from individual or guardian participants.

The survey adopted a multistage sampling method. First, 10 provinces/municipalities were selected based on China's Division of Central and Local Financial Governance and Expenditure Responsibilities in the Healthcare Sector, which stratifies the 31 provinces/municipalities into five layers [24]. In terms of location, socioeconomic development, and accessibility, 10 provinces/municipalities (3, 3, 1, 1, and 2 in each layer) were chosen, with their location and 2018 per capita GDP rank (e.g., 1/31) recorded in Figure 1. Second, in each province/municipality, a capital city or well-developed district and a non-capital city or less-developed district were selected. Third, two subdistricts/counties were chosen in each city or district, in which three or more immunization centers and the corresponding neighborhood committees were approached. The sample size was calculated under ILI prevalence assumptions, with an allowable error of 5% and disqualification rate of 10%.

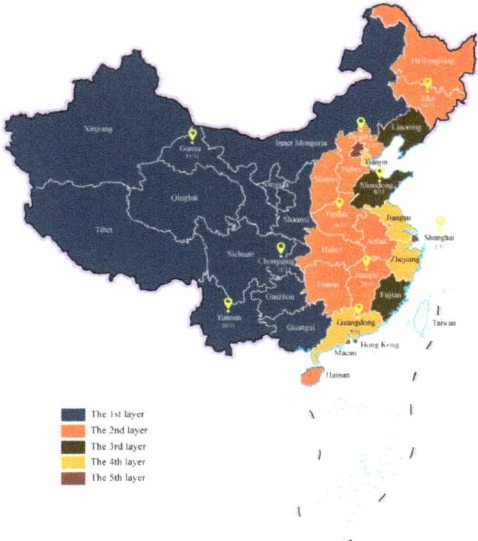

Figure 1. Ten provinces/municipalities selected for survey on the economic burden of influenza-like illness in China. In the survey, 10 provinces/municipalities (3, 3, 1, 1, and 2 in each layer) were chosen, including Beijing, Shanghai, Jilin, Yunnan, Shandong, Guangdong, Jiangxi, Gansu, Chongqing, and Henan. Their location and 2018 per capita GDP rank (e.g., 1/31) are marked in the figure.

3.2. Measures

The on-site survey was conducted by trained interviewers using a specially designed online questionnaire system on a portable Android device (PAD). The questionnaire was stored in advance in the PAD system, and interviewees would fill in the online questionnaire according to the answers of each respondent. Automatic logical proofreading was adopted in the online questionnaire to reduce input errors and missing values, and interview recordings were uploaded and spot-checked by quality-control personnel to find and correct problems in time. The structured online questionnaire collected: (1) sociodemographics; (2) whether the respondent had ILI in the past season; (3) healthcare-seeking behaviors after ILI; and (4) economic burden of the latest ILI in terms of direct (medical and non-medical) costs and indirect costs [25].

According to the WHO, body temperature ≥ 38 °C with either cough or sore throat was used in the present study to distinguish influenza from other respiratory illnesses [26]. For each interviewee (or their child aged 6–59 months) who reported ILI in the past season, direct medical costs were queried in terms of service type (outpatient service, inpatient service, and OTC medication) and co-payment in each service type; direct non-medical costs were inquired regarding aspects of transportation, nutrition/food, accommodation, and nursing-worker hiring; and indirect burden was obtained by multiplying the lost labor days of the respondents and their families and daily per capita household income of the respondents [25]. The reported direct medical and non-medical costs were adjusted for the provincial healthcare price index and consumer price index, respectively, according to the China Statistical Yearbook 2019 [27]. Total economic burden was calculated by summing up the adjusted values of direct medical cost, direct non-medical cost, and indirect cost for each respondent.

3.3. Statistical Analysis

We produced summary statistics of all respondents using frequencies and proportions for categorical variables, and means and standard deviations for continuous variables. The chi-square and Mann–Whitney tests were used to assess differences in sample characteristics. The economic burden values of ILI was displayed as means and 95% confidence intervals (CI) for those who reported ILI in the last influenza season.

In predicting the influencing factors of total economic burden, a two-part model was adopted because there were a large number of zeros in terms of total economic burden [28,29], and results are shown as coefficients and 95% CIs. The two-part model has been widely used in health-economics research [30,31]. In the first part of the regression, Y is a binary discrete dependent variable to estimate the probability of reporting ILI economic burden (if respondents report any economic burden of ILI, $Z' = 1$; otherwise, $Z' = 0$). We adopted the Probit model for regression and the maximum likelihood method for estimation, and the marginal effects of Part 1 are shown in Appendix A. The second part includes whether respondents truly received medical treatments and paid for them using ordinary least squares regression (If $Z' = 1$, respondents will be included in the second part of regression). We also took the log form of total economic burden, which obeyed the skewed distribution to capture the nonlinear property of the association.

The indicators of the two-part model were chosen in the light of previous literature [32–34]. We took age (different age groups for the three priority populations), gender (male and female), whether the only child in the family (only for the children group), household monthly per capita income (CNY 1000; CNY 1 = USD 0.144 on 13 August 2020), place of residence (urban and rural), region (western, central, and eastern) and basic medical insurance type (medical insurance for urban and rural residents, urban employee medical insurance, and without basic medical insurance) as possible influencing factors. We also controlled self-reported health status (good, fair, or poor), but we did not display the results because they are not easily observable for policy-makers.

We further used multivariate Tobit regression concentrating on boundary value 0 for all respondents to predict the influencing factors of total economic burden (in log form), and the results are shown in Appendix B. A two-sided *p*-value below 0.05 was considered statistically significant in the present study. All data were analyzed using Stata version 14.0 (Stata Corp., College Station, TX, USA).

4. Results

4.1. Study Sample Characteristics

A total of 12,252 valid questionnaires (6668 for children, 1735 for patients with chronic diseases, and 3849 for the elderly) were received, with an effective response rate of 99.80%. Table 2 shows the general characteristics of participants. Overall, 45.73% of children, 16.77% of chronic disease patients, and 12.70% of elderly people reported to have ILI in the past season. Among children, older children aged 3–5 years had a higher possibility of catching ILI than younger children ($p < 0.01$), while the only child in the family ($p < 0.01$) and children living in western areas ($p < 0.01$) were less likely to have ILI than those living in families with more than one child and those living in central or eastern China. Among chronic disease patients, those with a younger age were more likely to catch ILI than older adults ($p < 0.01$). Among the elderly, respondents with higher household monthly per capita income ($p < 0.05$), living in urban areas ($p < 0.01$), living in eastern areas ($p < 0.01$), or having urban employee medical insurance ($p < 0.01$) had a lower possibility of having ILI. In the three groups, respondents with fair or poor self-reported health status had higher risk of catching ILI than those with good self-reported health status ($p < 0.01$). We further compared the distribution of gender and age among the three groups with that recorded in the China Population and Employment Statistics Yearbook 2019 [35], and found similar results, indicating the national representativeness of the population collected in this study.

Table 2. Characteristics of 12,252 participants included in the analysis.

	Children Aged 6–59 Months			Chronic Disease Patients Aged 18–59 Years			Elderly Aged above 60 Years		
	n	ILI Cases, n (%)	p-Value	n	ILI Cases, n (%)	p-Value	n	ILI Cases, n (%)	p-Value
Total	6668	3049 (45.73)		1735	291 (16.77)		3849	489 (12.70)	
Age (years)			<0.01			<0.01			0.40
<2	3727	610 (16.37)		–	–		–	–	
3–5	2941	725 (24.65)		–	–		–	–	
18–39	–	–		72	24 (33.33)		–	–	
40–49	–	–		313	58 (18.53)		–	–	
50–59	–	–		1350	209 (15.48)		–	–	
60–69	–	–		–	–		2045	273 (13.35)	
70–79	–	–		–	–		1491	181 (12.14)	
≥80	–	–		–	–		313	35 (11.18)	
Gender			0.06			0.69			0.12
Female	3171	1412 (44.53)		1139	194 (17.03)		2334	281 (12.04)	
Male	3497	1637 (46.81)		596	97 (16.28)		1515	208 (13.73)	
The only child in the family			<0.01						
Yes	3038	1320 (43.45)		–	–		–	–	
No	3630	1729 (47.63)		–	–		–	–	
Household monthly per capita income (CNY 1000) [a]			0.62			0.24			<0.05
Mean (SD)	2.66 (2.76)	2.68 (2.69)		1.84 (2.41)	1.99 (2.31)		1.70 (1.61)	1.56 (1.86)	
Place of residence			0.33			0.94			<0.01
Rural	2814	1267 (45.02)		831	140 (16.85)		1742	255 (14.64)	
Urban	3854	1782 (46.24)		904	151 (16.7)		2107	234 (11.11)	
Region			<0.01			0.44			<0.01
Western	2219	793 (35.74)		602	99 (16.45)		1461	216 (14.78)	
Central	1932	1022 (52.90)		497	92 (18.51)		1035	136 (13.14)	
Eastern	2517	1234 (49.03)		636	100 (15.72)		1353	137 (10.13)	
Basic medical insurance type [b]			0.15			0.20			<0.01
Medical insurance for urban and rural residents	4081	1842 (45.14)		1212	193 (15.92)		2551	356 (13.96)	
Urban employee medical insurance	2380	1121 (47.10)		492	90 (18.29)		1189	118 (9.92)	
Without basic medical insurance	207	86 (41.55)		31	8 (25.81)		109	15 (13.76)	
Self-reported health status			<0.01			<0.01			<0.01
Good	5812	2536 (43.63)		596	74 (12.42)		1578	141 (8.94)	
Fair or poor	856	513 (59.93)		1139	217 (19.05)		2271	348 (15.32)	

[a] CNY 1 = USD 0.144 on 13 August 2020. [b] Basic medical insurance type in column refers to adult respondents.

4.2. Healthcare-Seeking Behaviors

Table 3 shows the distribution of healthcare-seeking behaviors among 3829 participants after the latest ILI by calculating the number of ILI cases leading to outpatient visits, hospitalization, and OTC medication. As the table indicates, most participants chose "Outpatient service only", "OTC medication only", or "Outpatient + OTC" after ILI, accounting for 84.29% of children, 84.53% of chronic disease patients, and 73.42% of elderly people.

Table 3. Healthcare-seeking behaviors of 3829 participants after influenza-like illness.

	Children Aged 6–59 Months		Chronic Disease Patients Aged 18–59 Years		Elderly Aged above 60 Years	
	n	%	n	%	n	%
Total	3049	100	291	100	489	100
Healthcare-seeking behaviors						
Outpatient service only	1162	38.11	100	34.36	159	32.52
Inpatient service only	46	1.51	4	1.37	26	5.32
OTC medication only [a]	316	10.36	69	23.71	123	25.15
Outpatient + Inpatient	172	5.64	10	3.44	40	8.18
Outpatient + OTC	1092	35.82	77	26.46	77	15.75
Inpatient + OTC	25	0.82	1	0.34	14	2.86
Outpatient + Inpatient + OTC	134	4.39	10	3.44	18	3.68
No treatment	102	3.35	20	6.87	32	6.54
Service types						
Outpatient service	2560	83.96	197	67.70	294	60.12
Inpatient service	377	12.36	25	8.59	98	20.04
OTC medication	1567	51.39	157	53.95	232	47.44

[a] OTC, over-the-counter.

More specifically, when ILI occurred in children, 38.11% of them only sought outpatient service, and 35.82% accepted a combination of outpatient treatment and OTC medication. There were also 102 children (3.35%) not receiving any medical services after ILI. In terms of service type, 83.96% of children received outpatient service after ILI, 12.36% had inpatient service, and 51.39% received OTC medication. As for chronic disease patients, 34.36% only sought outpatient service, and 26.46% received outpatient treatment and OTC medication. There were 20 chronic disease patients (6.87%) not receiving any medical services after ILI. In terms of service type, 67.70%, 8.59%, and 53.95% of chronic disease patients received outpatient service, inpatient service, and OTC medication, respectively. For the elderly, 32.52% of them only sought outpatient service, and 25.15% only received OTC medication. There were 32 elderly people (6.54%) not receiving any medical services. In terms of service type, 60.12%, 20.04%, and 47.44% of elderly people received outpatient service, inpatient service, and OTC medication, respectively.

4.3. Economic Burden of Influenza-Like Illness

Table 4 shows the economic burden of the three priority groups for the latest ILI episode during the 2018–2019 influenza season. As the results indicated, the economic burden of ILI for children was about CNY 1647, including reimbursed medical expenses of CNY 272, self-paid medical expenses of CNY 997, direct non-medical expenses of CNY 212, and indirect cost of CNY 166. The average economic burden for chronic disease patients was about CNY 951, including reimbursed medical expenses of CNY 335, self-paid medical expenses of CNY 386, direct non-medical expenses of CNY 102, and indirect cost of CNY 92. The elderly had a much higher average economic burden of about CNY 1796, including reimbursed medical expenses of CNY 766, self-paid medical expenses of CNY 778, direct non-medical expenses of CNY 162, and indirect cost of CNY 90. For children and chronic disease patients, outpatient and inpatient costs accounted for the vast majority of direct medical expenses, and nutrition/food and transportation costs accounted for most direct non-medical expenses. For the elderly, only inpatient costs accounted for the vast majority

Table 4. The economic burden of influenza-like illness for 3829 participants.

	Children Aged 6–59 Months		Chronic Disease Patients Aged 18–59 Years		Elderly Aged above 60 Years	
	Mean	95% CI [a]	Mean	95% CI	Mean	95% CI
Total direct medical cost (CNY) [b,e]	1269	(1168, 1370)	721	(512, 930)	1544	(1200, 1888)
Outpatient service	644	(595, 694)	239	(184, 293)	384	(281, 488)
Inpatient service	523	(454, 593)	394	(192, 595)	1053	(763, 1343)
OTC medication [f]	102	(93, 110)	89	(64, 113)	106	(75, 138)
Reimbursed direct medical cost (CNY) [b]	272	(234, 310)	335	(194, 477)	766	(568, 963)
Outpatient service	88	(67, 108)	85	(54, 116)	153	(95, 210)
Inpatient service	179	(151, 206)	239	(102, 375)	605	(426, 784)
OTC medication	6	(4, 8)	11	(6, 17)	8	(5, 12)
Self-paid direct medical cost (CNY) [b]	997	(919, 1074)	386	(295, 477)	778	(595, 961)
Outpatient service	556	(515, 597)	154	(114, 193)	232	(167, 296)
Inpatient service	345	(295, 395)	155	(75, 235)	448	(302, 595)
OTC medication	96	(88, 103)	77	(54, 101)	98	(67, 130)
Direct non-medical cost (CNY) [c]	212	(186, 238)	102	(31, 172)	162	(68, 256)
Transportation	79	(70, 87)	50	(−8, 109)	21	(8, 34)
Nutrition/food	107	(93, 121)	34	(18, 49)	96	(12, 180)
Accommodation	19	(12, 27)	18	(−2, 38)	40	(3, 76)
Nursing-worker hiring	8	(−5, 21)	0	(0, 0)	5	(−2, 12)
Indirect cost [d]	166	(152, 179)	92	(60, 125)	90	(57, 124)
Lost labor days of respondents' families	2	(1.9, 2.1)	0.7	(0.4, 1.0)	2	(1.5, 2.6)
Lost labor days of the respondents	–	–	1.1	(0.8, 1.5)	0.9	(0.5, 1.3)
Total economic costs	1647	(1527, 1768)	951	(671, 1159)	1796	(1413, 2179)

[a] CI, confidence interval. [b] Direct medical cost was adjusted for the provincial healthcare price index in the China Statistical Yearbook 2019.
[c] Direct non-medical cost was adjusted for the provincial consumer price index in the China Statistical Yearbook 2019. [d] Indirect cost was calculated based on the per capita GDP of each province in the China Statistical Yearbook 2019. [e] CNY 1 = USD 0.144 on 13 August 2020.
[f] OTC, over-the-counter.

of direct medical expenses, and nutrition/food and accommodation costs accounted for most direct non-medical expenses.

4.4. Influencing Factors of Total Economic Burden

Table 5 shows the two-part model results to predict the influencing factors of total economic burden (in log form), including age, gender, whether the only child in the family (only for children), household income, place of residence, region, and basic medical insurance type (see Appendix A for marginal effects of Part 1, and see Appendix B for the results of the multivariate Tobit regression).

In the first part of the regression, we found that among children, the probability of an economic burden of ILI occurring was higher for older children aged 3–5 years (Coef. = 0.37, 95% CI 0.31–0.43, $p < 0.05$), boys (Coef. = 0.06, 95% CI 0.00–0.12, $p < 0.05$), and those living in central (Coef. = 0.50, 95% CI 0.42–0.58, $p < 0.05$) and eastern (Coef. = 0.40, 95% CI 0.32–0.48, $p < 0.05$) areas compared with younger children, girls, or those living in western China. Among chronic disease patients, those with older age tended to have a lower probability of having an ILI economic burden ($p < 0.05$) compared with younger respondents who developed chronic diseases at an earlier age. Among the elderly, those living in eastern areas (Coef. = −0.25, 95% CI −0.38 − −0.12, $p < 0.05$) and those with urban employee medical insurance (Coef. = −0.21, 95% CI −0.36 − −0.07, $p < 0.05$) were less likely to have an economic burden for ILI than those living in western China or those with medical insurance for urban and rural residents.

In the second part, patients with higher household monthly per capita income reported a larger economic burden for ILI than those with lower income in the three groups ($p < 0.05$). Among children, the economic burden of ILI was smaller for older children aged 3–5 years (Coef. = −0.16, 95% CI −0.26 − −0.07, $p < 0.05$) compared with younger children, but larger for boys (Coef. = 0.15, 95% CI 0.05–0.25, $p < 0.05$), the only child in the family (Coef. = 0.26,

95% CI 0.16–0.36, $p < 0.05$), those living in central areas (Coef. = 0.15, 95% CI 0.02–0.28, $p < 0.05$), and those with uninsured caregivers (Coef. = 0.35, 95% CI 0.05–0.65, $p < 0.05$). Among chronic disease patients and the elderly, those living in urban areas and central areas tended to suffer from a lower economic burden for ILI ($p < 0.05$) compared with rural and western residents, and those with urban employee medical insurance had a higher economic burden for ILI than others covered by medical insurance for urban and rural residents.

Table 5. Two-part regression of total economic burden (in log form) for the three groups.

Factors [a]	Children		Chronic Disease Patients		Elderly	
	Part 1 Coef. (95% CI [b])	Part 2 Coef. (95% CI)	Part 1 Coef. (95% CI)	Part 2 Coef. (95% CI)	Part 1 Coef. (95% CI)	Part 2 Coef. (95% CI)
Age (years)						
<2	Ref.	Ref.	–	–	–	–
3–5	0.37 * (0.31, 0.43)	−0.16 * (−0.26, −0.07)	–	–	–	–
18–39	–	–	Ref.	Ref.	–	–
40–49	–	–	−0.47 * (−0.82, −0.12)	−0.55 (−1.29, 0.18)	–	–
50–59	–	–	−0.59 * (−0.91, −0.28)	−0.53 (−1.19, 0.14)	–	–
60–69	–	–	–	–	Ref.	Ref.
70–79	–	–	–	–	−0.07 (−0.18, 0.05)	0.05 (−0.33, 0.43)
≥80	–	–	–	–	−0.14 (−0.35, 0.06)	0.26 (−0.49, 1.01)
Gender						
Female	Ref.	Ref.	Ref.	Ref.	Ref.	Ref.
Male	0.06 * (0.00, 0.12)	0.15 * (0.05, 0.25)	−0.02 (−0.18, 0.13)	−0.22 (−0.59, 0.16)	0.10 (−0.01, 0.21)	−0.37 (−0.74, 0.00)
The only child in the family	−0.05 (−0.11, 0.02)	0.26 * (0.16, 0.36)	–	–	–	–
Household monthly per capita income (CNY 1000) [c]	−0.01 (−0.02, 0.01)	0.02 * (0.00, 0.04)	0.02 (−0.02, 0.05)	0.12 * (0.03, 0.20)	0.02 (−0.02, 0.06)	0.14 * (0.01, 0.26)
Place of residence						
Rural	Ref.	Ref.	Ref.	Ref.	Ref.	Ref.
Urban	−0.01 (−0.08, 0.06)	0.08 (−0.02, 0.19)	−0.05 (−0.21, 0.11)	−0.45 * (−0.85, −0.06)	−0.11 (−0.23, 0.00)	−0.65 * (−1.07, −0.23)
Region						
Western	Ref.	Ref.	Ref.	Ref.	Ref.	Ref.
Central	0.50 * (0.42, 0.58)	0.15 * (0.02, 0.28)	0.07 (−0.11, 0.25)	−0.52 * (−0.95, −0.08)	−0.12 (−0.25, 0.01)	−0.57 * (−1.00, −0.13)
Eastern	0.40 * (0.32, 0.48)	0.07 (−0.06, 0.20)	−0.06 (−0.24, 0.12)	−0.15 (−0.60, 0.29)	−0.25 * (−0.38, −0.12)	−0.19 (−0.66, 0.28)
Basic medical insurance type [d]						
Medical insurance for urban and rural residents	Ref.	Ref.	Ref.	Ref.	Ref.	Ref.
Urban employee medical insurance	0.04 (−0.03, 0.11)	0.06 (−0.05, 0.17)	0.05 (−0.13, 0.24)	0.60 * (0.14, 1.07)	−0.21 * (−0.36, −0.07)	0.56 * (0.05, 1.07)
Without basic medical insurance	−0.16 (−0.34, 0.02)	0.35 * (0.05, 0.65)	0.28 (−0.22, 0.78)	−1.07 (−2.19, 0.06)	−0.15 (−0.48, 0.18)	0.86 (−0.33, 2.04)

* Significant at the 5% level. [a] The results were controlled for self-reported health status. [b] CI, confidence interval. [c] CNY 1 = USD 0.144 on 13 August 2020. [d] Basic medical insurance type in column refers to adult respondents.

5. Discussion

To the best of our knowledge, this is the first study using a nationally representative sample from 10 provinces in China to investigate the economic burden of ILI among children, patients with chronic diseases, and the elderly. This study estimated the prevalence of self-reported ILI, ILI-related healthcare-seeking behaviors, the economic burden of ILI, and its influencing factors among children, chronic disease patients, and the elderly in China.

A high prevalence of ILI (45.73% of children, 16.77% of chronic disease patients, and 12.70% of elderly people) was found among high-risk groups, especially among children. The results were similar to those reported in previous studies [16,17]. As for the healthcare-seeking behaviors, "Outpatient service only", "OTC medication only", and "Outpatient + OTC" were most frequently chosen, consistent with a previous study in which 86% influenza patients aged 60 years and above received ambulatory care only [18]. The elderly were more likely to receive inpatient services, indicating that older ILI patients were at higher risk of becoming severe cases [3]. In addition, a larger portion of chronic disease patients and the elderly did not receive any medical services after ILI, reflecting the problem that adult high-risk groups did not attach much importance to their health conditions after ILI, and a previous study also revealed that financial protection was the most important cause of not seeking care [36]. In this case, adequate public education on influenza disease, especially during the influenza season, may help raise people's awareness of disease severity [37], and strengthened financial protection of health insurance can also help increase healthcare utilization, such as widened coverage of medical services and higher reimbursement rates [38].

After the occurrence of ILI, the economic burden of the elderly was the highest (CNY 1796), followed by children (CNY 1647) and chronic disease patients (CNY 951). It was found that outpatient service and OTC medication were most frequently chosen after ILI for the three groups, but the results of medical expenses demonstrated that once inpatient service was utilized in severe cases or patients with other complications, the medical burden of ILI would greatly increase in terms of both reimbursed expenses and self-paid expenses. Our estimates of ILI-related costs were higher than earlier estimates in China [16,17], similar to more recent estimates [22], but much lower than those reported in the United States, especially the lost productivity [13]. In the United States, studies found that indirect costs, including lost productivity from missed work days and lost lives, comprised a larger amount of influenza economic burden than hospitalization costs [12,13]. In the present study, direct medical and non-medical costs comprised a larger amount of economic burden of ILI, perhaps due to the fact that we only included lost productivity from missed work days in the indirect cost, and there are large gaps in labor costs between the two countries. Results derived from the present study on ILI economic burdens can help raise public awareness on the burdens and consequences of this important disease. Moreover, economic considerations are essential to effectively guide policy-making for influenza vaccination [39], so the direct and indirect economic costs of influenza at the national level are crucial to support national-level decision-making on the introduction of influenza vaccination as a public health project, complementary vaccination strategies, and/or expanding vaccination target groups [40].

There were several studies examining the incidence and economic burden of influenza at the hospital or provincial level in China. A population-based household survey conducted in 2007 in Guangdong Province found annual ILI incidence of 49.87% among children aged 1–4 years and 2.99% among the elderly aged >60 years, and the mean medical cost of one episode was CNY 172.5 for residents of all age groups [16]. A prospective study conducted in the 2011–2012 season among children <5 years in Suzhou reported that the mean direct and indirect costs per episode of influenza were CNY 777.4 for outpatient clinics and CNY 848.0 for emergency departments [19]. These results were similar to the ILI incidence and economic costs reported in the present study. As a rough estimate, the overall annual economic burden of ILI was about CNY 61.9 billion for children, CNY 25.0 billion for chronic disease patients, and CNY 38.0 billion for the elderly, based on the population size recorded in statistical yearbooks [27,35,41].

As for the co-payment of medical costs, the self-payment ratio and self-paid expenses were higher among children than chronic disease patients and the elderly due to the design of insurance schemes [42]. Moreover, compared with children and chronic disease patients, the elderly had a lower probability of catching ILI, but a higher economic burden after catching ILI. A previous study also found that young children and the elderly accounted for over 70% of the economic burden of influenza-associated hospitalizations in Jingzhou, China [22], indicating the importance of targeted interventions such as financed or re-imbursed influenza vaccination programs [13], early treatment of ILI [43], and a higher reimbursement rate for high-risk groups [38], especially elderly people with less income and a larger economic burden after ILI, as well as children with higher prevalence of ILI and a higher self-payment ratio for medical expenses.

For children, the two-part model indicated that older children had a higher probability of ILI economic burden occurring, but smaller economic burden after ILI, revealing that older children had higher incidence of ILI, while younger children may have had more severe conditions after occurring ILI. In addition, boys had a higher probability of an ILI economic burden occurring and a larger economic burden after ILI, which may be related to boys' lifestyles and potential son preference [44]. The economic burden after ILI was also larger for the only child in the family, as parents may switch investment from exclusively one child to others if they have more than one child [45]. As for adults, it was found that younger respondents who developed chronic diseases at an earlier age tended to have a higher probability of having an ILI economic burden compared with other chronic disease patients aged less than 60 years. Patients with a higher household income and adults with urban employee insurance reported larger economic costs after ILI in the three groups, but no significant difference was observed in the probability analysis (Part 1).

Regional or rural–urban differences were highlighted in the two-part analysis. For children, those living in central and eastern areas had higher probability of an ILI economic burden occurring, and those in central areas also had a higher economic burden after ILI. This was in line with previous findings on the economic burden of children with asthma (another respiratory disease) in China [46], which indicated that patients aged 0–14 years in central China had the highest use rate of medications, antibiotics, hematological tests, and chest X-rays. Reducing the unnecessary use of antibiotics and tests may help reduce young patients' ILI economic burden in western areas [46]. In comparison, chronic disease patients and the elderly living in western or rural areas tended to suffer from a higher economic burden after ILI. Given the lower lost productivity and direct expenditures in less-developed areas, it was expected that rural and western residents might have smaller economic burdens for ILI than urban or eastern residents [16]. However, a higher economic burden was observed among rural and western adult residents in this population-based survey, and this might be due to the higher hospitalization rate in rural (23.04% for rural and 8.25% for urban) and western (23.03% for western, 14.85% for central, and 6.75% for eastern) patients in this study. This revealed the substantial regional and rural–urban gaps in Chinese adult patients concerning ILI economic burden, especially the hospitalization burden, and joint efforts are needed to reduce the gap and strengthen the financial protection for rural and western residents.

The present study also had a few limitations. First, the economic burden was collected from ILI cases instead of confirmed influenza cases. As recommended by the WHO, ILI sentinel surveillance data can be used to estimate the disease burden of influenza for specific risk groups [47–49], which is less specific but sensitive and rapid than laboratory surveillance [50]. Therefore, ILI cases were used, given that nationwide laboratory surveillance was not available, and a population-based study could offer higher population representativeness. Second, part of the elderly surveyed in this study were recruited from community health centers, which may have resulted in selection bias. Nevertheless, given the high prevalence of chronic diseases among Chinese elderly [51], and the fact that community centers mainly provide primary care, the bias could be reduced. Third, self-reported responses may be subject to recalling bias, and self-reported data may be affected by the severity of flu. To minimize the bias, we conducted a face-to-face on-site survey so that interviewees were more cautious about their answers, trained interviewers would help them recall expenditures if they had any difficulty, and we asked for respondents' most recent influenza episode to minimize its effect. Fourth, in this cross-sectional survey, regression was performed only to show statistical correlations rather than inherent causal relations, which may have been subject to reverse causality. Fifth, in the regression, only a small number of respondents did not have any basic health insurance, making its coefficient not reliable enough, and future studies should be conducted to further detect the relationship between ILI economic burden and basic health insurance coverage. Despite these limitations, the nationally representative sample was large, with a diverse sociodemographic population, thus offering good generalizability for the three high-risk groups in China.

6. Conclusions

In conclusion, the prevalence of ILI was fairly high among the three priority groups in China, and outpatient service and/or OTC medication were most frequently chosen after ILI. The results highlighted the large economic burden of ILI, especially among two priority groups, including the elderly with less income and a larger economic burden after ILI, and children with a higher prevalence of ILI and a higher self-payment ratio for medical expenses. The financial burden of ILI on households can be viewed as an important healthcare issue, and it is time to adopt targeted interventions for children and the elderly, such as vaccinations and early treatment. At the same time, we should not ignore the regional and rural–urban differences of ILI economic burden in different priority groups. More importantly, this study can help decision-making on the introduction of influenza vaccination as a public health project in China for these high-risk groups by estimating the economic burden of influenza at the national level.

Author Contributions: Conceptualization, H.F. (Hai Fang), L.F., X.L., H.R., X.M., Z.H., S.L., and Z.P.; methodology, H.F. (Hai Fang)., L.F., X.L., H.R., X.M., Z.H., and S.L.; software, X.L. and H.F. (Hai Fang); formal analysis, X.L. and H.F. (Hai Fang); investigation, X.L., H.R., X.M., Z.H., S.L., R.J., H.Z., Y.L., J.W., H.F. (Huangyufei Feng), and Z.P.; writing—original draft preparation, X.L.; writing—review and editing, H.F. (Hai Fang), L.F., X.M., Z.H., S.L., and X.L.; funding acquisition, H.F. (Hai Fang). All authors have read and agreed to the published version of the manuscript.

Funding: This research was funded by the National Natural Science Foundation of China, grant numbers 71774006 and 71981320749.

Institutional Review Board Statement: The study was conducted according to the guidelines of the Declaration of Helsinki, and approved by the Peking University Institutional Review Board (protocol code IRB00001052-19076; date of approval 16 July 2019).

Informed Consent Statement: Informed consent was obtained from all subjects involved in the study.

Data Availability Statement: The data presented in this study are available on request from the corresponding author. The data are not publicly available due to some restrictions, and they are only available on reasonable request.

Acknowledgments: We would like to thank Beijing, Shanghai, Jilin, Yunnan, Shandong, Guangdong, Jiangxi, Gansu, Chongqing and Henan Provincial/Municipal Centers for Disease Control and Prevention; all participating community health centers; and community neighborhood committees for their contributions to this study.

Conflicts of Interest: The authors declare no conflict of interest.

Appendix A

Table A1. Two-part regression of total economic burden (in log form) for the three groups (reporting marginal effects of Part 1).

Factors [a]	Children Coef. (95% CI) [b]	Chronic Disease Patients Coef. (95% CI)	Elderly Coef. (95% CI)
Age (years)			
<2	Ref.	–	–
3–5	0.14 * (0.12, 0.16)	–	–
18–39	–	Ref.	–
40–49	–	−0.14 * (−0.26, −0.03)	–
50–59	–	−0.17 * (−0.28, −0.06)	–
60–69	–	–	Ref.
70–79	–	–	−0.01 (−0.03, 0.01)
≥80	–	–	−0.03 (−0.06, 0.01)
Gender			
Female	Ref.	Ref.	Ref.
Male	0.02 * (0.00, 0.05)	−0.01 (−0.04, 0.03)	0.02 (0.00, 0.04)

Table A1. Cont.

Factors [a]	Children Coef. (95% CI [b])	Chronic Disease Patients Coef. (95% CI)	Elderly Coef. (95% CI)
The only child in the family	−0.02 (−0.04, 0.01)	–	–
Household monthly per capita income (CNY 1000) [c]	0.00 (−0.01, 0.00)	0.00 (0.00, 0.01)	0.00 (0.00, 0.01)
Place of residence			
Rural	Ref.	Ref.	Ref.
Urban	0.00 (−0.03, 0.02)	−0.01 (−0.05, 0.03)	−0.02 (−0.04, 0.00)
Region			
Western	Ref.	Ref.	Ref.
Central	0.19 * (0.16, 0.22)	0.02 (−0.03, 0.06)	−0.03 (−0.05, 0.00)
Eastern	0.15 * (0.12, 0.18)	=0.01 (−0.06, 0.03)	−0.05 * (−0.07, −0.02)
Basic medical insurance type [d]			
Medical insurance for urban and rural residents	Ref.	Ref.	Ref.
Urban employee medical insurance	0.02 (−0.01, 0.04)	0.01 (−0.03, 0.06)	−0.04 * (−0.07, −0.01)
Without basic medical insurance	−0.06 (−0.13, 0.01)	0.07 (−0.05, 0.19)	−0.03 (−0.09, 0.04)

* Significant at the 5% level. [a] The results were controlled for self-reported health status. [b] CI, confidence interval. [c] CNY 1 = USD 0.144 on 13 August 2020. [d] Basic medical insurance type in column refers to adult respondents.

Appendix B

Table A2. Tobit regression of total economic burden (in log form) for the three groups.

Factors [a]	Children Coef.	95% CI [b]	Chronic Disease Patients Coef.	95% CI	Elderly Coef.	95% CI
Age (years)						
<2	Ref.		–	–	–	–
3–5	1.95 *	(1.60, 2.31)	–	–	–	–
18–39	–	–	Ref.		–	–
40–49	–	–	−4.17 *	(−7.12, −1.23)	–	–
50–59	–	–	−5.28 *	(−7.99, −2.57)	–	–
60–69	–	–	–	–	Ref.	
70–79	–	–	–	–	−0.64	(−1.72, 0.44)
≥80	–	–	–	–	−1.31	(−3.32, 0.70)
Gender						
Female	Ref.		Ref.		Ref.	
Male	0.44 *	(0.09, 0.79)	−0.25	(−1.57, 1.07)	0.88	(−0.17, 1.94)
The only child in the family	−0.12	(−0.48, 0.24)	–	–	–	–
Household monthly per capita income (CNY 1000) [c]	−0.03	(−0.10, 0.04)	0.15	(−0.11, 0.42)	0.23	(−0.16, 0.61)
Place of residence						
Rural	Ref.		Ref.		Ref.	
Urban	0.00	(−0.37, 0.38)	−0.57	(−1.95, 0.81)	−1.25 *	(−2.38, −0.11)
Region						
Western	Ref.		Ref.		Ref.	
Central	2.88 *	(2.42, 3.33)	0.44	(−1.11, 1.99)	−1.35 *	(−2.61, −0.09)
Eastern	2.31 *	(1.86, 2.75)	−0.60	(−2.15, 0.95)	−2.47 *	(−3.75, −1.19)
Basic medical insurance type [d]						
Medical insurance for urban and rural residents	Ref.		Ref.		Ref.	
Urban employee medical insurance	0.25	(−0.15, 0.64)	0.64	(−0.95, 2.23)	−1.91 *	(−3.32, −0.50)
Without basic medical insurance	−0.73	(−1.77, 0.30)	1.88	(−2.50, 6.26)	−1.25	(−4.46, 1.96)

* Significant at the 5% level. [a] The results were controlled for self-reported health status. [b] CI, confidence interval. [c] CNY 1 = USD 0.144 on 13 August 2020. [d] Basic medical insurance type in column refers to adult respondents.

References

1. Newall, A.T.; Chaiyakunapruk, N.; Lambach, P.; Hutubessy, R.C.W. WHO guide on the economic evaluation of influenza vaccination. *Influenza Other Respir. Viruses* **2018**, *12*, 211–219. [CrossRef]
2. World Health Organization. Influenza (Seasonal) Fact Sheet November 2018. Available online: http://www.who.int/mediacentre/factsheets/fs211/en/ (accessed on 20 April 2020).
3. Li, L.; Liu, Y.; Wu, P.; Peng, Z.; Wang, X.; Chen, T.; Wong, J.; Yang, J.; Bond, H.S.; Wang, L.; et al. Influenza-associated excess respiratory mortality in China, 2010-15: A population-based study. *Lancet Public Health* **2019**, *4*, 473–481. [CrossRef]
4. Osterholm, M.T.; Kelley, N.S.; Sommer, A.; Belongia, E.A. Efficacy and effectiveness of influenza vaccines: A systematic review and meta-analysis. *Lancet Infect. Dis.* **2012**, *12*, 36–44. [CrossRef]
5. Folland, S.; Goodman, A.C.; Stano, M. Epidemiology and Economics: HIV/AIDS in Africa. In *The Economics of Health and Health Care*, 7th ed.; Pearson Education: Cranbury, NJ, USA, 2012; pp. 531–548.
6. Wilder-Smith, A.; Longini, I.; Zuber, P.L.; Bärnighausen, T.; Edmunds, W.J.; Dean, N.; Spicher, V.M.; Benissa, M.R.; Gessner, B.D. The public health value of vaccines beyond efficacy: Methods, measures and outcomes. *BMC Med.* **2017**, *15*, 138. [CrossRef]
7. Chen, F.; Toxvaerd, F. The economics of vaccination. *J. Theor. Biol.* **2014**, *363*, 105–117. [CrossRef] [PubMed]
8. World Health Organization. Vaccines against influenza WHO position paper. *Wkly. Epidemiol. Rec.* **2012**, *87*, 461–476.
9. Technical guidelines for seasonal influenza vaccination in China (2019–2020). *Chin. J. Prev. Med.* **2020**, *54*, 21–36. (In Chinese) [CrossRef]
10. Yang, J.; Atkins, K.E.; Feng, L.; Pang, M.; Zheng, Y.; Liu, X.; Cowling, B.J.; Yu, H. Seasonal influenza vaccination in china: Landscape of diverse regional reimbursement policy, and budget impact analysis. *Vaccine* **2016**, *34*, 5724–5735. [CrossRef] [PubMed]
11. WHO. Immunization Schedule. Available online: http://www.who.int/immunization/monitoring_surveillance/data/en/ (accessed on 6 February 2021).
12. Molinari, N.A.; Ortega-Sanchez, I.R.; Messonnier, M.L.; Thompson, W.W.; Wortley, P.M.; Weintraub, E.; Bridges, C. The annual impact of seasonal influenza in the US: Measuring disease burden and costs. *Vaccine* **2007**, *25*, 5086–5096. [CrossRef] [PubMed]
13. Putri, W.C.W.S.; Muscatello, D.J.; Stockwell, M.S.; Newall, A.T. Economic burden of seasonal influenza in the United States. *Vaccine* **2018**, *36*, 3960–3966. [CrossRef] [PubMed]
14. Shrank, W.H.; DeParle, N.A.; Gottlieb, S.; Jain, S.H.; Orszag, P.; Powers, B.W.; Wilensky, G.R. Health Costs and Financing: Challenges and Strategies For A New Administration. *Health Aff.* **2021**, *2*, 235–242. [CrossRef]
15. de Francisco Shapovalova, N.; Donadel, M.; Jit, M.; Hutubessy, R. A systematic review of the social and economic burden of influenza in low- and middle-income countries. *Vaccine* **2015**, *33*, 6537–6544. [CrossRef]
16. Guo, R.; Zheng, H.; Li, J.; Sun, L.; Li, L.; Lin, J.; He, J. A population-based study on incidence and economic burden of influenza-like illness in south China, 2007. *Public Health* **2011**, *125*, 389–395. [CrossRef]
17. Guo, R.; Zheng, H.; Huang, L.; Zhou, Y.; Zhang, X.; Liang, C.; Lin, J.; He, J.; Zhang, J. Epidemiologic and economic burden of influenza in the outpatient setting: A prospective study in a subtropical area of China. *PLoS ONE* **2012**, *7*, e41403. [CrossRef]
18. Chen, J.; Li, Y.; Gu, B.; Yuan, Z. Estimation of the direct cost of treating people aged more than 60 years infected by influenza virus in Shanghai. *Asia Pac. J. Public Health* **2015**, *27*, NP936–946. [CrossRef]
19. Wang, D.; Zhang, T.; Wu, J.; Jiang, Y.; Ding, Y.; Hua, J.; Li, Y.; Zhang, J.; Chen, L.; Feng, Z.; et al. Socio-economic burden of influenza among children younger than 5 years in the outpatient setting in Suzhou, China. *PLoS ONE* **2013**, *8*, e69035. [CrossRef] [PubMed]
20. Zhang, X.; Zhang, J.; Chen, L.; Feng, L.; Yu, H.; Zhao, G.; Zhang, T. Pneumonia and influenza hospitalizations among children under 5 years of age in Suzhou, China, 2005-2011. *Influenza Other Respir. Viruses* **2017**, *11*, 15–22. [CrossRef] [PubMed]
21. Zhou, L.; Situ, S.; Huang, T.; Hu, S.; Wang, X.; Zhu, X.; Gao, L.; Li, Z.; Feng, A.; Jin, H.; et al. Direct medical cost of influenza-related hospitalizations among severe acute respiratory infections cases in three provinces in China. *PLoS ONE* **2013**, *8*, e63788. [CrossRef]
22. Yang, J.; Jit, M.; Leung, K.S.; Zheng, Y.; Feng, L.; Wang, L.; Lau, E.; Wu, J.; Yu, H. The economic burden of influenza-associated outpatient visits and hospitalizations in China: A retrospective survey. *Infect. Dis. Poverty* **2015**, *4*, 44. [CrossRef] [PubMed]
23. Lai, X.; Rong, H.; Ma, X.; Hou, Z.; Li, S.; Jing, R.; Zhang, H.; Peng, Z.; Feng, L.; Fang, H. Willingness to Pay for Seasonal Influenza Vaccination among Children, Chronic Disease Patients, and the Elderly in China: A National Cross-Sectional Survey. *Vaccines* **2020**, *8*, 405. [CrossRef] [PubMed]
24. The General Office of the State Council. Notice on the Reform Plan for the Division of Central and Local Financial Governance and Expenditure Responsibilities in the Healthcare Sector. Available online: http://www.gov.cn/zhengce/content/2018-08/13/content_5313489.htm (accessed on 11 January 2019).
25. Drummond, M.F.; O'Brien, B.; Stoddart, G.L.; Torrance, G.W. *Methods for the Economic Evaluation of Health Care Programmes*, 4th ed.; Oxford University Press: Oxford, UK, 2015.
26. Fitzner, J.; Qasmieh, S.; Mounts, A.W.; Alexander, B.; Besselaar, T.; Briand, S.; Brown, C.; Clark, S.; Dueger, E.; Gross, D.; et al. Revision of clinical case definitions: Influenza like illness and severe acute respiratory infection. *Bull. World Health Organ.* **2018**, *96*, 122–128. [CrossRef]
27. National Bureau of statistics. *China Statistical Yearbook 2019*; China Statistics Press: Beijing, China, 2019.
28. Cragg, J.G. Some Statistical Models for Limited Dependent Variables with Application to the Demand for Durable Goods. *Econometrica* **1971**, *5*, 829–844. [CrossRef]

29. Buntin, M.B.; Zaslavsky, A.M. Too much ado about two-part models and transformation? Comparing methods of modeling Medicare expenditures. *J. Health Econ.* **2004**, *3*, 525–542. [CrossRef]
30. Li, X.; Zhang, W. The impacts of health insurance on health care utilization among the older people in china. *Soc. Sci. Med.* **2013**, *4*, 59–65. [CrossRef] [PubMed]
31. Li, M.; Zhang, Y.; Zhang, Z.; Zhang, Y.; Zhou, L.; Chen, K. Rural-urban differences in the long-term care of the disabled elderly in china. *PLoS ONE* **2013**, *11*, e79955. [CrossRef] [PubMed]
32. Andersen, R.M.; Mccutcheon, A.; Aday, L.A.; Chiu, G.Y.; Bell, R. Exploring dimensions of access to medical care. *Health Serv. Res.* **1983**, *1*, 49–74.
33. Busch, S.H.; Duchovny, N. Family coverage expansions, impact on insurance coverage and health care utilization of parents. *J. Health Econ.* **2005**, *24*, 876–890. [CrossRef]
34. Heider, D.; Matschinger, H.; Müller, H.; Saum, K.U.; Quinzler, R.; Haefeli, W.E.; Wild, B.; Lehnert, T.; Brenner, H.; König, H.-H. Health care costs in the elderly in Germany: An analysis applying Andersen's behavioral model of health care utilization. *BMC Health Serv. Res.* **2014**, *14*, 71. [CrossRef] [PubMed]
35. Department of Population and Employment Statistics, National Bureau of Statistics of China. *China Population & Employment Statistics Yearbook 2019*; China Statistics Press: Beijing, China, 2019.
36. Anbari, Z.; Mohammadbeigi, A.; Mohammadsalehi, N.; Ebrazeh, A. Health expenditure and catastrophic costs for inpatient- and out-patient care in Iran. *Int. J. Prev. Med.* **2014**, *8*, 1023–1028.
37. Hickey, J.E.; Gagnon, A.J.; Jitthai, N. Knowledge about pandemic influenza preparedness among vulnerable migrants in Thailand. *Health Promot. Int.* **2016**, *1*, 124–132. [CrossRef]
38. Mazurenko, O.; Balio, C.P.; Agarwal, R.; Carroll, A.E.; Menachemi, N. The Effects of medicaid expansion under the ACA: A systematic review. *Health Aff.* **2018**, *6*, 944–950. [CrossRef]
39. WHO. *Guide for Standardization of Economic Evaluations of Immunization Programmes*, 2nd ed.; World Health Organization: Geneva, Switzerland, 2019.
40. WHO. *Manual for Estimating the Economic Burden of Seasonal Influenza*; World Health Organization: Geneva, Switzerland, 2016.
41. National Health Commission of the People's Republic of China. *China Health Statistics Yearbook 2019*; Peking Union Medical College Press: Beijing, China, 2019.
42. Zhou, Z.; Zhou, Z.; Gao, J.; Yang, X.; Yan, J.; Xue, Q.; Chen, G. The effect of urban basic medical insurance on health service utilisation in Shaanxi Province, China: A comparison of two schemes. *PLoS ONE* **2014**, *4*, e94909. [CrossRef] [PubMed]
43. Katzen, J.; Kohn, R.; Houk, J.L.; Ison, M.G. Early oseltamivir after hospital admission is associated with shortened hospitalization: A five-year analysis of oseltamivir timing and clinical outcomes. *Clin. Infect. Dis.* **2019**, *69*, 52–58. [CrossRef] [PubMed]
44. Barcellos, S.H.; Carvalho, L.S.; Lleras-Muney, A. Child Gender and Parental Investments in India: Are Boys and Girls Treated Differently? *Am. Econ. J. Appl. Econ.* **2014**, *6*, 157–189. [CrossRef] [PubMed]
45. Liu, J.; Duan, C.; Lummaa, V. Parent-offspring conflict over family size in current China. *Am. J. Hum. Biol.* **2017**, *3*, e22946. [CrossRef] [PubMed]
46. Wu, P.; Xu, B.; Shen, A.; He, Z.; Zhang, C.J.P.; Ming, W.K.; Shen, K. The economic burden of medical treatment of children with asthma in China. *BMC Pediatr.* **2020**, *1*, 386. [CrossRef] [PubMed]
47. WHO. *A Manual for Estimating Disease Burden Associated with Seasonal Influenza*; World Health Organization: Geneva, Switzerland, 2015.
48. Tadesse, M.; Mengesha, M.; Tayachew, A.; Belay, D.; Hassen, A.; Woyessa, A.B.; Zemelak, E.; Beyene, B.; Kassa, W.; Ayele, W.; et al. Burden and seasonality of medically attended influenza like illness (ILI) in Ethiopia, 2012 to 2017. *BMC Infect. Dis.* **2020**, *20*, 148. [CrossRef] [PubMed]
49. Perez, V.; Uddin, M.; Galea, S.; Monto, A.S.; Aiello, A.E. Stress, adherence to preventive measures for reducing influenza transmission and influenza-like illness. *J. Epidemiol. Community Health* **2012**, *66*, 605–610. [CrossRef]
50. WHO. *Recommended Surveillance Standards*, 2nd ed.; World Health Organization: Geneva, Switzerland, 1999.
51. Han, M.; Shi, X.; Cai, C.; Zhang, Y.; Xu, W. Evolution of non-communicable disease prevention and control in China. *Glob. Health Promot.* **2017**, *26*, 90–95. [CrossRef]

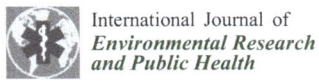

Article

Economic Role of Population Density during Pandemics—A Comparative Analysis of Saudi Arabia and China

Nadia Yusuf *[ ] and Lamia Saud Shesha [ ]

Economics Department, King Abdulaziz University, Jeddah 21551, Saudi Arabia; lshisha@kau.edu.sa
* Correspondence: nyusuf@kau.edu.sa

Abstract: As a novel infection with relatively high contagiousness, the coronavirus disease emerged as the most pertinent threat to the global community in the twenty-first century. Due to Covid-19's severe economic impacts, the establishment of reliable determining factors can help to alleviate future pandemics. While a population density is often cited as a major determinant of infectious cases and mortality rates, there are both proponents and opponents to this claim. In this framework, the study seeks to assess the role of population density as a predictor of Covid-19 cases and deaths in Saudi Arabia and China during the Covid-19 pandemic. With high infectivity and mortality being a definitive characteristic of overpopulated regions, the authors propose that Henry Kissinger's population reduction theory can be applied as a control measure to control future pandemics and alleviate social concerns. If high-density Chinese regions are more susceptible to Covid-19 than low-density Saudi cities, the authors argue that Neo-Malthusian models can be used as a basis for reducing the impacts of the coronavirus disease on the economic growth in countries with low population density. However, the performed correlation analysis and simple linear regression produced controversial results with no clear connection between the three studied variables. By assessing population density as a determinant of health crises associated with multiple socio-economic threats and epidemiological concerns, the authors seek to reinvigorate the scholarly interest in Neo-Malthusian models as a long-term solution intended to mitigate future disasters. The authors recommend that future studies should explore additional confounding factors influencing the course and severity of infectious diseases in states with different population densities.

Keywords: Covid-19; population density; Covid-19 mortality; economic recovery; population reduction; China; Saudi Arabia; Henry Kissinger

Citation: Yusuf, N.; Shesha, L.S. Economic Role of Population Density during Pandemics—A Comparative Analysis of Saudi Arabia and China. *Int. J. Environ. Res. Public Health* **2021**, *18*, 4318. https://doi.org/10.3390/ijerph18084318

Academic Editor: Dirga Kumar Lamichhane

Received: 5 March 2021
Accepted: 15 April 2021
Published: 19 April 2021

Publisher's Note: MDPI stays neutral with regard to jurisdictional claims in published maps and institutional affiliations.

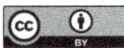

Copyright: © 2021 by the authors. Licensee MDPI, Basel, Switzerland. This article is an open access article distributed under the terms and conditions of the Creative Commons Attribution (CC BY) license (https://creativecommons.org/licenses/by/4.0/).

1. Introduction

A novel infection with high contagiousness, the coronavirus disease (Covid-19) emerged as the most pertinent threat to the global community in the twenty-first century. With a variety of transmission routes underlying the initial spread of the virus, globalization proved to be one of the key factors responsible for the unprecedented rise of infection cases across the world. The lack of evidence-based practice and empirical knowledge on the topic contributed to the ineffectiveness of certain preventive measures and delayed response in most states. As the Covid-19 pandemic paralyzed health systems and impaired national economies, most scholars focused on the short-term prospects of the encountered epidemiological crisis [1]. Seeking to mitigate anticipated economic consequences and ensure recovery of numerous industries, both governments and experts prioritized immediate solutions such as economic stimuli and mass vaccination. However, the importance of overpopulation, with high population density being one of its key functions, as a confounding factor of the pandemic's severity was largely overlooked. In this framework, the current research aims to evaluate the significance of population density as a determinant for high infection rates and mortality leading to the consequent economic slowdown in overpopulated countries. Furthermore, the authors analyze the validity of

Neo-Malthusian models informed by Henry Kissinger's population control theory under the outlined circumstances by comparing the development of the Covid-19 situation in Saudi Arabia and China.

Emerging in late 2019, the novel coronavirus infection affected the entirety of the world's population to a different degree. For the purposes of convenience and simplicity, both the infectious disease and the associated viral pathogen are addressed with the acronym Covid-19. With the first cases of Covid-19 being recorded in China's Hubei province, the severity of the acute respiratory syndrome caused by the SARS-CoV-2 strain of coronaviruses was not immediately apparent [2]. Recognizing the alarming incidence of new outbreaks outside of China, WHO promptly classified the evolving epidemiologic situation as a pandemic. Throughout spring and summer 2020, Covid-19 engulfed most sovereign states without distinction by their development rates, economic prosperity, or population size [3]. By July, the pandemic's epicenter shifted from its place of origin in China to countries located in Europe and the Americas. While several observers reported more than 14 million global cases and 607,746 deaths due to Covid-19 on 18 July, total Covid-19 cases exceeded 53 million and deaths reached 1.3 million by mid-November 2020 [4]. At the date of the research, the states with the highest recorded numbers of confirmed Covid-19 cases and deaths are the US, Brazil, and India. As the global number of cases exceeds 85 million, the number of fatal outcomes caused by the disease approaches 1.8 million.

Considering that countries at different stages of economic development have been reporting hundreds of thousands of Covid-19 cases and thousands of fatal outcomes on a daily basis, the situation is unlikely to be completely resolved in the upcoming months and years. By the time medical professionals started to identify instances of human-to-human transmission outside of China, the spread of Covid-19 was already out of control [5]. The collective outcome of the pandemic is not limited to immediate health concerns and deaths due to the fact that coronavirus's impacts encompass numerous spheres of life. Specifically, the implementation of social distancing and other measures aimed to reduce infection rates resulted in social disruptions and economic disturbances on a global scale [6]. The former became especially evident in regions with high population density as local authorities mandated shutdowns of entire industries while severely limiting citizens' ability to travel, work, and communicate [7]. Unsurprisingly, border closures and lockdowns amounted to a near-complete cessation of commercial and industrial activities in many regions. The resulting economic downturn can be adequately gauged by sharp declines in GDP growth rates as well as the shrinkage of previously robust markets [8].

As evident from the presented overview, the severity of detrimental impacts associated with Covid-19 necessitates the development of comprehensive long-term solutions that would help in mitigating socio-economic consequences of future epidemiologic crises. To this end, we performed a comparative analysis of Saudi Arabia and China, two non-democratic countries that successfully curtailed the spread of the coronavirus disease thanks to strict lockdown measures. The choice is further justified by the contrast in their respective population densities—the average for Saudi Arabia is 15.6 inhabitants per sq. km, and for China it is 148 inhabitants per sq. km. Although population density is an established demographic parameter, we approached the investigation from the socio-economic standpoint by assessing the predictive value of population density for a country's ability to cope with the pandemic [1,4]. Being intrinsically connected with urbanization rates and the economic growth, density levels could have a substantial impact on the country's capacity for economic recovery. The understanding of socio-economic and epidemiological consequences of overpopulation is integral for determining a long-term solution informed by population reduction models [8]. Accordingly, the study's contribution to the academia emerges from the assessment of population density as a determinant of the severity of health crises such as the Covid-19 pandemic. While overpopulation is associated with multiple socio-economic threats and epidemiological concerns, we seek to reinvigorate the scholarly interest in Neo-Malthusian models as a long-term solution intended to mitigate future disasters and health crises.

The current study begins with a literature review focusing on the development of the Covid-19 pandemic in Saudi Arabia and China which includes a detailed overview of the epidemiological, political, and economic circumstances in both countries. The subsequent subsection provides a background for using population density as a determinant of the epidemiological situations that can further inform the adoption of a Neo-Malthusian model to address further pandemics. Following the Methodology section that delineates the used quantitative techniques as well as the conceptual framework for qualitative analysis, the research continues with the Results and Discussion section. In the Conclusion section, the authors briefly outline the key findings of the study by reiterating the findings and commenting on the significance of the results in the context of the posed research question.

2. Literature Review
2.1. The Course of the Covid-19 Pandemic in Saudi Arabia

Centered on the Arabian Peninsula, The Kingdom of Saudi Arabia is one of the largest and most economically prosperous Middle Eastern states. The population of more than 34 million is unevenly spread across the vast area of 2,149,690 square kilometers resulting in a relatively low population density of 15 inhabitants per sq. km. The Kingdom boasts a robust economy with the highest GDP figures among other Middle Eastern nations. The development of the Covid-19 crisis in Saudi Arabia began with the official report of the first confirmed case on 2 March by the Kingdom's Ministry of Health [9]. In less than two months, the country experienced a substantial rise in Covid-19 cases with official reports indicating that 10,484 had been infected by 20 April 2020 [9]. As the country was engulfed by the pandemic, Saudi authorities prioritized awareness programs while seeking to contain the spread of Covid-19 with the help of curfews and social distancing measures [10]. To curtail the uncontrolled spread of Covid-19 among the population, the Saudi government introduced strict limitations on social gatherings, cultural activities, and other forms of close contact. The Muslim state resorted to completely closing mosques to minimize potential human-to-human transmissions [11]. The effectiveness of Saudi Arabia's anti-Covid-19 efforts is evidenced by the rapid decline in new cases and deaths by early summer 2020 [3]. By July, the Middle Eastern country started to revert harsh restrictions allowing citizens to engage in usual activities and even providing an opportunity for pilgrims to visit the city of Mecca.

There were no indications grounded on concrete evidence that would have suggested that statistics presented by the Saudi government are inaccurate or misleading. Although the reports on Covid-related infection rates and mortality rates are unlikely to be fabricated, it does not mean that the data provide an accurate representation of the pandemic's development. The key concern pertains to the fact that official reports account only for confirmed cases with the latter being closely correlated with the total number of performed PCR tests [12]. By the end of summer 2020, the Saudi data on Covid-19 was obtained by performing nearly 3.3 million tests which returned a 10% positive rate [13]. As the country's positive rate is within the boundaries set by the WHO, the confirmed cases and confirmed deaths could be reliably used by researchers. The total number of reported deaths does not raise questions as it is even higher than the global average. Another identified issue emerges as a result of the low population density and the complexity of performing testing in remote areas of Saudi Arabia, such as off-the-grid towns and communities in the Eastern Province [14]. The presence of closed-off communities with limited coverage of healthcare services is expected to skew the relationship between population density and Covid-19 statistics [9]. Importantly, the described problem is not localized within the MENA region as the logistical challenges of performing PCR tests on a global scale make it nearly impossible to assess the actual dynamics of the disease in any remote region of the world [6].

From the economic perspective, the Covid-19 pandemic both directly and indirectly disrupted a variety of Saudi Arabia's industries and sectors. While the nine-billion-dollar budget deficit in Q1 2020 was partially tied to disturbances in the global market for petroleum products, a sizable role was attributed to the coronavirus crisis [3]. Struggling to mitigate the disastrous effects of quarantine measures, Saudi Arabia's government stimulated the national economy by reducing spending and raising VAT. With the number of total confirmed cases and deaths approaching 360,000 and 6000, respectively, by the end of the year, Saudi Arabia incurred a budget deficit of $79 billion or nearly 300 billion SAR [14]. Considering that Covid-19 directly affects local businesses and indirectly influences global prices for crude oil, Saudi Arabia expects to reduce government expenses in 2021 to $263 billion to accommodate for the recession observed in the four quarters of 2020 [14,15].

2.2. The Course of the Covid-19 Pandemic in China

A country occupying the fourth largest landmass on the globe, PRC features a considerable population of 1.4 billion dispersed across sparsely populated rural regions and megacities such as Chongqing, Shanghai, and Beijing. The world's most populated state is subdivided into twenty-eight administrative regions as well as four centrally-controlled metropolitan areas. Although the total population density is 145 citizens per sq. km, the density of urban centers such as Shanghai and Beijing is considerably higher and approaches 4200 and 1300 per sq. km, respectively. Due to the fact that the Republic of China and regions such as Hong Kong followed distinctly different approaches towards registering Covid-related incidents and mitigating economic consequences, the research focuses on PRC, with both PRC and China being used interchangeably throughout the paper. While China has been at the forefront of numerous major epidemics throughout the past millennia, the most recent incidents include the 1968 Hong Kong flu, the 1997 bird flu, and the 2003 SARS epidemic [4]. The emergence of Covid-19 is deeply tied with PRC's Hubei province and, specifically, the city of Wuhan which is widely accepted as the location of the first outbreak. Notably, the government's hesitance to immediately recognize the epidemic resulted in the rapid spread of Covid-19 across all Chinese territories by 29 January 2020. As the severity of the novel coronavirus infection became evident, the authorities mandated the highest response level to curb the growing number of new Covid-19 cases. With the majority of early cases being restricted to Hubei, China reported nearly 25,000 cases and 700 deaths by early February 2020 [16]. The highest peak of the pandemic coincided with the Spring Festival which led scholars to believe that population migration and population aggregation patterns played an important role in the Covid-19 spread [17,18]. Moreover, Jiang et al. noted that the distance from the epicenter in the Wuhan province emerged as one of the key determinants for the epidemiological situation in Chinese provinces [19]. In the wake of the Covid-19 pandemic, PRC introduced increasingly strict social distancing measures as China's government enforced a strict quarantine in all provinces. Thanks to city-wide lockdowns and movement restrictions, China successfully contained the pandemic on its territories by March 2020 [4]. At the time of the study, the total number of confirmed cases and deaths was estimated at 86,000 and 4600, respectively.

However, the veracity of data and accuracy of reports presented by China's Communist Party had been the subject of critique for the entire duration of the pandemic. Scholars and governments questioned not only China's methods of containing the pandemic but also the validity of information on Covid-related morbidity and mortality [20,21]. The non-democratic country has been accused of publishing imprecise and even fabricated statistical data to preserve its image on domestic and international scenes. Despite the access to a robust economic base and nearly absolute control over media resources and industries, PRC was unable to conceal the existence of the problem. If not being completely truthful, the statistical records published by the government are expected to be somewhat accurate in depicting the proportional distribution of cases and deaths across regions [21]. Furthermore, the unfortunate incidents of suppressing whistleblowers in the healthcare system and authoritarian policies could have become the reason for data manipulations at the sub-national level [22]. As these manipulative reports by local governments consistently appeared in early 2020, PRC's Premier of the State Council Li Keqiang indirectly confirmed suspicions of the international community [20]. Despite the apparent lack of integrity and insufficient accuracy of Chinese official statistics on Covid-19, the problem is not limited to this Asian country. In fact, evidence of manipulation with official reports on Covid-19 morbidity and mortality can be found in most democratic countries such as the US and Germany [23]. Although there is a clear indication that global statistics regarding the spread and severity of the coronavirus pandemic is not entirely accurate at best and misleading at worst, the current scholarly consensus is to continue with caution when relying on governmental reports due to the possibility of manipulations [24].

Although PRC's anticipated economic growth in 2020 was estimated to be at 5.9%, Covid-19 had profound effects on all sectors including the transportation industry, tourism, banking, and others [1]. For example, the efforts to limit interprovincial movement led to the reduction of total train trips by 73% as compared to previous years and a considerable drop in sales of motor vehicles. During the period of harshest quarantine measures, China mandated the closure of businesses, industries, restaurants, and educational institutions [2]. Similar to Saudi Arabia's response to Covid-19, PRC mandated a near-complete shutdown of the tourism industry and curtailed all commercial flights in the country. Among the most controversial yet notable events was the extensive ban on the wildlife trade sector which reportedly amounted to more than $74 billion [25]. The singular focus on wildlife trade has both negative and positive economic connotations but most scholars recognize this decision as an effective response to the global pandemic [26,27]. In this context, international observers had estimated that PRC's economic growth would shrink to less than 2.3% in 2020 [28]. The timely implementation of anti-pandemic measures helped to alleviate the economic downturn in China as the expected growth for 2021 is likely to reach 8.4% [28].

2.3. Population Density and Covid-19

Considering the decisive role of human-to-human transmission for spreading the coronavirus disease, population density emerges as one of the most apparent factors influencing infection rates. From this perspective, numerous experts emphasize that people living in densely populated areas are more susceptible to being infected as opposed to the inhabitants of low-density rural regions [29,30]. The proponents of this theoretical approach indicate that countries with high population density, such as India and China, are likely to experience surges in Covid-19 cases and deaths. Several empirical inquiries have been made in Italy and Brazil regarding the potential feasibility of using population density as a determinant for Covid-19 spreading in different regions [31,32]. Although the opposing viewpoint on the issue will be discussed below, population density emerges as a crucial anthropogenic factor because the increasing frequency of interactions between people naturally contributes to high infection rates. Several authors provided plausible evidence pointing to the positive causative relationship between population density and the incidence of infectious diseases such as Covid-19 [33]. With people being more likely to engage in direct contact with others in crowded areas, the evidence further suggests that overpopulated cities and districts are prone to comparatively high infection rates [17,19]. Most authors agree that high-density cities provide conditions for crowding which offers an additional venue for viral transmission.

Despite the extensive empirical evidence indicating the significance of population density as a determinant of Covid-19 spread, the findings vary from country to country and from region to region. The pandemic lasted for less than 12 months by the time of this study but a comprehensive body of knowledge started to form with regard to the interrelation of socio-demographic factors and lockdown policies [34]. From this perspective, countries that implemented strict lockdown policies were expected to report lower infection rates and mortality rates in highly populated regions. As strict lockdown policies are especially effective in densely populated areas with expansive state control over the population, non-democratic nations showed the weakest causal relationships between the parameters investigates within the scope of the present research [35]. The described assumption does not deviate from the aforementioned claims because population density can still be used as a predicting factor during the early stages of an infectious outbreak as had been outlined in past studies. Moreover, countries with comparatively weak state control and disobedience among citizenry are those associated with the strongest positive correlation between population density and Covid-19 spread [32]. The strengths of causal relationships further vary across different cities and townships in the same country with the majority of reports confirming that low population density is tied to low infection rates [36]. There is no conclusive data on the relationship between population density and Covid-19 morbidity in sparsely populated regions.

Distinctly from the theory outlined above, certain researchers revealed that the Covid-19 pandemic does not always follow the expected pattern of high infection rates in densely populated regions. For example, Hamidi et al. [5] performed a meticulous analysis of Covid-19 cases and deaths in American counties with different population densities. While the authors concluded that density has no meaningful relationship with Covid-19 infection rates, high-density areas are considerably more likely to be associated with lower mortality rates. Several other authors confirm the described observation by explaining that people living in urbanized regions are better informed regarding social distancing measures and have access to superior health care than their rural-dwelling counterparts [37,38]. Additionally, skeptics note that metropolitan size and transportation links emerge as more significant determinants of Covid-19 infection rates and deaths than population density [39]. The skepticism is shared by scholars who accounted for lockdown policies because population density does not appear to be a significant determinant of Covid-19 incidence in some of the most densely populated countries of the world [33]. While multiple studies focusing on China provided inconclusive results, the authors recommended further investigation of the issue [35,40]. No such studies seeking to connect population density and Covid-19 mortality and morbidity were performed in Saudi Arabia to this day. The disagreement among scholars on the role played by population density in the development of pandemics is one of the principal motivators for the current research. Due to the inconclusive empirical data on the topic, it is crucial to investigate the practical significance of population density as a causative factor for newly emerging infectious diseases such as Covid-19 [41]. Previous studies emphasized the need of uncovering to what extent population density correlates with epidemiological variables such as infectivity rates and mortality rates in countries with strict lockdown policies. In this framework, the study seeks to assess the role of population density as a predictor of Covid-19 cases and deaths in Saudi Arabia and China after the peak of the Covid-19 pandemic in these two countries.

2.4. Kissinger's Malthusian Theory and Future Pandemics

Declassified in the 1990s, Henry Kissinger's 1974 report touched on the problem of worldwide population growth as a possible threat to the national interests of the US. The key idea of the document was that unchecked population growth in underdeveloped nations puts a strain on the global supply of food, minerals, and other resources. Whether due to possible civil disturbances or overconsumption of resources, the report recommended preemptively addressing the uncontrollable population growth by implementing population reduction strategies focused on promoting abortion, contraception, and family planning [42]. After being declassified, Kissinger's Malthusian theory was met with mixed responses from scholars who either proposed new Neo-Malthusian models or discarded the theory as unethical. With the recent addition of the global pandemic, the growing importance of social issues, famine, and environmental concerns revitalized the interest in population reduction as a viable long-term solution [43]. The recent examples of applying disincentives and coercion techniques informed by Neo-Malthusian models were reported in China and India. In line with China's one-child and two-child policies, there are multiple reports of coerced abortions, coerced sterilization, and country-wide propaganda efforts intended to control population growth [44]. While there are no such policies in India, authorities consistently pushed population reduction measures by indirectly penalizing families with more than two children [45]. Such methods were not widely used or considered for use in Saudi Arabia. Overall, the viability of Neo-Malthusian models to alleviate future pandemics remains understudied with nearly no data being available in regard to Covid-19.

The ongoing pandemic exacerbated socio-economic challenges encountered by the populations of rapidly developing non-democratic countries such as China and Saudi Arabia. As both China and Saudi Arabia enacted strict lockdown measures, less affluent citizens lost access to critical services and products which contributed to the already-existing lack of food security. Unable to survive without stable income, foreign workers and poor citizens experienced the devastating social impacts of an epidemiological emergency firsthand [46,47]. In this context, the Covid-19 pandemic showcased the need for robust private and public policies aimed at achieving food security and food sustainability. Although the governments of China and Saudi Arabia sought to prioritize health security, the lockdown measures were implemented at the expense of the least protected groups living in densely-populated regions. The absence of effective strategies for ensuring food provisioning and food security during health crises emerges as the critical concern for all nations who need to develop resilient systems for supplying and procuring food to the affected population [48]. In this framework, Neo-Malthusian models could provide a solution by informing comprehensive policies that would help to reduce population density and mitigate future medical disasters. Taking into account that the continuous population growth in Chinese territories is likely to be unsustainable from the long-term perspective, population density should be approached as one of the indicators guiding the gradual introduction of population reduction policies and initiatives [49]. Finally, the Covid-19 crisis highlighted the need for public programs that would not only address overpopulation but also tackle associated social concerns such as food security and sustainability [50].

With high infectivity and mortality being arguably a definitive characteristic of overpopulated regions, the authors propose that a Neo-Malthusian model informed by Henry Kissinger's population reduction theory can be applied as a control measure to control future pandemics [51]. In this framework, sparsely populated countries and regions can also benefit from policies informed by different population reduction frameworks. As the world's population will inevitably increase in the upcoming decades, the majority of regions that are currently sparsely populated are likely to be densely populated by the end of the twenty-first century [42]. Expected to surpass density levels at which pandemics can be effectively managed with lenient lockdown policies, many countries would have to either resort to strict lockdown policies, such as China's, or adopt a Neo-Malthusian model [21]. However, the viability of Neo-Malthusian models depends on a government's ability to manage its citizenry and implement potentially non-democratic policies. If the investigation uncovers that high-density Chinese regions are more susceptible to Covid-19 than low-density Saudi cities, Kissinger's Malthusian theory and Neo-Malthusian models can be used as a basis for reducing the impacts of future pandemics on the economic growth in the two countries. On the other hand, the absence of a causal relationship between population density and Covid-related morbidity and mortality in the studied countries would not invalidate the assumption that population reduction can be a viable solution for epidemiological, environmental, and social concerns. Within the scope of the described theoretical tenets, the study starts by assessing the role of population density as a predictor of Covid-19 cases and deaths in Saudi Arabia and China during the Covid-19 pandemic. Consequently, the investigation shifts towards the possibility of addressing the current and future epidemiological crises with the help of Neo-Malthusian theories. As a result, the current empirical study is informed by the following research question: What are the merits of using Neo-Malthusian models for reducing the impacts of pandemics on the economic growth in countries with low population density?

3. Methodology

Under the scope of the current study, the principal goal is to investigate the possibility of a correlational relationship between population density in Chinese and Saudi Arabian regions and Covid-related cases of infections and deaths. If the authors confirm the existence of correlation as was theorized, the consequent stages would pertain to modeling the linear relationship between population density and Covid-related deaths and cases as an independent variable and dependent variables, respectively. With infection rates and mortality being perceived as a possible function of population density, the authors consider the latter's significance for economic growth in the selected countries. Furthermore, the economic significance of the pandemic is analyzed through the lens of Kissinger's Malthusian theory. At this stage, there is no cohesive theoretical framework for describing the spread of highly infectious viral diseases in areas with different population densities and their impact on economic growth. Moreover, conflicting views on the topic necessitate additional research presenting a comparative analysis of high-density Chinese regions and low-density Saudi regions.

3.1. Data Used

Considering dependent variables for the study, the authors collected data for both infection cases and deaths caused by Covid-19 per 100,000 people for both countries with regions being selected as a unit of analysis. Furthermore, the research relies on the up-to-date dataset containing cumulative confirmed cases and mortalities for each province until 4 January 2021. Although the pandemic started and reached its peak at different timeframes in the two countries, the researchers are interested in comparing the results after the pandemic has been contained to a reasonable degree which justifies the choice of cumulative records for daily infection rates/mortality rates. Different reference dates would have no impact on the results because the study is focused on static data accumulated throughout a prolonged period as opposed to dynamic records. In the case of China, the dataset for 30 provinces, municipal areas, and territories was extracted from the JHU Covid-19 Resource Center [52]. To ensure normality, reports concerning Hubei were excluded due to the disproportionately high rates of infectivity and mortality as compared to other administrative units of PRC. On the other hand, the dataset for 13 provinces of Saudi Arabia was collected from the Covid-19 Dashboard operated by Saudi Arabia's MOH [53]. Both datasets contained full and up-to-date information pertaining to Covid-related deaths and Covid-19 cases in China and Saudi Arabia.

As the population density was chosen as the independent variable for the study, the authors calculated the demographic characteristic for each province by dividing the total number of residents by the land area of the respective province. With the province being the unit of analysis for the research, the population density represented with the number of citizens per sq. km was identified for China's 30 provinces and Saudi Arabia's 13 provinces. Specifically, the authors extracted the information regarding the total population for Chinese regions from the National Bureau of Statistics of China's database, with figures being the estimates for 2017 based on national sample surveys [54]. From the General Authority for Statistics' Demographic Survey, the authors obtained population figures for all Saudi provinces in 2016 [55]. The information from all databases for both countries was extracted and labeled for the consequent use with the R statistical software for correlation analysis and linear regression.

The author's primary goal is to identify a possible correlation between population density and Covid-related infection cases as well as mortality in administrative units of China and Saudi Arabia. After evaluating the existence and strength of correlation between variables, the following step includes modeling of simple linear regression data plots visualizing the linear relationship between the following variables: population density and Covid-19 cases in China; population density and Covid-19 mortality in China; population density and Covid-19 cases in Saudi Arabia, and; population density and Covid-19 mortality in Saudi Arabia. The obtained results are further reviewed and discussed through the lens of Kissinger's Malthusianism theory and its importance for economic growth in low-density and high-density regions.

3.2. Hierarchical Cluster Method

We employed the hierarchical cluster method to facilitate the comparison of Saudi and Chinese provinces based on the infection rates and population density. The average-linkage approach to the hierarchical agglomerative cluster analysis was deemed suitable for grouping distinct administrative regions for each of the investigated countries. The chosen technique helps to identify the groups of provinces with highest and lowest infection rates with regard to their respective population density figures [56]. The two-step clustering process pertained to the consecutive grouping of provinces based on the two dependent variables; consequently, we created clusters that would further incorporate the data on population density.

3.3. Pearson's Correlation

The authors calculate Pearson's two-tailed coefficient and R Square to establish nature as well as the strength of linear relationships between the two dependent variables and the independent variable. The computation is performed with the help of the standard formula for the product-moment correlation coefficient by separately using the datasets for China and Saudi Arabia. Furthermore, the null hypothesis test allows confirming the existence of a linear relationship in regard to the selected variables. After comparing the variance of variables with the help of Fisher's transformation and establishing the standard error, it is also possible to calculate the p-value for each pair of variables [57]. For the purposes of the study, $p < 0.05$ is the threshold of statistical significance. The formula used for the correlation equation is presented below.

$$r = \sum(x - mx)(y - my) \div \sqrt{\sum(x - mx)^2 \sum(y - my)^2}. \tag{1}$$

Apart from the main data set including all provinces and administrative regions of China and Saudi Arabia, correlation coefficients were additionally calculated for a separate model based on the average population density within both countries. In Saudi Arabia, population density is higher than the country-wide average of 15.6 people per sq. km in the following territories: Al Bahah, Al Qaseem, Jazan, Aseer, Ar Riyad, and Makkah al Mukarramah. The remaining geographic regions correspond to the vast swaths of sparsely inhabited land such as the Rub' al-Khali dessert. The median density for the group of densely populated territories is 38.4 per sq. km, and for the group of sparsely populated it is 6.2 per sq. km. As for PRC, the Heihe-Tengchong Line was employed as an accepted approach for demarcating highly-populated and sparsely-populated provinces in China. To ensure consistency, we also included Yunnan and Jilin to the following list of regions with population density being below the country average of 148 people per sq. km: Tibet, Qinghai, Xinjiang, Inner Mongolia, Gansu, Heilongjiang, and Ningxia. The median density for the group of sparsely populated territories to the West of the Heihe-Tengchong Line is 57.41 per sq. km, and for the group of densely populated it is 373.2 per sq. km.

3.4. Simple Linear Regression

Simple linear regression is performed to understand the underlying relationships between the chosen sets of variables for both countries. With the help of the regression line based on the standard formula for the method of least squares, the authors seek to illustrate the significance of population density as a determinant of Covid-19 cases and mortality over the observed period. The following mathematical equation underlies the process of modeling simple linear regression:

$$y = a + bx, \text{ with } b = \sum(x - \bar{x})(y - \bar{y}) \div \sum(x - \bar{x})^2. \tag{2}$$

Moreover, the simple linear regression provides an opportunity to model the aforementioned relationship with the intention of better understanding the role of the independent variable. To preserve the integrity of results, the authors ensure the following characteristics: normality, linearity, homoscedasticity, and independence of observations [57]. For the purposes of data analysis and computations, the R statistics software has been employed by the authors to process the extracted datasets for China and Saudi Arabia.

3.5. Conceptual Framework

The authors rely on empirical analysis of primary and secondary data to explore the possibility of applying Neo-Malthusian models to alleviate the detrimental impacts of future pandemics. Due to the absence of scholarly consensus on the role of population density as a determinant of Covid-19 morbidity and mortality, the present research performs a comparative analysis focusing on China and Saudi Arabia, two non-democratic states that have implemented strict lockdown policies to curb the pandemic. In this study, pragmatism was the chosen philosophical paradigm that helped to structure the scholarly inquiry in regard to the data collection and analysis for the purposes of answering the posed research question. The grounded theory underlies the comparative analysis by considering both primary and secondary data to investigate the studied problem and reach a plausible solution. The authors performed a comparative analysis of Saudi Arabia and China while using the resulting findings as a basis for exploring the possibility of applying Neo-Malthusian models for addressing future pandemics. With Saudi Arabia being sparsely populated and not engaged in population reduction programs, China emerges as a densely populated country that continuously relies on policies informed by Neo-Malthusianism. Throughout the 1970s, numerous scholars revisited the ideas proposed by Malthus in his 1798 essay [58,59]. Culminating with Kissinger's report, these studies concluded that current growth rates are unsustainable from the perspectives of food supply, environmental stress, and the availability of natural resources [45]. In this framework, a model informed by Neo-Malthusian principles could be used for the purposes of long-term population control in countries susceptible to these issues. Drawing from the aforementioned theories, the authors seek to analyze the viability of Neo-Malthusian models for minimizing the detrimental impacts of pandemics such as the Covid-19 pandemic.

4. Results and Discussion

By the time of the research, Saudi MOH reported the following cumulative figures from the pandemic's onset: 363,259 Covid-19 cases and 6265 deaths. In contrast, PRC confirmed 97,028 cumulative cases of Covid-19 infection and 4792 deaths by the same date. As China's population at 1.3 billion in 2017 is substantially larger than that of Saudi Arabia with 31.8 million inhabitants, the Covid-related figures were converted to represent incidence rates per 100,000 people. In the case of Saudi Arabia, 13 emirates substantially differ in population density as well as the number of reported cases and deaths, with Jazan being the most densely populated region of the country. On the other hand, among China's thirty administrative units selected for the research, the following cities feature the highest density: Shanghai, Tianjin, and Beijing.

By employing the hierarchical agglomerative cluster method based on the average-linkage approach, we initially classified the regions of Saudi Arabia and China based on the infection rates. The division into groups facilitated the consequent clustering process based on the population density in each of the aforementioned regions. The study population of 30 administrative regions in China was divided into groups as displayed on the dendrogram (see Figure 1). The first group includes Shanghai with estimated population density of 3814 inhabitants per sq. km and Covid-19 cases of 6.32 per 100,000. Tianjin and Beijing comprise the second group while the remaining regions form several smaller clusters corresponding to their estimated population density and Covid-19 cases. In the case of Saudi Arabia, 13 emirates were divided into multiple groups that included Eastern Province and Al Madinah Al Munawwarah, Ha'il and Najran, and others (see

Figure 2). The hierarchical clustering did not reveal any significant insights after classifying the emirates by the population density and Covi-19 cases.

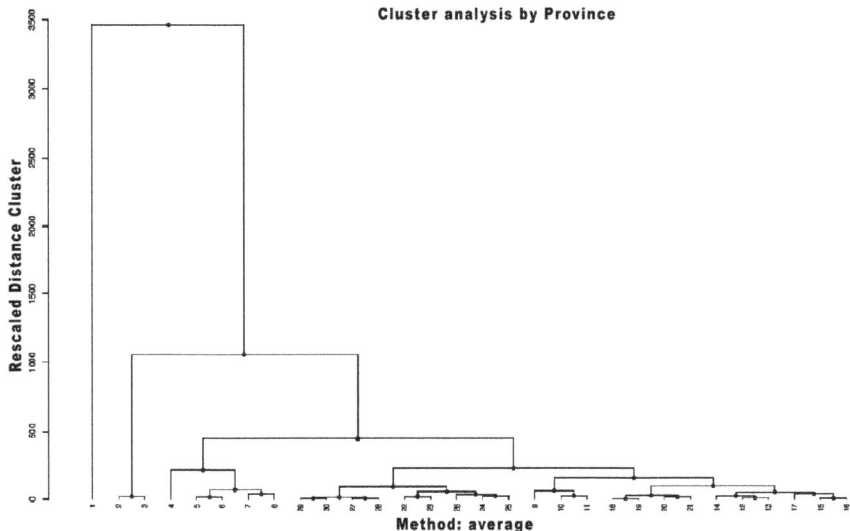

Figure 1. Cluster analysis of population density and Covid-19 cases for China's administrative regions.

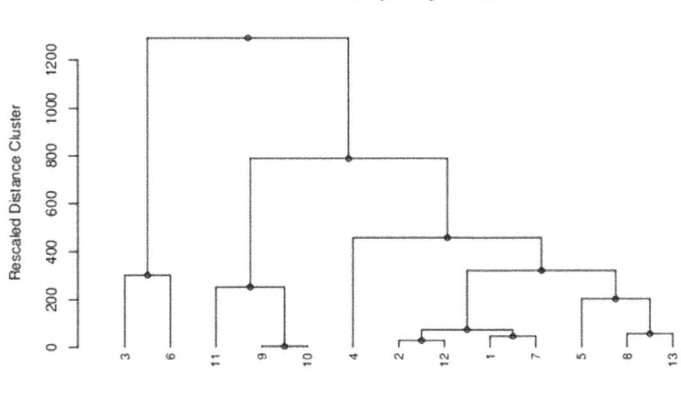

Figure 2. Cluster analysis of population density and Covid-19 cases for Saudi Arabia's administrative regions.

The preliminary analysis of data strongly suggests that Covid-19 infections in predominantly sparsely populated Saudi Arabia are not representative of population density figures. When excluding Hubei from the analysis, the opposite is evident in the case of China with high density being closely tied to the rise in Covid infections as seen in Figure 3. Notably, the mortality rate from Covid-19 appears to be higher in high-density areas of Saudi Arabia as compared to the lack of a meaningful connection in Chinese regions as depicted in Figure 4.

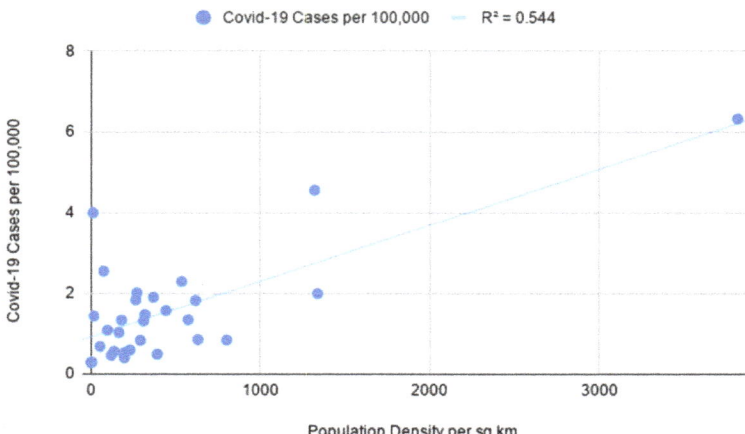

Figure 3. Simple linear regression with population density as an independent variable and Covid-19 cases as a dependent variable for China's administrative divisions.

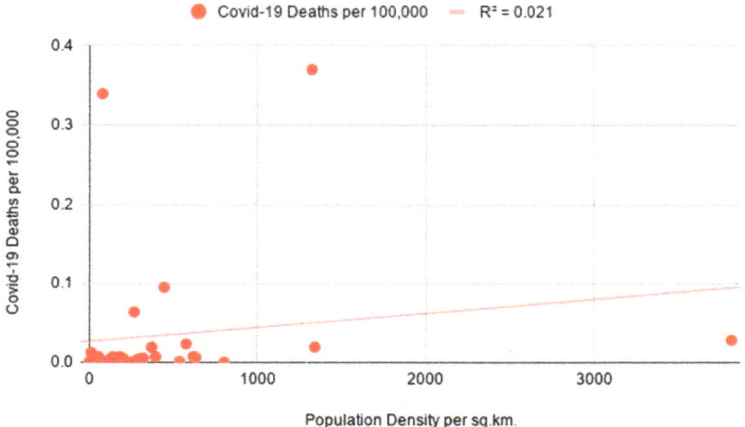

Figure 4. Simple linear regression with population density as an independent variable and Covid-19 deaths as a dependent variable for China's administrative divisions.

The following correlation coefficients are computed for independent and dependent variables for China's administrative regions: 0.73 for Covid-19 cases indicating a moderate positive correlation and 0.14 for Covid-19 deaths indicating a weak positive correlation. Furthermore, the coefficients for Saudi Arabia are as follows: −0.15 for Covid-19 cases indicating a weak negative correlation and 0.63 for Covid-19 deaths indicating a moderate positive correlation which is depicted in Figure 5. In the course of the significance test, the authors calculated p-values for China's Covid-19 infection rates and Saudi Arabia's mortality rates to be smaller than 0.05 at the chosen significance level, allowing us to reject the null hypothesis. As the p-value for China's mortality rates is 0.44 and the p-value for Saudi Arabia's infection rates is 0.64, the null hypothesis cannot be rejected and results should be considered not significant as p is larger than 0.05. As evident in Figure 6, the linear regression model for Saudi Arabia presents counter-intuitive results with a slight indication that higher population density could be a minor determinant for mortality rates as a result of Covid-19. The number of Covid-related deaths per 100,000 people in Saudi Arabia is not homogenous across all the regions. The empirical analysis shows that it is consistently higher in densely populated emirates as compared to sparsely populated ones. The latter is evidenced by Covid-19 mortality rates in the most overpopulated regions of the country—Jazan and Makkah Al Mukarramah. Interestingly, sparsely populated Eastern Province and Northern Borders reported unusually high mortality rates which can be explained by inconsistent diagnostic approaches in Saudi medical centers. While we do not have information on how Covid-related deaths were recorded in these emirates, the number of medical institutions could have been another determinant. Only in the case of China's infectivity rates, the obtained results align with a presumption that highly-dense areas are more prone to the spread of infectious diseases.

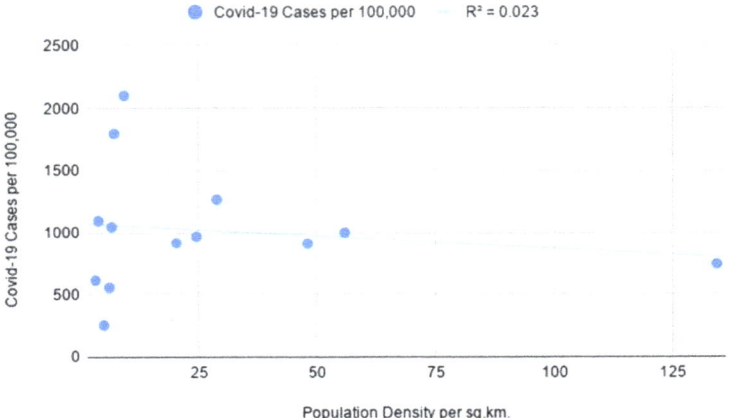

Figure 5. Simple linear regression with population density as an independent variable and Covid-19 cases as a dependent variable for Saudi Arabia's administrative divisions.

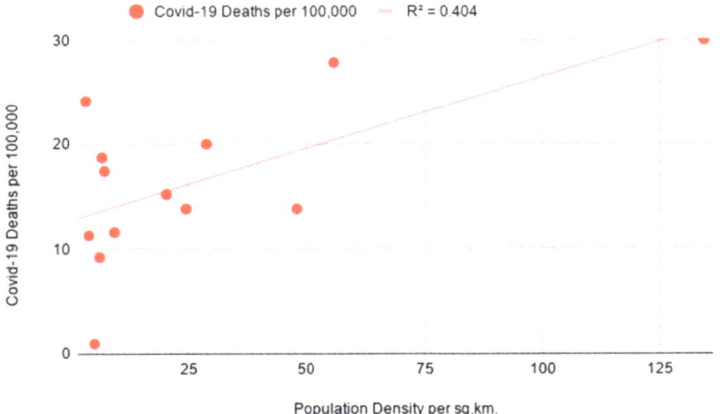

Figure 6. Simple linear regression with population density as an independent variable and Covid-19 deaths as a dependent variable for Saudi Arabia's administrative divisions.

At the R Square values of 0.54 (for China's infection rates) and 0.4 (for Saudi Arabia's mortality rates), the results indicate that the independent variable can partially explain the incidence of Covid-19 cases in China and the mortality rates in Saudi Arabia, respectively (Table 1). Low R Square values for China's infection rates (0.02) and Saudi Arabia's mortality rates (0.02) signify that the independent variable is not responsible for the majority of variations of the studied dependent variables. The lack of definitive and strong relationships between studied variables can be explained by the fact that population density is one of the many factors influencing the course of infectious diseases in different regions. Furthermore, the higher number of recorded Covid-19 deaths in Mecca and Jazan is possibly tied to superior diagnostic methods available in the metropolitan areas of the two regions. While Covid-related mortality rates in all Chinese regions are extremely low, the regression model for population density and infection cases aligns with the theory that the former can act as one of the determining factors for the latter. After separately assessing the data for densely-populated and sparsely-populated territories in both countries, the results proved to be largely not significant at $p < 0.05$. The sole exception pertained to Covid-19 cases in Chinese provinces to the east of the Heihe-Tengchong Line which indicated a relatively strong positive correlation with significant results at $p < 0.05$. The assessment of R Square values does not show considerable differences after separately analyzing the data for regions with different population density averages.

Table 1. Coefficients of determination and p-values.

		Saudi Arabia		China	
		Cases	Deaths	Cases	Death
All territories	R Square	0.02	0.4	0.54	0.02
	p-value	0.62	0.01	<0.00001	0.44
Densely populated regions	R Square	0.41	0.6	0.74	0.05
	p-value	0.16	0.06	<0.00001	0.32
Sparsely populated regions	R Square	0.53	0.07	0.04	0.01
	p-value	0.06	0.55	0.58	0.73

As evidenced by the results, the chosen methodology and data are prone to certain limitations that include the rapid development of the Covid-19 situation in different countries, the lack of conclusive data, and a non-uniform approach to recording and reporting Covid-related events. In this framework, a longitude time-series research would be uniquely suited to further explore the topic and provide robust evidence regarding the role of population density as a determinant of Covid-19 infection and mortality rates. Moreover, as the pandemic peaked at different periods in Saudi Arabia and China, the two countries relied on dramatically different approaches for reporting new cases, treating Covid-19 patients, and implementing anti-pandemic measures. From this perspective, future studies should account for distinctions in health systems as well as for numerous confounding factors such as pre-existing medical conditions.

The data analysis indicated that population density has no significant causal relationship with Covid-19 morbidity and mortality which suggests that other factors play a more significant role concerning the Covid-19 spread. The effectiveness of lockdown policies implemented by Saudi Arabia and China, two non-democratic regimes, may obscure the actual connection between the studied variables. In this framework, the existing evidence is not sufficient to conclude whether Covid-19 is a Malthusian event or not. Nevertheless, the concepts developed by Malthus and further explored in Kissinger's report may inform the solution to the ongoing environmental, social, and epidemiological crises. As the population growth puts a strain on the global supply of resources, this includes the ability of countries to provide healthcare services to the ever-increasing population. By considering various population reduction strategies, governments would be able to align with the requirement of sustainable development. Despite the fact that Neo-Malthusianism remains a highly controversial theory, its implementation can indirectly contribute to the resolution of pertinent problems such as food shortages and epidemics [60]. The latter is evident in the case of China which has been arguably effective in addressing the Covid-19 outbreak while also practicing several population control measures [16,17,21]. Finally, the authoritarian qualities of both governments presented an opportunity to maintain strict lockdown policies which suggest the potential for adopting a form of Neo-Malthusianism to preserve China's and Saudi Arabia's economic growth in the aftermath of the pandemic. Population density can be considered as one of the numerous determinants associated with health crises such as the Covid-19 pandemic. Taking into account socio-economic threats and epidemiological concerns arising as a result of overpopulation, a combined work of scholars and professionals is necessary to propose effective Neo-Malthusian models that would act as a long-term solution for future disasters and health crises.

Considering that the research did not provide uniform evidence that population density has a strong positive relationship with Covid-19 cases and deaths, population control informed by Neo-Malthusian models is likely to be rather ineffective as a direct Covid control measure. As seen in the example of densely populated regions of China, the ensuing economic recovery was primarily tied to centrally-planned policies and effective quarantine measures implemented by the government. From another perspective, Covid-19 events in low-density regions of Saudi Arabia are preeminently tied to other confounding factors that should be further explored in future studies. Furthermore, both global prices for crude oil and Covid-19 are responsible for Saudi Arabia's economic decline in 2020. As China and Saudi Arabia managed to achieve meaningful economic recovery after containing the coronavirus, Kissinger's Malthusian theory of population reduction is likely to be ineffective as a control measure for future pandemics. Population reduction approaches should be further explored after identifying other major determinants for Covid-19 infection and mortality along with population density.

5. Conclusions

The Covid-19 pandemic emerged as the most significant crisis of the twenty-first century that continues challenging health experts and economists across the world to find suitable solutions to the ever-increasing number of epidemiological, social, and environmental concerns. Due to the infection's rapid spread across the globe, the existing evidence and knowledge base are constrained by the lack of data. In this context, the pandemic's economic impact remains largely understudied as many potential determinants of Covid-19 infection and mortality rates remain hidden. The role of population density as a factor contributing to the course of an emerging infectious disease is somewhat controversial with several authors presenting contrasting viewpoints on the topic. The current study did not uncover a meaningful and conclusive causal relationship between the studied variables suggesting that population density does not explain variations in Covid-related mortality and infection rates. Although Covid-19 does not appear to be a Malthusian event, the possibility of using Neo-Malthusian models to address future pandemics should be explored further. Furthermore, the findings indicate that the role of population density could be obscured by other factors such as statistical inaccuracies and lockdown policies. There is a need for additional studies on the importance of strict lockdown policies in non-democratic nations as an effective anti-pandemic measure. In the case of population control, Neo-Malthusianism remains a viable solution to the problems posed by the uncontrolled population growth that should be further investigated. Although a moderate positive correlation was observed between the independent variable and China's infection rates and Saudi Arabia's mortality rates, the results are inconclusive due to the potential impact of other factors. In the case of China and Saudi Arabia, the analysis of Covid-19 cases and deaths in comparison to the population density of different regions did not reveal any conclusive evidence that population control can be used as a Covid control measure. However, the analysis indicates that Neo-Malthusian models could be considered by non-democratic governments to implement long-term policies that would facilitate economic recovery in the post-pandemic period. The research reveals that the severity of health crises such as the Covid-19 pandemic is closely tied to an array of social and economic problems. To ensure food security and sustainability consistently threatened by overpopulation, the authors recommend to prioritize scholarly investigations of Neo-Malthusian models as possible solutions intended to mitigate future disasters and health crises. Future research is necessary to investigate population control policies as a possible approach to alleviating the economic impact of global pandemics.

Author Contributions: Conceptualization, N.Y.; methodology, N.Y.; software, N.Y.; validation, N.Y. and L.S.S.; formal analysis, N.Y.; investigation, L.S.S.; resources, N.Y. and L.S.S.; data curation, L.S.S.; writing—original draft preparation, N.Y.; writing—review and editing, N.Y. and L.S.S. All authors have read and agreed to the published version of the manuscript.

Funding: This research received no external funding.

Institutional Review Board Statement: Not applicable.

Informed Consent Statement: Not applicable.

Data Availability Statement: The datasets pertaining to Covid-19 cases and mortality used in the current study were obtained from Saudi Arabia's MOH (https://covid19.moh.gov.sa/, accessed on 6 January 2021) and JHU Covid-19 Resource Center (https://coronavirus.jhu.edu/data/new-cases, accessed on 6 January 2021). Other demographic datasets were extracted from China's Bureau of Statistics (https://data.stats.gov.cn/, accessed on 6 January 2021) and Saudi Arabia's General Authority for Statistics (https://www.stats.gov.sa/, accessed on 6 January 2021).

Acknowledgments: The authors are grateful to the anonymous reviewers for providing valuable insights on the discussed topics.

Conflicts of Interest: The authors declare no conflict of interest.

References

1. Bagchi, B.; Chatterjee, S.; Ghosh, R.; Dandapat, D. Impact of COVID-19 on Global Economy. In *Coronavirus Outbreak and the Great Lockdown*; Springer: Singapore, 2020; pp. 15–26.
2. Khan, N.; Faisal, S. Epidemiology of Corona Virus in the World and Its Effects on the China Economy. *SSRN Electron. J.* **2020**. [CrossRef]
3. Abodunrin, O.; Oloye, G.; Adesola, B. Coronavirus pandemic and its implication on global economy. *Int. J. Arts Lang. Bus. Stud.* **2020**, *4*, 13–23.
4. Copiello, S.; Grillenzoni, C. The spread of 2019-nCoV in China was primarily driven by population density. Comment on "Association between short-term exposure to air pollution and COVID-19 infection: Evidence from China" by Zhu et al. *Sci. Total Environ.* **2020**, *744*, 141028. [CrossRef] [PubMed]
5. Hamidi, S.; Sabouri, S.; Ewing, R. Does Density Aggravate the COVID-19 Pandemic? *J. Am. Plan. Assoc.* **2020**, *86*, 495–509. [CrossRef]
6. Imtyaz, A.; Haleem, A.; Javaid, M. Analysing governmental response to the COVID-19 pandemic. *J. Oral Biol. Craniofac. Res.* **2020**, *10*, 504–513. [CrossRef]
7. Hsu, J. Population Density Does Not Doom Cities to Pandemic Dangers. Scientific American. 2020. Available online: https://www.scientificamerican.com/article/population-density-does-not-doom-cities-to-pandemic-dangers/ (accessed on 6 January 2021).
8. Nicola, M.; Alsafi, Z.; Sohrabi, C.; Kerwan, A.; Al-Jabir, A.; Iosifidis, C.; Agha, M.; Agha, R. The socio-economic implications of the coronavirus pandemic (COVID-19): A review. *Int. J. Surg.* **2020**, *78*, 185–193. [CrossRef]
9. AlMofada, S.K.; Alherbisch, R.J.; AlMuhraj, N.A.; Almeshary, B.N.; Alrabiah, B.; Al Saffan, A.; Baseer, M.A. Knowledge, Attitudes, and Practices Toward COVID-19 in a Saudi Arabian Population: A Cross-Sectional Study. *Cureus* **2020**, *12*, e8905. [CrossRef]
10. Alahdal, H.; Basingab, F.; Alotaibi, R. An analytical study on the awareness, attitude and practice during the COVID-19 pandemic in Riyadh, Saudi Arabia. *J. Infect. Public Health* **2020**, *13*, 1446–1452. [CrossRef] [PubMed]
11. Alrasheed, H.; Althnian, A.; Kurdi, H.; Al-Mgren, H.; Alharbi, S. COVID-19 Spread in Saudi Arabia: Modeling, Simulation and Analysis. *Int. J. Environ. Res. Public Health* **2020**, *17*, 7744. [CrossRef] [PubMed]
12. Al-Khani, A.M.; Khalifa, M.A.; Almazrou, A.; Saquib, N. The SARS-CoV-2 pandemic course in Saudi Arabia: A dynamic epidemiological model. *Infect. Dis. Model.* **2020**, *5*, 766–771. [CrossRef] [PubMed]
13. Adly, H.M.; Aljahdali, I.A.; Garout, M.A.; Khafagy, A.A.; Saati, A.A.; Saleh, S.A.K. Correlation of COVID-19 Pandemic with Healthcare System Response and Prevention Measures in Saudi Arabia. *Int. J. Environ. Res. Public Health* **2020**, *17*, 6666. [CrossRef] [PubMed]
14. Nereim, V.; Abu Omar, A.; Martin, M. Saudi Arabia Plans Spending Cuts in 2021 as Economy Recovers. Bloomberg. 2020. Available online: https://www.bloomberg.com/news/articles/2020-12-15/saudi-arabia-sticks-to-spending-cuts-as-2021-budget-announced (accessed on 6 January 2021).
15. Barry, M.; Ghonem, L.; AlSharidi, A.; Alanazi, A.; Alotaibi, N.; Al-Shahrani, F.; Majid, F.; Bahammam, A. Coronavirus disease-2019 pandemic in the Kingdom of Saudi Arabia: Mitigation measures and hospital preparedness. *J. Nat. Sci. Med.* **2020**, *3*. [CrossRef]

16. Kraemer, M.U.G.; Yang, C.-H.; Gutierrez, B.; Wu, C.-H.; Klein, B.; Pigott, D.M.; Du Plessis, L.; Faria, N.R.; Li, R.; Hanage, W.P.; et al. The effect of human mobility and control measures on the COVID-19 epidemic in China. *Science* **2020**, *368*, 493–497. [CrossRef] [PubMed]
17. Zeng, P.; Sun, Z.; Chen, Y.; Qiao, Z.; Cai, L. COVID-19: A Comparative Study of Population Aggregation Patterns in the Central Urban Area of Tianjin, China. *Int. J. Environ. Res. Public Health* **2021**, *18*, 2135. [CrossRef] [PubMed]
18. Zheng, Y.; Huang, J.; Yin, Q. What Are the Reasons for the Different COVID-19 Situations in Different Cities of China? A Study from the Perspective of Population Migration. *Int. J. Environ. Res. Public Health* **2021**, *18*, 3255. [CrossRef] [PubMed]
19. Jiang, X.; Wei, W.; Wang, S.; Zhang, T.; Lu, C. Effects of COVID-19 on Urban Population Flow in China. *Int. J. Environ. Res. Public Health* **2021**, *18*, 1617. [CrossRef] [PubMed]
20. Adiguzel, F.S.; Cansunar, A.; Corekcioglu, G. Truth or Dare? Detecting Systematic Manipulation of COVID-19 Statistics. *J. Politi-Inst. Politi-Econ.* **2020**, *1*, 543–557. [CrossRef]
21. You, C.; Deng, Y.; Hu, W.; Sun, J.; Lin, Q.; Zhou, F.; Pang, C.H.; Zhang, Y.; Chen, Z.; Zhou, X.-H. Estimation of the time-varying reproduction number of COVID-19 outbreak in China. *Int. J. Hyg. Environ. Health* **2020**, *228*, 113555. [CrossRef]
22. Abazi, V. Truth Distancing? Whistleblowing as Remedy to Censorship during COVID-19. *Eur. J. Risk Regul.* **2020**, *11*, 375–381. [CrossRef]
23. Held, K.S. COVID-19 Statistics and Facts: Meaningful or a Means of Manipulation? *J. Am. Physicians Surg.* **2020**, *25*, 3.
24. Lin, T.P.H.; Wan, K.H.; Huang, S.S.; Jonas, J.B.; Hui, D.S.C.; Lam, D.S.C. Death tolls of COVID-19: Where come the fallacies and ways to make them more accurate. *Glob. Public Health* **2020**, *15*, 1–6. [CrossRef]
25. Ribeiro, J.; Bingre, P.; Strubbe, D.; Reino, L. Coronavirus: Why a permanent ban on wildlife trade might not work in China. *Nat. Cell Biol.* **2020**, *578*, 217. [CrossRef]
26. Koh, L.P.; Li, Y.; Lee, J.S.H. The value of China's ban on wildlife trade and consumption. *Nat. Sustain.* **2021**, *4*, 2–4. [CrossRef]
27. Roe, D.; Lee, T.M. Possible negative consequences of a wildlife trade ban. *Nat. Sustain.* **2021**, *4*, 5–6. [CrossRef]
28. Yao, K. POLL-China's Economic Growth Seen Hitting 44-Year Low in 2020, Bounce 8.4% in 2021. NASDAQ, 2020. Available online: https://www.nasdaq.com/articles/poll-chinas-economic-growth-seen-hitting-44-year-low-in-2020-bounce-8.4-in-2021-2020-10-27 (accessed on 6 January 2021).
29. Bhadra, A.; Mukherjee, A.; Sarkar, K. Impact of population density on Covid-19 infected and mortality rate in India. *Model. Earth Syst. Environ.* **2021**, *7*, 623–629. [CrossRef] [PubMed]
30. Carozzi, F.; Provenzano, S.; Roth, S. *Urban Density and COVID-19*; Institute of Labor Economics: Bonn, Germany, 2020.
31. Coccia, M. Factors determining the diffusion of COVID-19 and suggested strategy to prevent future accelerated viral infectivity similar to COVID. *Sci. Total Environ.* **2020**, *729*, 138474. [CrossRef]
32. Pequeno, P.; Mendel, B.; Rosa, C.; Bosholn, M.; Souza, J.L.; Baccaro, F.; Barbosa, R.; Magnusson, W. Air transportation, population density and temperature predict the spread of COVID-19 in Brazil. *PeerJ* **2020**, *8*, e9322. [CrossRef]
33. Kodera, S.; Rashed, E.A.; Hirata, A. Correlation between COVID-19 Morbidity and Mortality Rates in Japan and Local Population Density, Temperature, and Absolute Humidity. *Int. J. Environ. Res. Public Health* **2020**, *17*, 5477. [CrossRef]
34. Garland, P.; Babbitt, D.; Bondarenko, M.; Sorichetta, A.; Tatem, A.J.; Johnson, O. The COVID-19 pandemic as experienced by the individual. *arXiv* **2020**, arXiv:2005.01167.
35. Sun, Z.; Zhang, H.; Yang, Y.; Wan, H.; Wang, Y. Impacts of geographic factors and population density on the COVID-19 spreading under the lockdown policies of China. *Sci. Total Environ.* **2020**, *746*, 141347. [CrossRef]
36. Tzampoglou, P.; Loukidis, D. Investigation of the Importance of Climatic Factors in COVID-19 Worldwide Intensity. *Int. J. Environ. Res. Public Health* **2020**, *17*, 7730. [CrossRef] [PubMed]
37. Adlakha, D.; Sallis, J.F. Activity-friendly neighbourhoods can benefit non-communicable and infectious diseases. *Cities Health* **2020**, 1–5. [CrossRef]
38. Kadi, N.; Khelfaoui, M. Population density, a factor in the spread of COVID-19 in Algeria: Statistic study. *Bull. Natl. Res. Cent.* **2020**, *44*, 1–7. [CrossRef]
39. Sy, K.T.L.; White, L.F.; Nichols, B.E. Population density and basic reproductive number of COVID-19 across United States counties. *MedRxiv* **2020**. [CrossRef]
40. Byass, P. Eco-epidemiological assessment of the COVID-19 epidemic in China, January–February 2020. *Glob. Health Action* **2020**, *13*. [CrossRef]
41. Arif, M.; Sengupta, S. Nexus between population density and novel coronavirus (COVID-19) pandemic in the south Indian states: A geo-statistical approach. *Environ. Dev. Sustain.* **2020**, 1–29. [CrossRef]
42. Pham, N.M.; Huynh, T.L.D.; Nasir, M.A. Environmental consequences of population, affluence and technological progress for European countries: A Malthusian view. *J. Environ. Manag.* **2020**, *260*, 110143. [CrossRef] [PubMed]
43. Cullather, N. "Stretching the Surface of the Earth": The Foundations, Neo-Malthusianism and the Modernising Agenda. *Glob. Soc.* **2014**, *28*, 104–112. [CrossRef]
44. Pan, G. China and Birth Control. In *Socio-Biological Implications of Confucianism*; Springer: Berlin/Heidelberg, Germany, 2015; pp. 55–61.
45. Follett, C. *Neo-Malthusianism and Coercive Population Control in China and India*; Policy Analysis; Cato Institute: Washington, DC, USA, 2020.

46. Ma, N.L.; Peng, W.; Soon, C.F.; Hassim, M.F.N.; Misbah, S.; Rahmat, Z.; Yong, W.T.L.; Sonne, C. Covid-19 pandemic in the lens of food safety and security. *Environ. Res.* **2021**, *193*, 110405. [CrossRef] [PubMed]
47. Béné, C. Resilience of local food systems and links to food security—A review of some important concepts in the context of COVID-19 and other shocks. *Food Secur.* **2020**, *12*, 805–822. [CrossRef]
48. Agovino, M.; Cerciello, M.; Gatto, A. Policy efficiency in the field of food sustainability. The adjusted food agriculture and nutrition index. *J. Environ. Manag.* **2018**, *218*, 220–233. [CrossRef] [PubMed]
49. Ali, I.; Alharbi, O.M. COVID-19: Disease, management, treatment, and social impact. *Sci. Total. Environ.* **2020**, *728*, 138861. [CrossRef] [PubMed]
50. Gatto, A.; Drago, C.; Ruggeri, M. On the Frontline—Sustainability and Development Research Amidst the COVID-19 Pandemic. 2020. Available online: https://www.researchsquare.com/article/rs-103974/v1 (accessed on 6 January 2021). [CrossRef]
51. LaRouche, L.H.; Zepp-LaRouche, H. *There Are No Limits to Growth*; Executive Intelligence Review: Leesburg, VA, USA, 2015.
52. Johns Hopkins Coronavirus Resource Center. Global Map. Available online: https://coronavirus.jhu.edu/map.html (accessed on 6 October 2020).
53. Ministry of Health. COVID 19 Dashboard: Saudi Arabia. 2020. Available online: https://covid19.moh.gov.sa/ (accessed on 6 January 2021).
54. National Bureau of Statistics of China. National Data. 2020. Available online: https://data.stats.gov.cn/english/ (accessed on 6 January 2021).
55. GAStat. Demography Survey 2016. 2016. Available online: https://www.stats.gov.sa/sites/default/files/en-demographic-research-2016_2.pdf (accessed on 6 January 2021).
56. Kassambara, A. Practical Guide to Cluster Analysis in R: Unsupervised Machine Learning. STHDA, 2017. Available online: https://xsliulab.github.io/Workshop/week10/r-cluster-book.pdf (accessed on 6 January 2021).
57. Bewick, V.; Cheek, L.; Ball, J. Statistics review 7: Correlation and regression. *Crit. Care* **2003**, *7*, 451–459. [CrossRef] [PubMed]
58. Frey, M. Neo-Malthusianism and development: Shifting interpretations of a contested paradigm. *J. Glob. Hist.* **2011**, *6*, 75–97. [CrossRef]
59. Bashford, A.; Levine, P. (Eds.) *The Oxford Handbook of the History of Eugenics*; OUP USA: New York, NY, USA, 2010.
60. Sengupta, R.P.; Chaudhuri, C. COVID-19: Neo-Malthusianism, Ecological Links, and Challenges for Humanity. *Int. J. Ecol. Environ. Sci.* **2020**, *46*, 141–154.

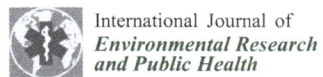 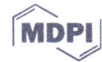

Article

Can Socioeconomic, Health, and Safety Data Explain the Spread of COVID-19 Outbreak on Brazilian Federative Units?

Diego Galvan [1,2,3,*], Luciane Effting [4], Hágata Cremasco [4] and Carlos Adam Conte-Junior [1,2,3]

[1] COVID-19 Research Group, Center for Food Analysis (NAL), Technological Development Support Laboratory (LADETEC), Cidade Universitária, Rio de Janeiro, RJ 21941-598, Brazil; conte@iq.ufrj.br
[2] Laboratory of Advanced Analysis in Biochemistry and Molecular Biology (LAABBM), Department of Biochemistry, Federal University of Rio de Janeiro (UFRJ), Cidade Universitária, Rio de Janeiro, RJ 21941-909, Brazil
[3] Nanotechnology Network, Carlos Chagas Filho Research Support Foundation of the State of Rio de Janeiro (FAPERJ), Rio de Janeiro, RJ 20020-000, Brazil
[4] Chemistry Department, State University of Londrina (UEL), Londrina, PR 86057-970, Brazil; luciane.effting@uel.br (L.E.); hagata@uel.br (H.C.)
* Correspondence: diegogalvann@gmail.com or diegogalvann@iq.ufrj.br

Received: 19 October 2020; Accepted: 14 November 2020; Published: 30 November 2020

Abstract: Infinite factors can influence the spread of COVID-19. Evaluating factors related to the spread of the disease is essential to point out measures that take effect. In this study, the influence of 14 variables was assessed together by Artificial Neural Networks (ANN) of the type Self-Organizing Maps (SOM), to verify the relationship between numbers of cases and deaths from COVID-19 in Brazilian states for 110 days. The SOM analysis showed that the variables that presented a more significant relationship with the numbers of cases and deaths by COVID-19 were influenza vaccine applied, Intensive Care Unit (ICU), ventilators, physicians, nurses, and the Human Development Index (HDI). In general, Brazilian states with the highest rates of influenza vaccine applied, ICU beds, ventilators, physicians, and nurses, per 100,000 inhabitants, had the lowest number of cases and deaths from COVID-19, while the states with the lowest rates were most affected by the disease. According to the SOM analysis, other variables such as Personal Protective Equipment (PPE), tests, drugs, and Federal funds, did not have as significant effect as expected.

Keywords: coronavirus disease; artificial neural networks; SARS-CoV-2; ventilator; index development index; developing country

1. Introduction

In December 2019, cases of acute pneumonia in the city of Wuhan, China, called attention due to the speed of contagion [1]. The virus that caused this pneumonia in affected individuals is the SARS-CoV-2, the causative agent of the novel coronavirus (COVID-19). The number of cases quickly evolved into a pandemic, decreed by the World Health Organization (WHO) on 11 March 2020. Currently, a few months after the first cases, this disease has been plaguing the world [2].

At the moment, the pandemic epicenter is in Latin America, with Brazil, Argentina, Colombia, Peru, Mexico, and Chile being the most representative countries, concentrating more than 10 million cases. Brazil already has more than 5 million cases and 150,000 deaths, ranking third in the world in the number of cases and deaths by COVID-19, behind only to the United States and India [3].

Intense efforts by the scientific community are focused on finding drugs to treat [4] and develop a vaccine for the disease [5]. Other research tries to understand how the disease has spread around the world. Some factors can influence the spread of the virus, including the disregard of preventive measures adopted by the government by population [6], climatic [7–9], comorbidities [10,11], hospital structure, prepared professionals, personal protective equipment, and financial resources [4].

In order to monitor the pandemic, it is necessary to collect information on the most significant possible number of factors that can influence the disease's dissemination behavior and, with this, establish a relationship that allows to affirm which measures delay the spread of COVID-19. Statistical tools have been used to study the behavior of epidemics for years; this area treats, analyzes, and obtains information from large datasets that cannot be analyzed by traditional systems [12].

Artificial Neural Networks (ANNs) are tools that have been gaining scientific relevance to perform pattern recognition, classification, or prediction tasks. ANN is a non-linear computational model attempting to simulate human brain structure and decision-making [13]. Its architecture is inspired by biological neural networks and consists of simple processing units that store empirical knowledge through a learning process [14].

Among the most common types of neural networks are the Feed-Forward Neural Network (FFNN), the Convolutional Neural Network (CNN), and the Recursive Neural Network (RNN). FFNNs are the most common type of ANN in practical applications, consisting of one or more hidden layers of perceptrons (neurons) that require supervised training. The input data of the desired sample datasets and the output results are sent to the network several times until the error in the output is minimized [13].

Traditionally, several types of neural networks exist with various techniques such as Autoregression (AR) [15,16], Moving Average (MA) [17,18], Exponential Smoothing (ES) [19], Hybrid Methods (HM) [20–22], and Autoregressive Integrated Moving Average (ARIMA) [23]. They have been used to predict the dependent variable in a time series [15–23]. Among these techniques, unsupervised neural networks of the type Self-Organizing Maps model has mostly outperformed others in precision and accuracy [14].

Self-Organizing Maps (SOM) or Kohonen Map is a method for the analysis of multivariate data used for pattern recognition and classification, which may be taken as a non-linear generalization of principal component analysis [24]. The SOM algorithm consists of input nodes and a grid of computational connected nodes (neurons), which compete among themselves for activation as the one that most closely resembles the input vector. If the input data exhibit some similarity across the input classes, the neurons will organize themselves, showing similarity patterns in a grid [13,25].

SOM has already been used successfully for data mining in several areas of knowledge [24,26–30], like food science [26,28,29], fuels [27], monitoring chemical reactions [24,30], and other applications [25,31,32]. Recently, SOM was used to verify the spatial relationship of the COVID-19 spread in countries and states in Mexico [31]. Most published papers have the main theme of the modelling or prediction of the spread of COVID-19 [2,9,33–36]. In our literature searches, we did not evidence reports that simultaneously consider the historical data on the number of cases/deaths from COVID-19 with possible external factors that affect the spread of the virus through a spatial analysis by pattern recognition.

In a previous study, we demonstrated that the spread of COVID-19 varies according to Brazilian regions, states, and cities. However, it was not possible to allege the reason for this behavior. In this study, 14 possible factors that can affect the spread of COVID-19 were analyzed jointly by SOM. This analysis will verify which variables may be essential and will point out possible variables that had the most significant effect on each Brazilian state.

2. Theoretical Foundations

The Kohonen algorithm was proposed by Teuvo Kohonen in 1982 [14]. In SOM, there is no given output target, the objective of the algorithm is to find a set of neurons to represent the cluster, but with topological restrictions [31]. The learning process begins with the random initialization of the synaptic weights vector of each neuron. In sequence, three key steps are developed for the formation of the feature map: Competition, cooperation, and synaptic adaptation [24].

The following is a brief description of the Kohonen algorithm, as described previously by Haykin [14]. The function is chosen to represent the topological neighborhood in the following equation.

$$h_{j,i} = \exp(-d_{j,i}^2/2\sigma^2)$$

where σ is the effective radius of the topological neighborhood, and $d_{j,i}$ is the lateral distance between the winning neuron i and the excited neuron j, defined through Euclidean distance. Over the training epochs, there is a reduction in the size of the neighborhood due to an exponential decay, described by the equation.

$$\sigma(n) = \sigma_0 \exp(-n/\tau_1) \quad n = 0, 1, 2, \ldots$$

where σ_0 is the effective radius in the initialization of the algorithm, τ_1 is the time constant, with $\tau_1 = 1000/\log \sigma_0$ being recommended, and n is the number of training epochs.

During the adaptive process, the synaptic weight vector ($\mathbf{w}_j$) of the j neuron in the grid must be modified concerning the input vector $\mathbf{x}$. The modification process is a modification of the Hebb learning postulate, described by the equation.

$$\mathbf{w}_j(n+1) = \mathbf{w}_j(n) + (\eta)h_{j,i(x)}(\mathbf{x} - \mathbf{w}_{j(n)})$$

where $\eta(n)$ is the learning rate, which is variable and decreases during the training epochs, n. The learning rate decrease may be modelled by an exponential decay, as described in the equation. In this equation, η_0 is the initial learning rate, and τ_2 is another time constant; the recommended values are, respectively, 0.1 and 1000:

$$\eta(n) = \eta_0 \exp(-n/\tau_2)$$

3. Methodology

3.1. Dataset

The dataset used in the study by neural networks was obtained from websites of Brazilian government agencies or institutions, available for download. Before the SOM analysis, the variables that would constitute the study were selected. All variables related to socioeconomic, health, and safety factors that could explain the dissemination of COVID-19 in Brazil were included in our research. They were made available and updated daily by institutional sites of the Brazilian federal government.

Initially, data for all variables were converted and expressed as rates for each 100,000 inhabitants. For the conversion, we used data from the Brazilian population estimated in 2019 by the Instituto Brasileiro de Geografia e Estatística – IBGE (Brazilian Institute of Geography and Statistics); the public agency responsible for conducting censuses and organizing information related to the country's geosciences and social, demographic, and economic statistics [37]; available in https://www.ibge.gov.br/.

The numbers of cases and accumulated deaths by COVID-19 were analyzed for 16 epidemiological weeks. According to the international convention, each week starts on Sunday and ends on Saturday. The information represents the numbers recorded from 26 February to 13 June, 2020 (110 days), a period that corresponds from the 9th to the 24th epidemiological week of the year, first COVID-19 case record in Brazil. The data were obtained from the website of the Ministério da Saúde—MS (Ministry of Health) of Brazil, the government sector responsible for the administration and maintenance of public health in the country, updated daily with information about the COVID-19 pandemic in the country [38]; available in https://covid.saude.gov.br/.

The Federal Government of Brazil transfers financial resources, supplies, and equipment for structuring health services in the country to combat or treat patients affected by COVID-19. The MS frequently updates a panel of inputs considered essential, distributed to each Brazilian state: Influenza vaccination—H1N1 and H3N2 (distributed and applied), drugs (chloroquine and oseltamivir), COVID-19 tests (rapid and reverse-transcriptase polymerase chain reaction—RT-PCR), hand sanitizer per liter, and Personal Protective Equipment—PPE (surgical masks, N95 mask, gowns, gloves, glasses, face shield, caps, and sneakers) [39]. These data were obtained on June 13, 2020, at https://covid-insumos.saude.gov.br/paineis/insumos/painel.php.

The destination of Federal funds transferred to each federative unit (Brazilian states) is monitored and presented on the Federal Government website [40], available in https://www.tesourotransparente.gov.br/visualizacao/painel-de-monitoramentos-dos-gastos-com-covid-19. The data used in this study represent the sum of all transfers made until 13 June 2020. For better visualization, the values were converted from the real (R$) to the US dollar (US$) by the quotation of R$ 5.05 equals to US$ 1.00, referring to 12 June 2020, provided by the Banco Central do Brasil—BCB (Central Bank of Brazil) [41], available in https://www.bcb.gov.br/.

Health data from public and private institutions, such as the number of physicians, nurses, ventilators, and Intensive Care Unit (ICU) beds for COVID-19 in each state, were obtained from the IBGE [42]; available in https://mapasinterativos.ibge.gov.br/covid/saude/.

Finally, the data referring to the Human Development Index (HDI) of each state for the year 2015 (last census registered in the country) were obtained from the Atlas do Desenvolvimento Humano do Brasil—ADHB (Human Development Atlas of Brazil), a public institution that provides information about human development in Brazil [43]; available in http://www.atlasbrasil.org.br/2013/pt/download/base/.

3.2. Data Analysis by Artificial Neural Network

The Kohonen Map routine developed was carried out in Matlab software (MathWorks, Natick, MA, USA) according to the algorithm previously described in Haykin [14] and Cremasco et al. [26]. The datasets were evaluated using three different approaches. In the first step, two SOM analyses were conducted to verify the distribution of the numbers of cases and deaths from COVID-19 in Brazilian regions and states. In the second step, the distribution of 14 variables for the Brazilian states was verified: ICU beds, ventilators, physicians, nurses, PPE, hand sanitizer, rapid test, PCR test, vaccines distributed, vaccines applied, chloroquine tablets, oseltamivir capsules, HDI, and federal funds distribution.

The SOM setup was a hexagonal topology of 8 × 8 and 4 × 4 for 27 Brazilian states and five regions, respectively, for the number of cases and deaths from COVID-19 (**first step**); 8 × 8 for 27 Brazilian states with 14 variables (**second step**) with 7000 training epochs to ensure convergence of the average quantization error. The initial neighborhood relationship was 3.5, decreasing to 0.07, with an initial learning rate of 0.1, decaying exponentially with the training epochs to 9.11×10^{-5}. It was used a computer Intel® Core™ i7-4790 CPU© 3.60 GHz, 32 GB RAM, and 250 GB HDD.

In order to obtain a better representation, the values collected after the SOM analysis were transposed through the color scale to the Brazilian cartographic map for each variable. This procedure was adopted to facilitate the interpretation of unfamiliar people with the Kohonen map. The original SOM output weight maps for the 14 variables generated are displayed in the Supplementary Material in Figures S1–S14.

3.3. Spearman's Correlation Test

The Spearman's rank correlation coefficient is adopted to determine the correlation between variables. It analyzes how well the association between two variables can be defined using a monotonic function. The correlation matrix was performed using the package "corrplot" in the Software R Core Team (Vienna, Austria) [44].

4. Tests and Results

Figure 1 shows the number of cases and deaths accumulated by Brazilian states and regions per 100,000 inhabitants. All states belonging to the South (S) and Central-West (CW) regions of the country had the lowest rates of cases and deaths by COVID-19 recorded, an average of 180 cases and 4 deaths per 100,000 inhabitants. Most of the Brazilian states with the highest rates of cases and deaths belong to the North (N) region, an average of 954 cases and 43 deaths per 100,000 inhabitants, mainly represented by Acre (AC), Amapá (AP), Amazonas (AM), Pará (PA), and Roraima (RR).

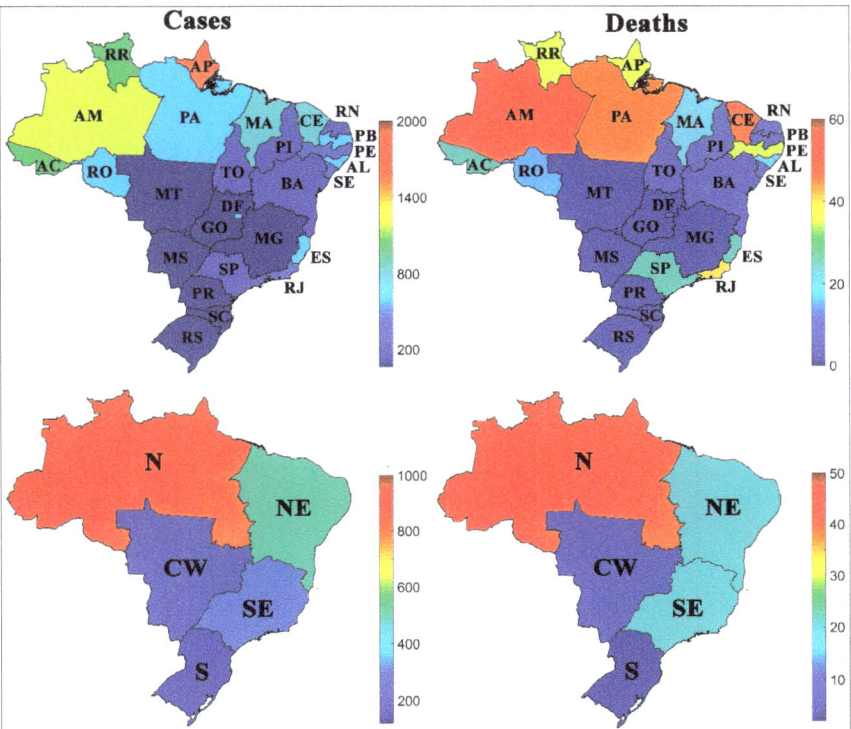

Figure 1. Geographical distribution of cases and deaths by COVID-19 in Brazilian states (above) and regions (below) per 100,000 inhabitants.

Some states in the Brazilian Northeast (NE) and Southeast (SE) also had high rates of cases and deaths when compared to the other states in the South (S) and Central-West (CW) regions. The Northeast (NE) is the second region with the highest rate of cases and deaths, an average of 527 cases and 24 deaths per 100,000 inhabitants, the states in this region that were most aggravated by the disease were Ceará (CE), Maranhão (MA), and Pernambuco (PE). The Southeast (SE) is the third region with the highest rate of cases and deaths, with an average of 338 cases and 23 deaths by COVID-19, with Espírito Santo (ES), Rio de Janeiro (RJ), and São Paulo (SP) being the most representative states in the region.

The neural network demonstrated that the spread of COVID-19 in Brazil has heterogeneous behavior; see Figure 1. It is essential to understand this behavior. The North of the country was more affected by COVID-19 than the South. The Northeast and Southeast differ in case rates but have similar death rates. In this sense, possible factors were evaluated that may explain the reason for this behavior and point out which measures are more relevant in the fight against COVID-19 in each Brazilian state.

After the training phase of the SOM network, we generated the topological map of the 14 variables evaluated together, which represents the distribution of each federative unit in Brazil, according to the winning neuron; see Figure 2. In the topological map, each federative unit is associated with a respective winning neuron, that is, the one that best represents in the analysis. The SOM network classifies the input data as clusters that can be formed by one or more neurons. The definition of clusters is characterized by the presence of empty neurons between the groups. Nearby clusters share some similarity, that is, the greater the Euclidean distance, the greater the difference in behavior.

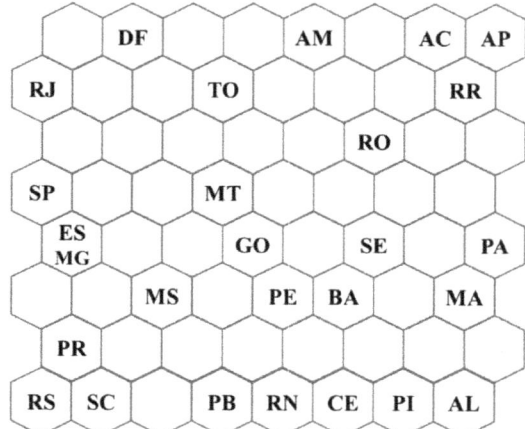

Figure 2. Distribution of Brazilian federative units according to the winning neuron. Where: Acre—AC; Alagoas—AL; Amapá—AP; Amazonas—AM; Bahia—BA; Ceará—CE; Distrito Federal—DF; Espírito Santo—ES; Goiás—GO; Maranhão—MA; Mato Grosso—MT; Mato Grosso do Sul—MS; Minas Gerais—MG; Pará—PA; Paraíba—PB; Paraná—PR; Pernambuco—PE; Piauí—PI; Roraima—RR; Rondônia—RO; Rio de Janeiro—RJ; Rio Grande do Norte—RN; Rio Grande do Sul—RS; Santa Catarina—SC; São Paulo—SP; Sergipe—SE; Tocantins—TO.

We identified the formation of some clusters by evaluating the topological map. Among some of the clusters formed, we highlight the one formed in the lower-left corner of the map in Figure 2, represented by the states of the Southern region of the country, which contain the federative units: Paraná (PR), Rio Grande do Sul (RS), and Santa Catarina (SC). This cluster contains the federal units and the region of the country with the lowest rates of deaths and cases by COVID-19, as shown in Figure 1. Another cluster formed that we can highlight is composed of some states in the North region of the country, represented by the states of Acre (AC), Amapá (AP), and Roraima (RR), presented in the upper-right corner of the map. This cluster represents the region and some of the federative units with the highest rates of deaths and cases due to COVID-19 in the country. This same analysis can be done for the other formed clusters.

To verify the applicability of SOM analysis, we compared the results obtained with another unsupervised method. Thus, we evaluated the ability to group the data obtained using the Hierarchical Cluster Analysis (HCA) method. The results obtained with the HCA were very similar to those obtained with the SOM algorithm. The dataset presents different patterns according to the region in which the Brazilian states are located. In other words, most states in the North and Northeast regions formed a cluster, while most federative units in the Central-West, South, and Southeast formed another cluster. The graphic output generated by the HCA method is shown in Figure S15 of the Supplementary Material.

In general, the topological map of the SOM network made it possible to state that the socioeconomic, health and safety data demonstrate that the spread of COVID-19 in the country varies according to the Brazilian federative units. However, only the topological map does not allow to state which of the 14 variables evaluated may be the main responsible for explaining the spread of COVID-19 in the country. Thus, we used weight maps in the following discussions. In order to obtain a better representation, the values collected from the weight maps were transposed through the color scale to the Brazilian cartographic map for each variable. However, when doing the transposition procedure, we lose the neighborhood relationship. In Figures S1–S14 of the Supplementary Material, the original outputs of the weight maps for each variable in the SOM network are shown.

The 14 variables were evaluated jointly by ANN. However, for better results visualization and discussion, the weight maps were divided into four blocks and grouped according to similarities: (i) Available hospital infrastructure; (ii) inputs and tests available; (iii) drugs available; and (iv) financial resources,

The first set of variables is shown in Figure 3, composed of the rates of ICU beds, ventilators, physicians, and nurses per 100,000 inhabitants. In general, it is observed that the states that belong to the South, Southeast, and Central-West regions of Brazil had higher rates than the North and Northeast. There is evidence that these variables influence the rates of cases and deaths in each Brazilian state, and it can be said that the states with the lowest rates of ICU, respirators, physicians, and nurses, have the highest rates of cases and deaths from COVID-19.

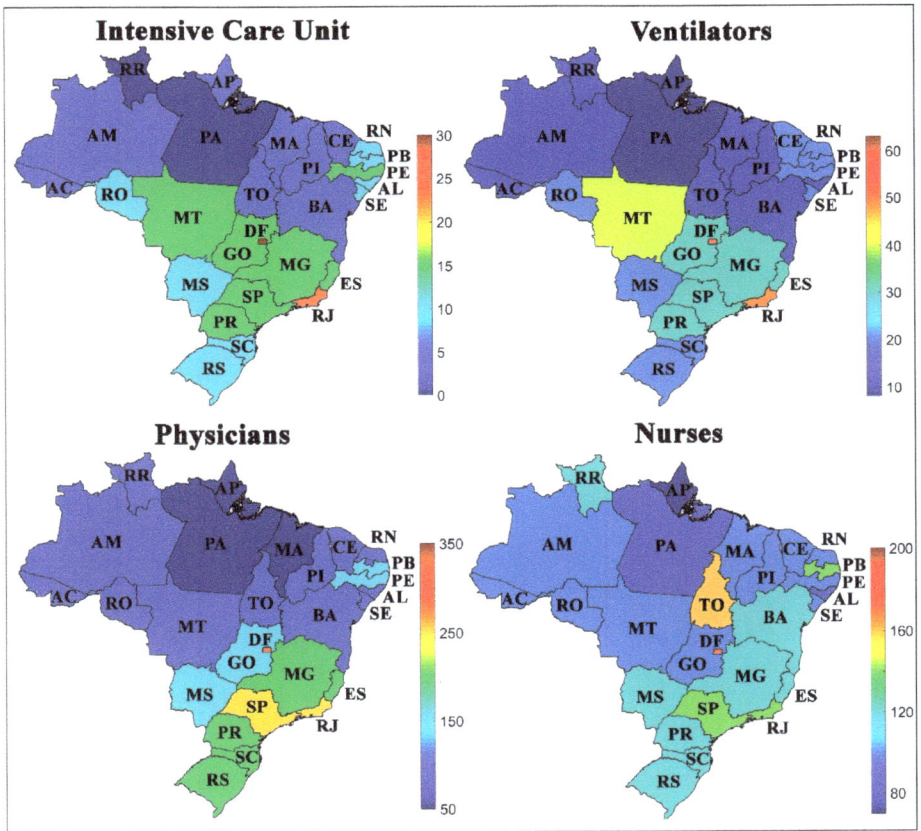

Figure 3. Geographical distribution of Intensive Care Unit (ICU) bed, ventilators, physicians and nurses in Brazilian states per 100,000 inhabitants.

It is also evident that these were not the only relevant factors. The state of Rio de Janeiro (RJ), for example, has high rates of ICU beds, respirators, physicians, and nurses and despite this, it has a higher death rate than other states in the North region, such as Acre (AC), Amapá (AP), and Roraima (RR).

The second set of variables presented in Figure 4 represents the inputs destined to each state by the Federal Government to combat and control the spread of COVID-19, composed by PPE, hand sanitizer, rapid test, and PCR test per 100,000 inhabitants. In general, the PPE and hand sanitizer rates distributed for each state did not have a direct relationship with the rates of cases or deaths by COVID-19 according to the SOM analysis.

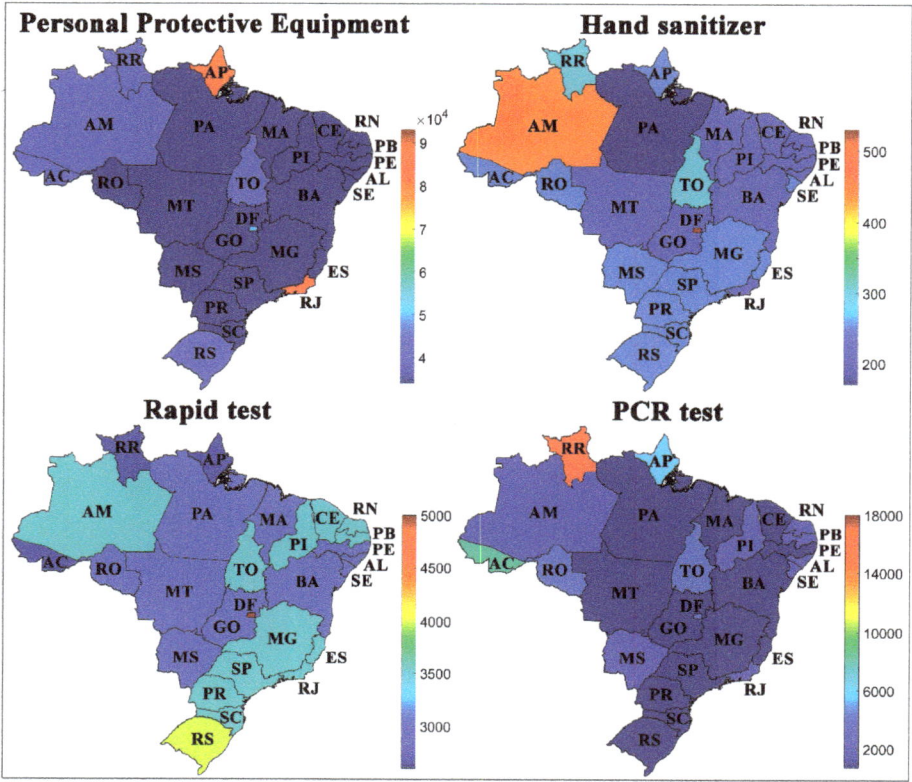

Figure 4. Geographical distribution of Personal Protective Equipment (PPE), hand sanitizer, rapid tests, and PCR tests available to Brazilian states per 100,000 inhabitants.

The states of Amapá (AP) and Rio de Janeiro (RJ), for example, had the highest rates of PPE distributed, and Amazonas (AM) had the highest rates of liters of hand sanitizer distributed per 100,000 inhabitants; however, these three states present higher rates of cases and deaths when compared to other Brazilian states.

It is important to note that the data refer to the distributed quantity of inputs, and it is not possible to estimate which portion was used by hospitals or the population, or even say if they were used correctly. The cultural factor also interferes in these variables, mainly concerning the education and awareness of the local population about the use of these inputs [45].

The disease tests in the country have been carried out homogeneously, as shown in Figure 4. This homogeneity is considered an important aspect and demonstrates that differences do not influence the data collected regarding the number of cases in the form of confirmation of the disease, which could question the reliability of the data. The states that had the highest test rates available were the Distrito Federal (DF), Rio Grande do Sul (RS), and Roraima (RR), which belong to the Central-West, South, and North regions, respectively, i.e., the most and least affected regions by COVID-19 in the country.

Rapid tests are cheaper, less reliable, and can result in false positives or negatives, while the PCR test is reliable but expensive and time-consuming [46]. It is necessary to adopt a balance between rapid tests and PCR; for example, if PCR test indices are higher, it will not be possible to follow the spread in a short period, while rapid tests, when misused, can generate mistaken information.

Previous measures as vaccines and drugs against diseases with similar symptoms, such as influenza H1N1 and H3N2, can facilitate the diagnosis of COVID-19, since they are relevant information during the patient's anamnesis. These procedures allow faster and more efficient identification of the disease, which makes the adopted treatments more assertive and precocious [47]. Another measure that focuses on significant discussions in the scientific community is the use of drugs against the coronavirus [48]. Among several drugs, the Brazilian Federal Government has invested and passed on chloroquine tablets to the states.

The third set of variables in Figure 5 consists of influenza vaccines distributed and applied, and drugs distributed by states per 100,000 inhabitants. The states of the North region, such as Amazonas (AM), Roraima (RR), Pará (PA), and Acre (AC), had a more significant disparity than the other states in the rates of vaccines applied and distributed. At first, this behavior could be related to health factors, shown in Figure 3. However, this disparity would also be observed in the Northeast region. Other intrinsic factors may include geographic and logistical factors that make distribution and access to the population a challenge to receive the vaccine.

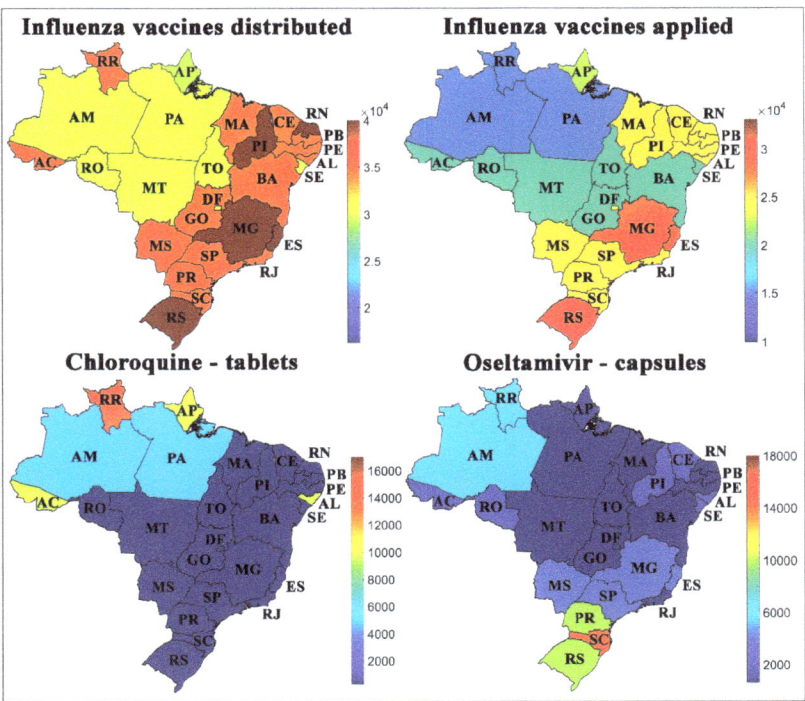

Figure 5. Geographical distribution of influenza vaccines distributed, influenza vaccines applied, chloroquine tablets, and oseltamivir capsules available in Brazilian states per 100,000 inhabitants.

As far as we know, there is no drug with proven efficiency against SARS-CoV-2; some drugs have been evaluated to combat or alleviate the disease's symptoms [48]. Recent studies demonstrate that dexamethasone welcomes the preliminary treatment of critically ill patients with COVID-19 [49]. Recently, the Food and Drug Administration (FDA) revoked emergency use authorization for chloroquine and hydroxychloroquine in patients with COVID-19 [50].

Figure 5 shows the chloroquine rates distributed by the Federal Government per 100,000 inhabitants. Chloroquine tablets were more widely distributed in the states of the North region, which has higher rates of deaths and cases of COVID-19 in Brazil. The possibility of greater distribution of chloroquine in these states may have occurred as an attempt to treat the disease symptoms when there were no restrictions on its use.

The oseltamivir rates distributed by the Federal Government per 100,000 inhabitants is shown in Figure 5. This drug is commonly used to treat symptoms caused by the influenza virus and is administered when there is still no confirmed diagnosis of COVID-19 [51]. Oseltamivir was more widely distributed in the Southern and Northern states of Brazil; however, it is not possible to establish a direct relationship with the rates of cases and deaths by COVID-19 using SOM analysis.

The last set of variables evaluated comprises the HDI and the distribution of federal funds destined to each state. According to Figure 6, the destination of Federal funds was more significant for some states in the North, the region which has the highest rates of cases and deaths due to COVID-19. More resources destined for this region can be guided by the scenario of cases and deaths registered.

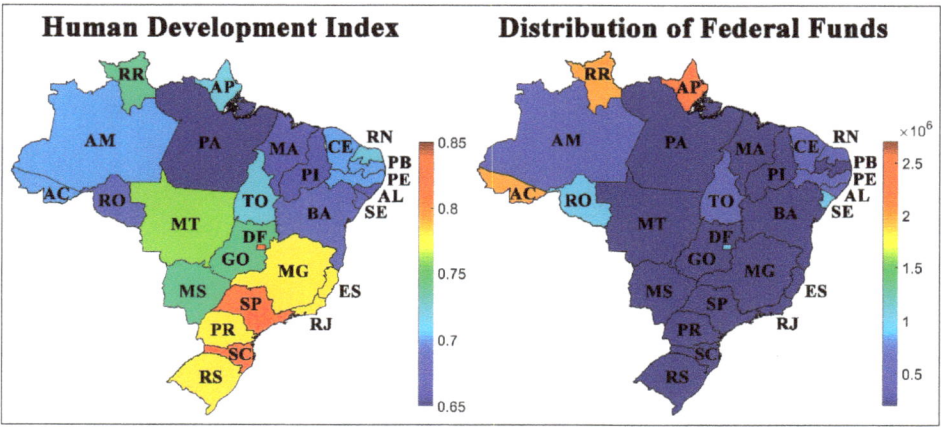

Figure 6. Geographical distribution by Index Development Index (HDI) and Federal funds destined to combat COVID-19 in Brazilian states per 100,000 inhabitants.

The highest HDI values are in the Central-West, South, and Southeast regions, with the Federal District (DF), Santa Catarina (SC), and São Paulo (SP) being the highest values in the country. It is also worth mentioning that the most affected states by COVID-19 have some of the lowest HDIs in the country, showing problems that some of these states have in fundamental areas of the population service.

Figure 7 shows the Spearman's correlation test adopted to determine the correlation among variables. The test demonstrated that the influenza vaccine applied, ICU, ventilators, physicians, nurses, and HDI were the most correlated significant variables, all positive correlations, while chloroquine had a negative correlation with all these variables. The HDI is directly related to essential aspects of the population, such as family income, education level, health, among other factors; therefore, the correlation with the HDI was already expected, since it takes into account important aspects of health for its determination. Other variables evaluated showed minor correlations, while PPE did not correlate with any other variable.

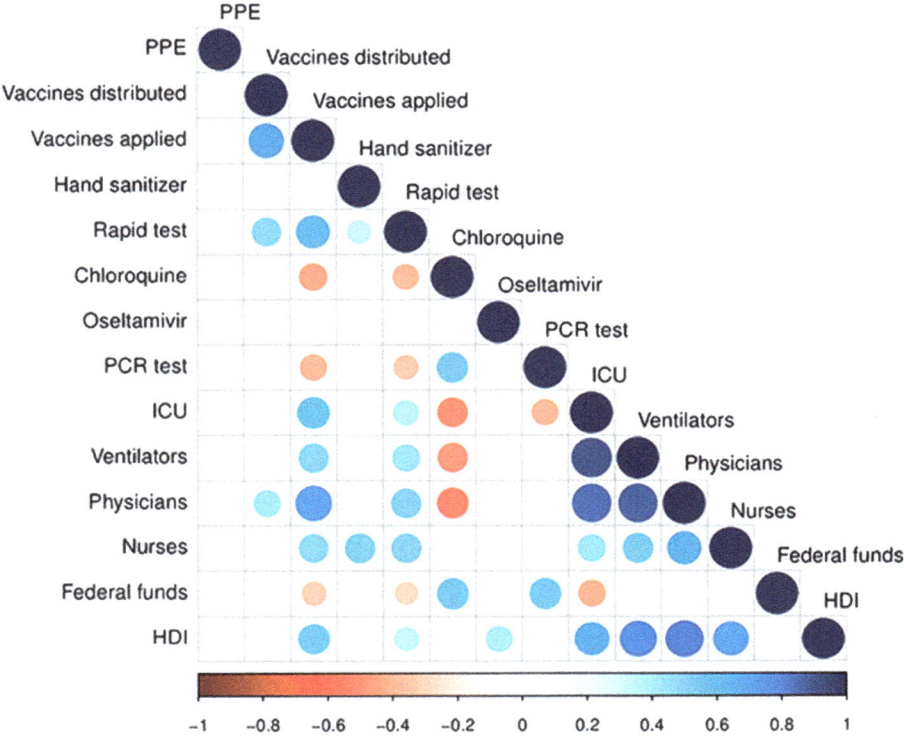

Figure 7. Spearman correlation coefficients for the 14 evaluated variables. Correlations with p-value > 0.05 are considered insignificant.

5. Discussion

Considering the importance of understanding the spread of the virus, many studies have been presented in recent months related to different aspects of the pandemic, with the application of computational intelligence tools to model and predict the spread of the disease [34].

In our study, we gave the data a differentiated approach from the reported works. It is not common to find simultaneous studies with historical data on the number of COVID-19 cases, related to external factors, that affect the spread of the virus through spatial analysis [31]. For this, we used unsupervised pattern recognition to analyze some variables, among many others, that may be related to the disease spread.

Brazil is one of the most affected countries by the pandemic and by the tremendous socioeconomic, territorial, climatic differences, among the country's federative units. We understand that it may be interesting to try to establish spread patterns of the virus in the country. Thus, once the relationship of these factors with the spread and lethality of the disease has been identified, we hope that our study can assist in the analysis of the data that have been generated by institutions and, consequently, assist in directing decision-making on practical combat actions.

It is important to note that our analysis does not aim to point out or compare which were the best actions adopted to contain the spread of COVID-19, so we approached each variable according to the significance indicated by the SOM analysis.

Based on SOM's clustering skills, we were able to spatially group similar federative units in terms of the number of cases and deaths by COVID-19 with data on the distribution of financial resources, equipment, health professionals and HDI, represented by a color scale. Thus, SOM's ability to cluster, made it possible to cluster together with the federal units that are behaving similarly and, therefore, can benefit from similar strategies to deal with the virus spread.

The SOM analysis allowed us to raise some hypotheses about the spread of the virus in Brazil. In general, the analysis indicated that the spread of the disease has a direct relationship with quite heterogeneous socioeconomic, health, and safety variations in the national territory; see topological map in Figure 2.

In Figure 2, we can see that the spread of the disease in Brazilian states has been differentiated and regionalized. Interestingly, the network separated the most and least regions affected by COVID-19. We found that there was a separation pattern, in which all the Southern federative units are located at the bottom left of the map (PR, RS, and SC), while the Southeast states (SP, RJ, MG, and ES) and the Central-West (MS, MT, DF, and GO) are in the upper left corner of the map. In the North and Northeast regions, the federative units were classified on the right side of the map.

For better visualization, we invite readers to check the original output weight maps of the variables in the Supplementary Material. Weight maps represent the overlap of the topological map (Figure 2) and allow us to evaluate the behavior of each variable for the segmentation of the federative units. Analyzing the weight maps for the 14 variables extracted from the SOM network, it was possible to show which were the main responsible for differentiating the states, regarding the number of cases and deaths by COVID-19 in Brazil by socioeconomic, health, and safety data.

According to the 14 weight maps, the HDI was one of the essential variables for the distribution obtained (Figure 6 and Figure S13). The analysis indicated that the federal units with the lowest HDI were considerably more affected by the pandemic and that they had greater difficulty in combating the spread of the virus. Meanwhile, the best-prepared Brazilian federations with higher HDI values were more capable of deal with the pandemic.

Possibly, the HDI was the main measure responsible for the separation due to its high correlation with the other variables. It is noteworthy that this index relates to health (life expectancy), education (adult literacy index and levels of education), and income (GDP—gross domestic product—per capita). Thus, it is possible to observe the correlation of the HDI in Figure 7, with other variables, such as ICU (Figure S1), ventilators (Figure S2), doctors (Figure S3), and nurses (Figure S4).

Another important variable that allowed us to assess the behavior of the spread of COVID-19 in Brazil was the influenza vaccine rates of doses distributed and applied, highly correlated according to the Spearman correlation test (Figure 7). According to Figure 6, Figures S9 and S10, we show that the federative units with the highest rates of vaccines applied had lower rates of cases and deaths from COVID-19, as pointed out by the SOM analysis. Although this procedure is not effective against SARS-CoV-2, this measure may have facilitated clinical diagnosis and made the treatment of affected patients by COVID-19 faster and more accurate, and may have reflected in the number of cases and deaths in these regions and federative units.

Other measures adopted in the country, such as the use of drugs as chloroquine and oseltamivir, did not allow to evaluate the spread of COVID-19, as shown in Figure 5 and the weight maps of the variables in Figures S11 and S12. The SOM analysis indicated that the federative units in the North and Northeast regions had higher rates of chloroquine tablets distribution but more cases and deaths from the disease were registered. On the other hand, oseltamivir capsules had higher distribution rates in the Southern and Northern states, representing the regions more and less affected by the disease, which means that this variable, the spread of COVID-19 was similar.

We evidence that PPE (Figure S5) and hand sanitizer (Figure S6) rates distributed for each state did not have a direct relationship with the rates of cases or deaths by COVID-19 when considering the SOM analysis (Figure 4). It is known that these measures directly influence the control of the COVID-19 dissemination [45]; in this sense, we show that the SOM analysis allowed us to verify that although these items have been distributed to federative units, the population has not followed the measures adopted or made use of these items properly. Figure 7 reinforces this hypothesis since the

PPE did not correlate with any other variable. Thereby, government agencies must further encourage the use of available items.

Among the other less expressive variables evaluated, we show that the rapid test (Figure S8), PCR test (Figure S9), and distribution of Federal funds (Figure S14) did not present an obvious behavior that would allow explaining the spread of COVID-19 using the numbers of cases and deaths in the country, according to the SOM analysis indicated.

6. Conclusions

Unsupervised Artificial Neural Networks of the Self-Organizing Map type have demonstrated that the spread of the coronavirus has heterogeneous behavior and varies among Brazilian regions and states. According to the analysis, among the 14 variables evaluated, the factors responsible for the highest relationship with the numbers of cases and deaths by COVID-19 in Brazilian states were: Rates of influenza vaccine applied, ICU beds, ventilators, physicians, nurses, and HDI, positively correlated according to the Spearman's correlation test. In general, the lowest rates of cases and deaths by COVID-19 were recorded in the Brazilian states with the highest rates of influenza vaccine applied, ICU beds, respirators, physicians, and nurses, per 100,000 inhabitants, which consequently has some of the highest HDI in the country.

As a future work, we intend to integrate the SOM algorithm to analyze the spatial and temporal aspects of the COVID-19 spread in a unified way to obtain a complete view and solution to the problem. In addition, to analyze the possibility of applying SOM in other diseases that have affected Brazil, caused by dengue virus, Chikungunya virus, Zika virus, and yellow fever virus.

Supplementary Materials: The following are available online at http://www.mdpi.com/1660-4601/17/23/8921/s1, Figure S1: Weight maps overlaid by topological maps for variable Intensive Care Unit (ICU) by Brazilian federative unit. Figure S2: Weight maps overlaid by topological maps for variable Ventilators by Brazilian federative unit. Figure S3: Weight maps overlaid by topological maps for variable Physicians by Brazilian federative unit. Figure S4: Weight maps overlaid by topological maps for variable Nurses by Brazilian federative unit. Figure S5: Weight maps overlaid by topological maps for variable Personal Protective Equipment by Brazilian federative unit. Figure S6: Weight maps overlaid by topological maps for variable Hand sanitizer by Brazilian federative unit. Figure S7: Weight maps overlaid by topological maps for variable Rapid test by Brazilian federative unit. Figure S8: Weight maps overlaid by topological maps for variable PCR test by Brazilian federative unit. Figure S9: Weight maps overlaid by topological maps for variable Influenza vaccines distributed by Brazilian federative unit. Figure S10: Weight maps overlaid by topological maps for variable Influenza vaccines applied by Brazilian federative unit. Figure S11: Weight maps overlaid by topological maps for variable Chloroquine tablets by Brazilian federative unit. Figure S12: Weight maps overlaid by topological maps for variable Oseltamivir capsules by Brazilian federative unit. Figure S13: Weight maps overlaid by topological maps for variable Human Development Index (HDI) by Brazilian federative unit. Figure S14: Weight maps overlaid by topological maps for variable Distribution of Federal funds by Brazilian federative unit. Figure S15: Dendrogram of an HCA for Brazilian Federative Units.

Author Contributions: D.G.: Conceptualization, formal analysis, investigation, methodology, software, validation, visualization, writing—review and editing. L.E.: Conceptualization, formal analysis, investigation, methodology, software, validation, visualization, writing—review and editing. H.C.: Conceptualization, formal analysis, investigation, methodology, software, validation, visualization, writing—review and editing. C.A.C.-J.: Methodology, writing—review and editing, supervision, project administration, funding acquisition. All authors have read and agreed to the published version of the manuscript.

Funding: The authors are thankful for the financial support provided by the Fundação Carlos Chagas Filho de Amparo à Pesquisa do Estado do Rio de Janeiro (FAPERJ), D.G.: [grant number E-26/200.062/2020, E-26/010.000.984/2019, and E-26/010.000148/2020]. http://www.faperj.br/. The funders had no role in study design, data collection and analysis, decision to publish, or preparation of the manuscript.

Conflicts of Interest: The authors have declared that no competing interests exist.

References

1. Wells:, C.R.; Sah, P.; Moghadas, S.M.; Pandey, A.; Shoukat, A.; Wang, Y.; Wang, Z.; Meyers, L.A.; Singer, B.H.; Galvani, A.P. Impact of international travel and border control measures on the global spread of the novel 2019 coronavirus outbreak. *Proc. Natl. Acad. Sci. USA* **2020**, *117*, 7504–7509. [CrossRef] [PubMed]

2. Gatto, M.; Bertuzzo, E.; Mari, L.; Miccoli, S.; Carraro, L.; Casagrandi, R.; Rinaldo, A. Spread and dynamics of the COVID-19 epidemic in Italy: Effects of emergency containment measures. *Proc. Natl. Acad. Sci. USA* **2020**, *117*, 10484–10491. [CrossRef] [PubMed]
3. WHO. WHO Coronavirus Disease (COVID-19) Dashboard. Available online: https://covid19.who.int/ (accessed on 22 June 2020).
4. Sanders, J.M.; Monogue, M.L.; Jodlowski, T.Z.; Cutrell, J.B. Pharmacologic Treatments for Coronavirus Disease 2019 (COVID-19): A Review. *JAMA J. Am. Med. Assoc.* **2020**, *323*, 1824–1836. [CrossRef] [PubMed]
5. AminJafari, A.; Ghasemi, S. The possible of immunotherapy for COVID-19: A systematic review. *Int. Immunopharmacol.* **2020**, *83*. [CrossRef] [PubMed]
6. Zhang, R.; Li, Y.; Zhang, A.L.; Wang, Y.; Molina, M.J. Identifying airborne transmission as the dominant route for the spread of COVID-19. *Proc. Natl. Acad. Sci. USA* **2020**, *117*, 14857–14863. [CrossRef]
7. Xu, H.; Yan, C.; Fu, Q.; Xiao, K.; Yu, Y.; Han, D.; Wang, W.; Cheng, J. Possible environmental effects on the spread of COVID-19 in China. *Sci. Total Environ.* **2020**, *731*. [CrossRef]
8. Rosario, D.K.A.; Mutz, Y.S.; Bernardes, P.C.; Conte-Junior, C.A. Relationship between COVID-19 and weather: Case study in a tropical country. *Int. J. Hyg. Environ. Health* **2020**, 113587. [CrossRef]
9. Lin, S.; Fu, Y.; Jia, X.; Ding, S.; Wu, Y.; Huang, Z. Discovering Correlations between the COVID-19 Epidemic Spread and Climate. *Int. J. Environ. Res. Public Health* **2020**, *17*, 7958. [CrossRef]
10. Al-Quteimat, O.M.; Amer, A.M. The Impact of the COVID-19 Pandemic on Cancer Patients. *Am. J. Clin. Oncol.* **2020**, *43*, 452–455. [CrossRef]
11. Schofield, J.; Leelarathna, L.; Thabit, H. COVID-19: Impact of and on Diabetes. *Diabetes Ther.* **2020**, *11*, 1429–1435. [CrossRef]
12. Butt, C.; Gill, J.; Chun, D.; Babu, B.A. Deep learning system to screen coronavirus disease 2019 pneumonia. *Appl. Intell.* **2020**, 1–7. [CrossRef]
13. De Carvalho Rocha, W.F.; Do Prado, C.B.; Blonder, N. Comparison of chemometric problems in food analysis using non-linear methods. *Molecules* **2020**, *25*, 3025. [CrossRef] [PubMed]
14. Haykin, S. *Neural Networks: A Comprehensive Foundation*; Prentice Hall: New York, NY, USA, 2001; ISBN 978-0-02-352761-6.
15. Jiang, C.; Jiang, M.; Xu, Q.; Huang, X. Expectile regression neural network model with applications. *Neurocomputing* **2017**, *247*, 73–86. [CrossRef]
16. Castañeda-Miranda, A.; Castaño, V.M. Smart frost control in greenhouses by neural networks models. *Comput. Electron. Agric.* **2017**, *137*, 102–114. [CrossRef]
17. Arora, S.; Taylor, J.W. Rule-based autoregressive moving average models for forecasting load on special days: A case study for France. *Eur. J. Oper. Res.* **2018**, *266*, 259–268. [CrossRef]
18. Hassan, M.M.; Huda, S.; Yearwood, J.; Jelinek, H.F.; Almogren, A. Multistage fusion approaches based on a generative model and multivariate exponentially weighted moving average for diagnosis of cardiovascular autonomic nerve dysfunction. *Inf. Fusion* **2018**, *41*, 105–118. [CrossRef]
19. Barrow, D.; Kourentzes, N.; Sandberg, R.; Niklewski, J. Automatic robust estimation for exponential smoothing: Perspectives from statistics and machine learning. *Expert Syst. Appl.* **2020**, *160*, 113637. [CrossRef]
20. Amo Baffour, A.; Feng, J.; Taylor, E.K. A hybrid artificial neural network-GJR modeling approach to forecasting currency exchange rate volatility. *Neurocomputing* **2019**, *365*, 285–301. [CrossRef]
21. Castañeda-Miranda, A.; Castaño-Meneses, V.M. Smart frost measurement for anti-disaster intelligent control in greenhouses via embedding IoT and hybrid AI methods. *Meas. J. Int. Meas. Confed.* **2020**, *164*. [CrossRef]
22. Pradeepkumar, D.; Ravi, V. Soft computing hybrids for FOREX rate prediction: A comprehensive review. *Comput. Oper. Res.* **2018**, *99*, 262–284. [CrossRef]
23. Castañeda-Miranda, A.; Castaño-Meneses, V.M. Internet of things for smart farming and frost intelligent control in greenhouses. *Comput. Electron. Agric.* **2020**, *176*, 105614. [CrossRef]
24. Galvan, D.; Cremasco, H.; Gomes Mantovani, A.C.; Bona, E.; Killner, M.; Borsato, D. Kinetic study of the transesterification reaction by artificial neural networks and parametric particle swarm optimization. *Fuel* **2020**, *267*, 1–9. [CrossRef]
25. Clark, S.; Sisson, S.A.; Sharma, A. Tools for enhancing the application of self-organizing maps in water resources research and engineering. *Adv. Water Resour.* **2020**, *143*, 103676. [CrossRef]

26. Cremasco, H.; Borsato, D.; Angilelli, K.G.; Galão, O.F.; Bona, E.; Valle, M.E. Application of self-organising maps towards segmentation of soybean samples by determination of inorganic compounds content. *J. Sci. Food Agric.* **2016**, *96*, 306–310. [CrossRef]
27. Kimura, M.; Savada, F.Y.; Tashima, D.L.M.; Romagnoli, É.S.; Chendynski, L.T.; Silva, L.R.C.; Borsato, D. Application of the self-organizing map in the classification of natural antioxidants in commercial biodiesel. *Biofuels* **2018**, 1–6. [CrossRef]
28. Cremasco, H.; Galvan, D.; Angilelli, K.G.; Borsato, D.; de Oliveira, A.G. Influence of film coefficient during multicomponent diffusion–KCL/NaCL in biosolid for static and agitated system using 3D computational simulation. *Food Sci. Technol.* **2019**, *39*, 173–181. [CrossRef]
29. Silva, L.R.C.; Angilelli, K.G.; Cremasco, H.; Romagnoli, É.S.; Galão, O.F.; Borsato, D.; Moraes, L.A.C.; Mandarino, J.M.G. Application of self-organising maps towards segmentation of soybean samples by determination of amino acids concentration. *Plant Physiol. Biochem.* **2016**, *106*, 264–268. [CrossRef]
30. Sanchez, J.L.; Pereira, S.B.G.; Tanamati, A.; Tanamati, A.A.C.; Bona, E. Monitoring industrial hydrogenation of soybean oil using self-organizing maps. *Emir. J. Food Agric.* **2019**, *31*, 779–787. [CrossRef]
31. Melin, P.; Monica, J.C.; Sanchez, D.; Castillo, O. Analysis of Spatial Spread Relationships of Coronavirus (COVID-19) Pandemic in the World using Self Organizing Maps. *Chaos Solitons Fractals* **2020**, *138*, 109917. [CrossRef]
32. Kebonye, N.M.; Eze, P.N.; Kingsley, J.; Gholizadeh, A.; Dajčl, J.; Drábek, O.; Němeček, K.; Borůvka, L. A combined self-organizing map artificial neural networks and conditional Gaussian simulation technique for mapping potentially toxic element hotspots in polluted mining soils. *J. Geochem. Explor.* **2020**, 106680. [CrossRef]
33. Moghadas, S.M.; Shoukat, A.; Fitzpatrick, M.C.; Wells, C.R.; Sah, P.; Pandey, A.; Sachs, J.D.; Wang, Z.; Meyers, L.A.; Singer, B.H.; et al. Projecting hospital utilization during the COVID-19 outbreaks in the United States. *Proc. Natl. Acad. Sci. USA* **2020**, *117*, 9122–9126. [CrossRef] [PubMed]
34. Haghshenas, S.S.; Pirouz, B.; Haghshenas, S.S.; Pirouz, B.; Piro, P.; Na, K.S.; Cho, S.E.; Geem, Z.W. Prioritizing and analyzing the role of climate and urban parameters in the confirmed cases of COVID-19 based on artificial intelligence applications. *Int. J. Environ. Res. Public Health* **2020**, *17*, 3730. [CrossRef]
35. Al-Anzi, B.S.; Alenizi, M.; Al Dallal, J.; Abookleesh, F.L.; Ullah, A. An overview of the world current and future assessment of novel COVID-19 trajectory, impact, and potential preventive strategies at healthcare settings. *Int. J. Environ. Res. Public Health* **2020**, *17*, 7016. [CrossRef] [PubMed]
36. Eltoukhy, A.E.E.; Shaban, I.A.; Chan, F.T.S.; Abdel-Aal, M.A.M. Data analytics for predicting covid-19 cases in top affected countries: Observations and recommendations. *Int. J. Environ. Res. Public Health* **2020**, *17*, 7080. [CrossRef] [PubMed]
37. IBGE. Estimated Brazilian Population for 2019. Available online: https://covid.saude.gov.br/ (accessed on 13 June 2020).
38. MS Coronavirus Pandemic Data in Brazil. Available online: https://covid.saude.gov.br/ (accessed on 13 June 2020).
39. Federal Government Federal Government of Brazil Transfers Financial Resources. Available online: https://covid-insumos.saude.gov.br/paineis/insumos/painel.php (accessed on 13 June 2020).
40. Federal Government Covid-19 Spending Monitoring Panel. Available online: https://www.tesourotransparente.gov.br/visualizacao/painel-de-monitoramentos-dos-gastos-com-covid-19 (accessed on 13 June 2020).
41. BCB Dollar Exchange Rate. Available online: https://www.bcb.gov.br/ (accessed on 13 June 2020).
42. IBGE. Interactive Health Maps in Brazil. Available online: https://mapasinterativos.ibge.gov.br/covid/saude/ (accessed on 13 June 2020).
43. ADHB. Brazilian Human Development Database. Available online: http://www.atlasbrasil.org.br/2013/pt/download/base/ (accessed on 13 June 2020).
44. Taiyun, W.; Simko, V. *R Package "Corrplot": Visualization of a Correlation Matrix*; CRAN, Germany; R Core Team: Vienna, Austria, 2017.
45. Ranney, M.L.; Griffeth, V.; Jha, A.K. Critical Supply Shortages—The Need for Ventilators and Personal Protective Equipment during the Covid-19 Pandemic. *N. Engl. J. Med.* **2020**, *382*, e41. [CrossRef] [PubMed]

46. Carter, L.J.; Garner, L.V.; Smoot, J.W.; Li, Y.; Zhou, Q.; Saveson, C.J.; Sasso, J.M.; Gregg, A.C.; Soares, D.J.; Beskid, T.R.; et al. Assay Techniques and Test Development for COVID-19 Diagnosis. *ACS Cent. Sci.* **2020**, *6*, 591–605. [CrossRef]
47. Liu, X.; Liu, C.; Liu, G.; Luo, W.; Xia, N. Theranostics COVID-19: Progress in diagnostics, therapy and vaccination. *Theranostics* **2020**, *10*, 7821–7835. [CrossRef]
48. Wu, R.; Wang, L.; Kuo, H.-C.D.; Shannar, A.; Peter, R.; Chou, P.J.; Li, S.; Hudlikar, R.; Liu, X.; Liu, Z.; et al. An Update on Current Therapeutic Drugs Treating COVID-19. *Curr. Pharmacol. Rep.* **2020**, *6*, 56–70. [CrossRef]
49. NDPH Low-Cost Dexamethasone Reduces Death by Up to One Third in Hospitalised Patients with Severe Respiratory Complications of COVID-19. Available online: https://www.recoverytrial.net/news/low-cost-dexamethasone-reduces-death-by-up-to-one-third-in-hospitalised-patients-with-severe-respiratory-complications-of-covid-19 (accessed on 20 June 2020).
50. FDA Coronavirus (COVID-19) Update: FDA Revokes Emergency Use Authorization for Chloroquine and Hydroxychloroquine. Available online: https://www.fda.gov/news-events/press-announcements/coronavirus-covid-19-update-fda-revokes-emergency-use-authorization-chloroquine-and (accessed on 20 June 2020).
51. Li, I.W.; Hung, I.F.; To, K.K.; Chan, K.H.; Wong, S.S.Y.; Chan, J.F.; Cheng, V.C.; Tsang, O.T.; Lai, S.T.; Lau, Y.L.; et al. The natural viral load profile of patients with pandemic 2009 influenza A(H1N1) and the effect of oseltamivir treatment. *Chest* **2010**, *137*, 759–768. [CrossRef]

Publisher's Note: MDPI stays neutral with regard to jurisdictional claims in published maps and institutional affiliations.

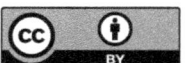

© 2020 by the authors. Licensee MDPI, Basel, Switzerland. This article is an open access article distributed under the terms and conditions of the Creative Commons Attribution (CC BY) license (http://creativecommons.org/licenses/by/4.0/).

MDPI
St. Alban-Anlage 66
4052 Basel
Switzerland
Tel. +41 61 683 77 34
Fax +41 61 302 89 18
www.mdpi.com

International Journal of Environmental Research and Public Health Editorial Office
E-mail: ijerph@mdpi.com
www.mdpi.com/journal/ijerph

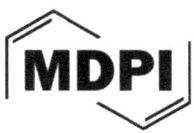

www.ingramcontent.com/pod-product-compliance
Lightning Source LLC
LaVergne TN
LVHW070157120526
838202LV00013BA/1330